Essentials
of
Human
Physiology
for
Pharmacy

CRC PRESS
PHARMACY
EDUCATION
SERIES

Essentials *of* Human Physiology *for* Pharmacy

LAURIE KELLY

CRC PRESS

Boca Raton London New York Washington, D.C.

Library of Congress Cataloging-in-Publication Data

Kelly, Laurie J.
   Essentials of human physiology for pharmacy / by Laurie J. Kelly
        p. ; cm. — (CRC Press pharmacy education series)
   Includes bibliographical references and index.
   ISBN 1-56676-997-3 (alk. paper)
   1. Human physiology. 2.Pharmacy. I. Title. II. Series.
   [DNLM: 1. Physiological Processes. 2. Pharmaceutical Preparations. 3.
Pharmacy—methods. QT 4 K29e 2004]
   QP34.5K45 2004
   612—dc22   2003070029

Visit the CRC Press Web site at www.crcpress.com

© 2004 by CRC Press LLC

No claim to original U.S. Government works
International Standard Book Number 1-56676-997-3
Library of Congress Card Number 2003070029
Printed in the United States of America 1 2 3 4 5 6 7 8 9 0
Printed on acid-free paper

Dedication

To my sister, Kit, my nieces,
Katie and Danielle,
and
especially to Tat, whose love and support
mean everything in the world to me.

∞×9

Preface

This textbook is designed to provide the fundamentals of human physiology to students of pharmacy and other health sciences. An important goal of this book is to enhance students' perceptions of the relevance of physiology to pharmacy practice. The book includes important concepts in physiology described in sufficient detail so that the student may integrate and understand these principles and then be able to apply them in subsequent coursework in pharmacology and therapeutics. Furthermore, this text contains frequent and specific references to pharmacotherapeutics and the practice of pharmacy designed to facilitate students' understanding of basic physiological concepts and their pertinence to their chosen profession.

The book begins with an overview of the fundamental aspects of cell membrane physiology with particular emphasis on nerve cell function. This is followed by a detailed discussion of the two major regulatory systems in the body: the nervous system, including the brain, spinal cord, pain, and autonomic nervous system; as well as the endocrine system. The book then continues with in-depth presentations of the muscular, cardiovascular, respiratory, digestive, and renal systems. An important focus throughout this textbook is how tissue and organ function is regulated in order to maintain homeostasis.

The intent of this book is to present the material in a manner as clear and concise as possible. Study objectives are provided at the beginning of each chapter to help students focus on important principles and mechanisms. Whenever possible, information is provided in the form of bulleted lists, tables, figures, or flow charts. Finally, subsections of *pharmacy applications* separate from the text serve to relate a given concept in physiology to the practice of pharmacy.

Laurie J. Kelly
Massachusetts College of Pharmacy and Health Sciences

Acknowledgments

Thanks to Althea Chen, who prepared the illustrations for this book, and to Gail Williams, who prepared the tables.

Pharmacy Applications

Application	Chapter
Homeostatic functions of drugs	1
Lipid solubility and drug elimination	2
Hydrophilic drugs bind to receptors	2
Intravenous solutions	2
Local anesthetics	4
Centrally acting drugs	6
Antihistamines and the blood–brain barrier	6
Spinal anesthesia	7
Epidural anesthesia	7
Alpha-one adrenergic receptor antagonists	9
Sympathomimetic drugs	9
Cholinomimetic drugs	9
Muscarinic receptor antagonists	9
Therapeutic effects of calcitonin	10
Therapeutic effects of corticosteroids	10
Antiarrhythmic drugs	13
Diuretics and cardiac output	14
Cardiac glycosides and cardiac output	14
Antihypertensive drugs	15
Nitroglycerin and angina	15
Antiplatelet drugs	16
Anticoagulant drugs	16
Infant respiratory distress syndrome	17
Pharmacological treatment of asthma	17
Drug-induced hypoventilation	17
Anticholinergic side effects in the digestive system	18
Drug-induced gastric disease	18
Pharmacological treatment of gastric ulcers	18
Physiological action of diuretics	19
Drug-related nephropathies	19

Contents

chapter one

Physiology and the concept of homeostasis

Study objectives

- Define the internal environment
- Understand the importance of homeostasis
- Describe the overall function of each of the three major components of the nervous system
- Compare the general functions of the nervous system and the endocrine system
- Explain the mechanism of negative feedback
- Describe the potential role of medications in the maintenance of homeostasis

1.1   Introduction

Physiology is the study of the functions of the human body. In other words, the mechanisms by which the various organs and tissues carry out their specific activities are considered. Emphasis is often placed on the processes that control and regulate these functions. In order for the body to function optimally, conditions within the body, referred to as the *internal environment*, must be very carefully regulated. Therefore, many important variables, such as body temperature, blood pressure, blood glucose, oxygen and carbon dioxide content of the blood, as well as electrolyte balance, are actively maintained within narrow physiological limits.

1.2   Homeostasis

This maintenance of relatively constant or steady-state internal conditions is referred to as *homeostasis*. It is important because the cells and tissues of the body will survive and function efficiently only when these internal conditions are properly maintained. This is not to say that the internal

Table 1.1 Contribution of Organ Systems to the Maintenance of Homeostasis

Organ System	Function
Nervous system	Regulates muscular activity and glandular secretion; responsible for all activities associated with the mind
Endocrine system	Regulates metabolic processes through secretion of hormones
Muscular system	Allows for body movement; contributes to thermoregulation
Circulatory system	Transports nutrients, O_2, waste, CO_2, electrolytes, and hormones throughout the body
Respiratory system	Obtains oxygen and eliminates carbon dioxide; regulates acid-base balance (pH)
Gastrointestinal tract	Digests food to provide nutrients to the body
Renal system	Eliminates waste products from the body; regulates blood volume and blood pressure; regulates acid-base balance (pH)

environment is fixed or unchanging. The body is constantly faced with a changing external environment as well as with events and activities occurring within it that may alter the balance of important variables. For example, most metabolic reactions within cells consume oxygen and glucose. These substances must then be replaced. In addition, these reactions produce metabolic wastes including carbon dioxide and urea, which must then be eliminated. Therefore, it is more accurate to say that the internal environment is in a *dynamic steady state* — one that is constantly changing, but in which optimal conditions are physiologically maintained.

All of the organ systems in the body, except the reproductive system, contribute to the maintenance of homeostasis (see Table 1.1). For example, the gastrointestinal tract digests foods to provide nutrients to the body. The respiratory system obtains oxygen and eliminates carbon dioxide. The circulatory system transports all of these materials and others from one part of the body to another. The renal system eliminates wastes and plays a role in regulating blood volume and blood pressure.

The study of physiology includes study not only of how each of these systems carries out its functions, but also of the mechanisms involved that regulate these activities in order to maintain homeostasis under a variety of conditions. For example, the body's needs are very different during a resting state compared to that of exercise. How do organ systems adjust their activities in response to varied levels of physical exertion or when confronted with altered internal and external environments? In order to maintain homeostasis, the body must be able to monitor and sense changes in the internal environment. It must also be able to compensate, or make adjustments, for these changes.

Two regulatory systems in the body influence the activity of all the other organ systems so that homeostasis is ultimately maintained:

- Nervous system
- Endocrine system

The *nervous system* has three functional components (see Figure 1.1):

- Sensory division of the peripheral nervous system
- Central nervous system
- Motor division of the peripheral nervous system

Many different types of sensory receptors are located throughout the body. These receptors monitor the status of the internal environment or that of the surroundings. *Sensory receptors* are sensitive to specific types of stimuli and measure the value of a physiological variable. For example, *arterial baroreceptors* measure blood pressure and *chemoreceptors* measure the oxygen and carbon dioxide content of the blood. The information detected by these sensors then travels by way of *afferent* neuronal pathways to the *central nervous system* (CNS). The CNS is the *integrative portion* of the nervous system and consists of the (1) brain and the (2) spinal cord.

The brain receives, processes, and stores sensory input; generates thoughts; and determines the reactions that the body should perform in

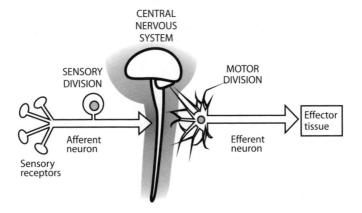

Figure 1.1 Functional components of the nervous system. The sensory division of the peripheral nervous system is sensitive to changes in the internal and external environment. The information gathered by this component is transmitted to the CNS where it is processed, integrated, and interpreted. The CNS then determines the appropriate response to this input. This response is carried out by the transmission of nerve impulses in the motor division of the peripheral nervous system to the effector tissues.

response to this input. The spinal cord is important in processing reflexes. It is within this integration area of the nervous system that the actual value of a physiological variable as measured by a sensory receptor is compared to its set point or optimal value. One or more compensatory responses are then determined.

The third component of the nervous system is the *motor division*. Appropriate signals are transmitted from the CNS to various body parts or *effector tissues* by way of *efferent* neuronal pathways. These effector tissues, which include organs, muscles, and glands, carry out the appropriate physiological responses to bring the variable back to within its normal limits.

The other regulatory system in the body contributing to the maintenance of homeostasis is the *endocrine system*, which carries out its effects by secreting *hormones*. These hormones are transported in the blood to the specific tissues upon which they exert their effects. In general, the nervous system primarily regulates muscular activity and glandular secretion and the endocrine system primarily regulates metabolic activity in the body's cells. However, these two systems may work together in the regulation of many organs, as well as influence each other's activity.

1.3   Negative feedback

Most of the body's *compensatory homeostatic mechanisms* function by way of *negative feedback*. This is a response that causes the level of a variable to change in a direction opposite to that of the initial change. For example, when blood pressure increases, the arterial baroreceptors are stimulated and an increased number of nerve impulses are transmitted to the CNS through afferent pathways. The region of the brain regulating the cardiovascular system responds to this sensory input by altering efferent nerve activity to the heart. The result is a decrease in heart rate and therefore a decrease in blood pressure back to its baseline value (see Figure 1.2). In general, when a physiological variable becomes too high or too low, a control system elicits a negative feedback response consisting of one or a series of changes that returns the variable to within its normal physiological range. These compensatory mechanisms operating via negative feedback allow the body to maintain homeostasis effectively.

Interestingly, one of the greatest stressors on the body, and therefore challenges to the maintenance of homeostasis, is increased physical activity or exercise. During intense exercise, glucose utilization can be increased up to 20-fold; skeletal muscle pH drops dramatically; several liters of water can be lost in the form of sweat; and core body temperature can increase to as high as 106°F. These profound disturbances must be compensated for in order to ensure cell survival. An important focus throughout this textbook will be how tissue and organ system function is regulated under various normal physiological conditions and, where appropriate, under abnormal pathophysiological conditions. Furthermore, discussions of how basic physiological principles may be applied to the practice of pharmacy are included.

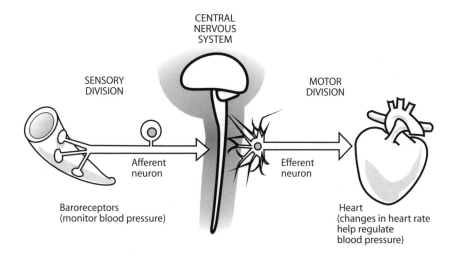

Figure 1.2 Negative feedback. These types of responses are employed throughout the body in order to maintain homeostasis. In this example, any change in blood pressure, which is monitored within the circulatory system and processed within the CNS, will cause reflex changes in heart rate. The change in heart rate will be in the opposite direction of the change in blood pressure: if blood pressure increases, then heart rate decreases; if blood pressure decreases, then heart rate increases. In this way, blood pressure is adjusted back to its normal value.

Pharmacy application: homeostatic functions of drugs

Diseases are generally divided into two categories: those in which the pathophysiology involves internal failure of some normal physiological process and those that originate from some external source such as bacterial or viral infection. In either case, one or more variables in the internal environment will be disrupted. Therefore, many of the medications currently in use are designed to assist the body in the maintenance of homeostasis when its own regulatory mechanisms fail to do so. For example, angiotensin-converting enzyme (ACE) inhibitors, such as enalapril, and beta-blockers, such as propranolol, lower blood pressure in patients with idiopathic (unexplained) hypertension (elevated blood pressure). Glibenclamide, which increases cellular sensitivity to insulin and decreases hepatic glucose production, maintains blood glucose within the normal range in patients with type II diabetes mellitus. Diuretics such as furosemide decrease blood volume and therefore reduce cardiac workload in patients with congestive heart failure. In each of these disorders, pharmacological intervention is necessary for the given organ system to function efficiently and effectively in order to maintain the health of the patient.

Bibliography

1. *AHFS Drug Information 2000,* American Society of Health-System Pharmacists, Bethesda, MD, 2000.
2. Papanek, P.E., Exercise physiology and the bioenergetics of muscle contraction, in *Physiology Secrets,* Raff, H., Ed., Hanley and Belfus, Inc., Philadelphia, 1999, chap. 8.
3. Sherwood, L., *Human Physiology from Cells to Systems,* 4th ed., Brooks/Cole, Pacific Grove, CA, 2001.
4. Silverthorn, D., *Human Physiology: An Integrated Approach,* 2nd ed., Prentice-Hall, Upper Saddle River, NJ, 2001.

chapter two

Plasma membrane

Study objectives

- Describe the function of each component of the plasma membrane
- Understand the physiological importance of the permeability barrier created by the plasma membrane
- Describe the factors that affect diffusion
- Explain how osmosis takes place
- Understand the clinical significance of the osmotic pressures of solutions
- Describe the factors that affect mediated transport
- Compare and contrast facilitated diffusion and active transport

2.1   Introduction

Each cell is surrounded by a plasma membrane that separates the cytoplasmic contents of the cell, or the intracellular fluid, from the fluid outside the cell, the extracellular fluid. An important homeostatic function of this plasma membrane is to serve as a *permeability barrier* that insulates or protects the cytoplasm from immediate changes in the surrounding environment. Furthermore, it allows the cell to maintain a cytoplasmic composition very different from that of the extracellular fluid; the functions of neurons and muscle cells depend on this difference. The plasma membrane also contains many enzymes and other components such as antigens and receptors that allow cells to interact with other cells, neurotransmitters, blood-borne substances such as hormones, and various other chemical substances, such as drugs.

2.2   Structure and function of plasma membrane

The major components of the plasma membrane include:

- Phospholipids
- Cholesterol

- Proteins
- Carbohydrates

The basic structure of the plasma membrane is formed by *phospholipids* (Figure 2.1), which are one of the more abundant of the membrane components. Phospholipids are *amphipathic* molecules that have polar (water-soluble) and nonpolar (water-insoluble) regions. They are composed of a phosphorylated glycerol backbone, which forms a hydrophilic polar head group and a nonpolar region containing two hydrophobic fatty acid chains. In an aqueous environment such as the body, these molecules are arranged in a formation referred to as the *lipid bilayer* consisting of two layers of phospholipids. The polar region of the molecule is oriented toward the outer surface of the membrane where it can interact with water; the nonpolar, hydrophobic fatty acids are in the center of the membrane away from the water. The functional significance of this lipid bilayer is that it creates a *semipermeable barrier*. Lipophilic, or nonwater-soluble, substances can readily cross the membrane by simply passing through its lipid core. Important examples of these substances include gases, such as oxygen and carbon dioxide, and fatty acid molecules, which are used to form energy within muscle cells.

Most hydrophilic, or water-soluble, substances are repelled by this hydrophobic interior and cannot simply diffuse through the membrane. Instead, these substances must cross the membrane using specialized transport mechanisms. Examples of lipid-insoluble substances that require such mechanisms include nutrient molecules, such as glucose and amino acids, and all species of ions (Na^+, Ca^{++}, H^+, Cl^-, and HCO_3^-). Therefore, the plasma membrane plays a very important role in determining the composition of the intracellular fluid by selectively permitting substances to move in and out of the cell.

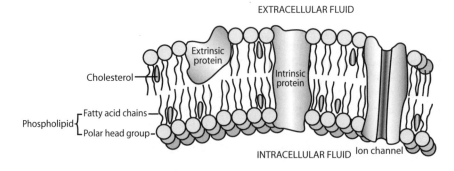

Figure 2.1 Structure of the plasma membrane. The plasma membrane is composed of a bilayer of phospholipid molecules. Associated with this bilayer are intrinsic proteins embedded within and spanning the membrane as well as intrinsic proteins found on the external or internal surface of the membrane. Molecules of cholesterol are found in the inner, nonpolar region of the membrane.

Pharmacy application: lipid solubility and drug elimination

The lipid solubility of many substances can change when physiological conditions vary. For example, the surrounding pH can determine whether a molecule is in a protonated form (positively charged, lipid insoluble) or in an unprotonated form (uncharged, lipid soluble). As discussed, charged substances do not readily cross the membrane, as do uncharged substances. This principle regarding lipid solubility is used in the treatment of an overdose of phenobarbital, a barbiturate used for sedation and seizure disorders. At the normal blood pH of 7.4, the phenobarbital molecules are 50% protonated and 50% unprotonated. Only the uncharged form can cross cell membranes to leave the blood and enter the kidney for excretion in the urine. Treatment with sodium bicarbonate increases the pH of the blood causing many of the protonated phenobarbital molecules to lose their proton and become unprotonated. Therefore, an alkaline environment increases the percentage of uncharged phenobarbital molecules; increases the lipid solubility of these molecules; and facilitates their elimination by the kidneys.

Another important aspect of the lipid bilayer is that the phospholipids are not held together by chemical bonds. This enables molecules to move about freely within the membrane, resulting in a structure that is not rigid in nature, but instead, very fluid and pliable. Also contributing to membrane fluidity is the presence of *cholesterol*. Cholesterol has a steroid nucleus that is lipid soluble. Therefore, these molecules are found in the interior of the membrane lying parallel to the fatty acid chains of the phospholipids (see Figure 2.1). As such, they prevent the fatty acid chains from packing together and crystallizing, which would decrease membrane fluidity.

Membrane fluidity is very important in terms of function in many cell types. For example, skeletal muscle activity involves shortening and lengthening of muscle fibers. Furthermore, as white blood cells leave the blood vessels and enter the tissue spaces to fight infection, they must squeeze through tiny pores in the wall of the capillary requiring significant deformation of the cell and its membrane. Finally, in all cells, many processes that transport substances across the plasma membrane require the embedded proteins to change their conformation and move about within the bilayer. In each case, in order for the cell membrane, or the entire cell, to change its shape, the membrane must be very fluid and flexible.

Proteins are also associated with the lipid bilayer and essentially float within it. Intrinsic proteins are embedded within and span the membrane, and extrinsic proteins are found on the internal or external surface of the membrane (see Figure 2.1). These proteins provide a variety of important cellular functions by forming the following structures:

- Channels
- Carrier molecules
- Enzymes
- Chemical receptors
- Antigens

Some proteins may form *channels* through the cell membrane that allow small, water-soluble substances such as ions to enter or leave the cell. Other proteins may serve as *carrier molecules* that selectively transport larger water-soluble molecules, such as glucose or cellular products, across the membrane. Regulators of specific chemical reactions, *enzymes* are extrinsic proteins found on the internal (e.g., adenylate cyclase) or external (e.g., acetylcholinesterase) surfaces of the membrane. *Chemical receptors* are found on the outer surface of the cell membrane and selectively bind with various endogenous molecules as well as with drugs. Through receptor activation, many substances unable to enter the cell and cause a direct intracellular effect may indirectly influence intracellular activity without actually crossing the membrane. Other proteins found on the external surface of the plasma membrane are *antigens*. These molecules serve as cell "markers" that allow the body's immune system to distinguish between its own cells and foreign cells or organisms such as bacteria and viruses.

The plasma membrane contains a small amount of carbohydrate (2 to 10% of the mass of the membrane) on the outer surface. This carbohydrate is found attached to most of the protein molecules, forming glycoproteins, and to some of the phospholipid molecules (<10%), forming glycolipids. Consequently, the external surface of the cell has a carbohydrate coat, or glycocalyx.

These carbohydrate moieties have several important functions, including:

- Repelling negatively charged substances: many of the carbohydrates are negatively charged, creating an overall negative charge on the surface of the cell that repels negatively charged extracellular molecules.
- Cell-to-cell attachment: the glycocalyx of one cell may attach to the glycocalyx of another cell, which causes the cells to become attached.
- Receptors: carbohydrates may also serve as specific membrane receptors for extracellular substances such as hormones.
- Immune reactions: carbohydrates play a role in the ability of cells to distinguish between "self" cells and foreign cells.

Pharmacy application: hydrophilic drugs bind to receptors

Many substances within the body, including hormones and neurotransmitters, are hydrophilic and therefore incapable of entering the cells to carry out their effects directly. Instead, they bind to their specific receptors on the cell surface. This receptor binding then elicits a series of intracellular events that alter cell function and cell metabolism. Often instances occur in which it would be advantageous to enhance or to inhibit these activities; therefore, drugs may be designed to bind to these specific receptors. A drug that binds to and stimulates a receptor and mimics the action of the endogenous chemical substance is referred to as a receptor *agonist*. An example is albuterol sulfate, a selective beta$_2$-adrenergic receptor agonist, which causes dilation of the airways in a patient experiencing an asthmatic attack. A drug that binds to and blocks a receptor, preventing the action of the endogenous substance, is referred to as a receptor *antagonist*. An example in this case is cimetidine hydrochloride, which inhibits histamine H$_2$ receptors on parietal cells in the stomach, thus reducing gastric acid output. This medication is used to treat patients with a peptic ulcer or gastroesophageal reflux disease (GERD).

2.3 Membrane transport

The lipid bilayer arrangement of the plasma membrane renders it selectively permeable. Uncharged or nonpolar molecules, such as oxygen, carbon dioxide, and fatty acids, are lipid soluble and may permeate through the membrane quite readily. Charged or polar molecules, such as glucose, proteins, and ions, are water soluble and impermeable, unable to cross the membrane unassisted. These substances require protein channels or carrier molecules to enter or leave the cell.

2.4 Passive diffusion through the membrane

Molecules and ions are in constant motion and the velocity of their motion is proportional to their temperature. This passive movement of molecules and ions from one place to another is referred to as *diffusion*. When a molecule is unevenly distributed across a permeable membrane with a higher concentration on one side and a lower concentration on the opposite side, there is said to be a *concentration gradient* or a concentration difference. Although all of the molecules are in motion, the tendency is for a greater number of molecules to move from the area of high concentration toward the area of low concentration. This uneven movement of molecules is referred to as *net*

Table 2.1 Factors Influencing Rate of Diffusion of a Substance

Factor	Rate of diffusion
↑ Concentration gradient	↓
↑ Permeability of membrane	↓
↑ Surface area of membrane	↓
↑ Molecular weight of substance	↓
↑ Thickness of membrane	↓

diffusion. The net diffusion of molecules continues until the concentrations of the substance on both sides of the membrane are equal and the subsequent movement of molecules through the membrane is in a *dynamic equilibrium.* In other words, the number of molecules moving in one direction across the membrane is equal to the number of molecules moving in the opposite direction. At this point, although the diffusion of molecules continues, no further *net* diffusion takes place.

The rate of diffusion of a substance is influenced by several factors (see Table 2.1). It is proportional to the concentration gradient; the permeability of the membrane; and the surface area of the membrane. For example, as the permeability of the membrane increases, the rate of diffusion increases. It is inversely proportional to the molecular weight of the substance and the thickness of the membrane. Larger molecules diffuse more slowly.

The movement of ions, in particular, depends not only on a concentration gradient but also on an *electrical gradient.* Positively charged ions (cations) are attracted to a negatively charged area and negatively charged ions (anions) are attracted to a positively charged area. Ions of a similar charge tend to repel each other and oppose diffusion.

2.5 Osmosis

Water is a small polar molecule that can easily diffuse across plasma membranes through small intermolecular spaces. *Osmosis* is the net movement of water through a semipermeable membrane down its own concentration gradient from an area of high water concentration to an area of low water concentration. In other words, water moves toward an area of higher *solute* concentration. The solute particles may be thought of as "drawing" the water toward them. Therefore, the *osmotic pressure* of a solution is the pressure or force by which water is drawn into the solution through a semipermeable membrane. The magnitude of this pressure depends on the number of solute particles present. An increase in the number of particles in the solution results in an increase in the osmotic pressure and, therefore, an increase in the movement of water toward it.

The plasma membrane is *semipermeable* because it is not permeable to all solute particles present. As a result, it maintains a concentration difference for many ions and molecules across itself, although water crosses the membrane freely in either direction. The movement of water in and out of the cell will occur whenever there is a difference in osmotic pressure between the intracelluar fluid and the extracellular fluid. For example, an increase in the osmotic pressure of the extracellular fluid (more solute, lower water concentration) will cause water to leave the cell by osmosis. On the other hand, a decrease in the osmotic pressure in the extracellular fluid (less solute, higher water concentration) will cause water to enter the cells.

Pharmacy application: intravenous solutions

Intravenous (i.v.) solutions are commonly administered to patients in hospitals, long-term care facilities, and ambulances. They are used primarily to replace body fluids and to serve as a vehicle for injecting drugs into the body. The advantages of this pharmaceutical dosage form include the rapid onset of action, the ability to treat patients unable to take medication orally and the ability to administer a medication unavailable in any other dosage form.

Intravenous solutions must be isosmotic (same osmotic pressure) with red blood cells. If red blood cells were to be exposed to an i.v. solution that was hypoosmotic (lower osmotic pressure), water would move into the cells causing them to swell and possibly lyse. If red blood cells were to be exposed to a hyperosmotic i.v. solution (higher osmotic pressure), water would move out of the cells causing them to dehydrate and shrink. Both of these conditions would damage the red blood cells and disrupt function.

Patient discomfort is another important consideration. The stinging caused by a hypoosmotic or hyperosmotic i.v. solution is not experienced with one that is isosmotic. Intravenous injections are often prepared with 0.9% sodium chloride or 5% dextrose, both of which are approximately isosmotic with red blood cells.

2.6   Mediated transport

In the process of *mediated transport*, carrier proteins embedded within the plasma membrane assist in the transport of larger polar molecules into or out of the cell. When a given substance attaches to a specific binding site on the carrier protein, the protein undergoes a conformational change such that this site with the bound substance moves from one side of the plasma membrane to the other. The substance is then released. Mediated transport displays three important characteristics influencing its function:

- Specificity
- Competition
- Saturation

Carrier proteins display a high degree of *specificity*. In other words, each of these proteins may bind only with select substances that "fit" into its binding site. Another characteristic is *competition*; different substances with similar chemical structures may be able to bind to the same carrier protein and therefore compete for transport across the membrane. The third characteristic displayed by mediated transport is *saturation*. The greater the number of carrier proteins utilized at any given time, the greater the rate of transport is. Initially, as the concentration of a substance increases, the rate of transport increases; however, a finite number of carrier proteins exist in a given cell membrane. Once all these proteins are utilized in the transport process, any further increase in the concentration of the substance no longer increases the rate of transport because it has reached its maximum. At this point, the process is saturated.

Mediated transport has two forms:

- Facilitated diffusion
- Active transport

With *facilitated diffusion*, carrier proteins move across the membrane in either direction and will transport a substance down its concentration gradient. In other words, substances are moved from an area of high concentration to an area of low concentration — a passive process that requires no energy. An example of a substance transported by facilitated diffusion is glucose, which is a large polar molecule. Because cells are constantly utilizing glucose to form ATP, a concentration gradient is always available for diffusion into the cell.

With *active transport*, energy is expended to move a substance against its concentration gradient from an area of low concentration to an area of high concentration. This process is used to accumulate a substance on one side of the plasma membrane or the other. The most common example of active transport is the sodium–potassium pump that involves the activity of Na^+–K^+ ATPase, an intrinsic membrane protein. For each ATP molecule hydrolyzed by Na^+–K^+ ATPase, this pump moves three Na^+ ions out of the cell and two K^+ ions into it. As will be discussed further in the next chapter, the activity of this pump contributes to the difference in composition of the extracellular and intracellular fluids necessary for nerve and muscle cells to function.

Bibliography

1. *AHFS Drug Information 2000*, American Society of Health-System Pharmacists, Bethesda, MD, 2000.
2. Bell, D.R., *Core Concepts in Physiology*, Lippincott–Raven Publishers, Philadelphia, 1998.
3. Costanzo, L., *Physiology*, W.B. Saunders, Philadelphia, 1998.
4. Guyton, A.C. and Hall, J.E., *Textbook of Medical Physiology*, 10th ed., W.B. Saunders, Philadelphia, 2000.

5. Hunt, M.L., Jr., *Training Manual for Intravenous Admixture Personnel*, 5th ed., Baxter Healthcare Corp., 1995.
6. Lombard, J.H. and Rusch, N.J., Cells, nerves and muscles, in *Physiology Secrets*, Raff, H., Ed., Hanley and Belfus, Inc., Philadelphia, 1999, chap. 1.
7. Rhoades, R. and Pflanzer, R., *Human Physiology*, 4th ed., Brooks/Cole, Pacific Grove, CA, 2003.
8. Sherwood, L., *Human Physiology from Cells to Systems*, 4th ed., Brooks/Cole, Pacific Grove, CA, 2001.

chapter three

Membrane potential

Study objectives

- Define membrane potential
- Describe how the resting membrane potential is developed and maintained
- Compare the distribution and permeability differences of ions across the cell membrane
- Describe how differences in ion distribution and permeability contribute to the resting membrane potential
- Explain the role of the Na^+–K^+ ATPase pump in this process

3.1   Introduction

Intracellular fluid and extracellular fluid are electrically neutral solutions, in that each has an equal number of positively and negatively charged ions. A simple but important concept is that these opposite charges are attracted to each other and ions of the same charge repel each other. In an unstimulated or resting cell, a slight accumulation of negative charges (–) on the internal surface of the plasma membrane is attracted to an equal number of positive charges (+) that have accumulated on the external surface of the membrane. Therefore, all cells at rest are electrically *polarized*; that is, the inside of the cell is slightly negative relative to the outside. This separation of charge across the plasma membrane is referred to as the *membrane potential*.

The magnitude of the membrane potential depends primarily on the number of opposite charges separated by the membrane. The greater the separation of charge then, the greater the membrane potential is. Because the actual number of charges involved is quite small, the potential is measured in millivolts (mV). Furthermore, the sign (+ or –) of the potential is defined by the predominant charge on the internal surface of the cell membrane. Therefore, the membrane potential under resting conditions is negative. As will be discussed, nerve cells and muscle cells rely on changes in this membrane potential for their functions. In other words, changes in the membrane potential convey information to these types of cells.

3.2   Development of resting membrane potential

In a typical unstimulated neuron, the *resting membrane potential* is approximately –70 mV. The development of this potential depends on the *distribution* and *permeability* of three ions: (1) sodium (Na^+); (2) potassium (K^+); and (3) anions (A^-) (see Table 3.1 and Figure 3.1). These ions are unevenly distributed between the intracellular fluid (ICF) and the extracellular fluid (ECF) and each has a different degree of permeability across the plasma membrane. Sodium ions are found in a greater concentration in the ECF and K^+ ions are found in a greater concentration in the ICF; A^- refers to large anionic proteins found only within the cell. Under resting conditions, most mammalian plasma membranes are approximately 50 to 75 times more permeable to K^+ ions than they are to Na^+ ions. The anions are impermeable at all times. It is due to these underlying conditions that the resting membrane potential is generated and maintained.

When permeable, the movement of Na^+ and K^+ ions in and out of the cell depends on two factors:

- Concentration gradient
- Electrical gradient

Consider a condition in which the membrane is permeable only to potassium. Because potassium is in a greater concentration inside the cell, the K^+ ions initially diffuse out of the cell down their *concentration gradient*. As a result, an excess of these positively charged ions would accumulate in the ECF along the external surface of the plasma membrane. Attracted to these positive charges, the impermeable A^- ions would remain inside the cell along the internal surface of the plasma membrane. This outward movement of positive charges creates a negative membrane potential because the inside of the cell is now negative relative to the outside. However, as the positively charged K^+ ions continue to diffuse outward, an electrical gradient begins to develop that also influences the diffusion of K^+ ions.

The K^+ ions that moved out of the cell down their concentration gradient have caused an excess of (+) charges to accumulate on the external surface

Table 3.1 Concentration and Permeability of Ions Responsible for Membrane Potential in a Resting Nerve Cell

| Ion | Concentration (millimoles/liter) | | Relative permeability |
	Extracellular fluid	Intracellular fluid	
Na+	150	15	1
K+	5	150	50–75
A–	0	65	0

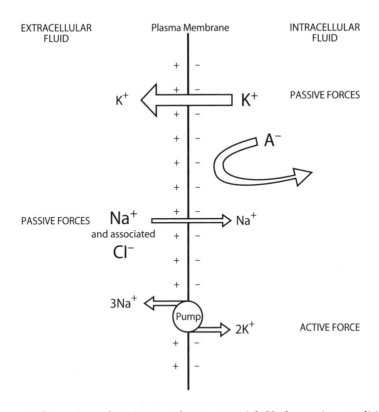

Figure 3.1 Generation of resting membrane potential. Under resting conditions, potassium (K$^+$) is significantly more permeable than sodium (Na$^+$) and the negatively charged intracellular anions (A$^-$) are impermeable. Therefore, the abundant outward movement of K$^+$ ions down their concentration gradient exerts a powerful effect, driving the membrane potential toward the equilibrium potential for potassium (–90 mV). However, the slight inward movement of Na$^+$ ions, which would tend to drive the membrane potential toward the equilibrium potential for sodium (+60 mV), renders the membrane potential somewhat less negative. The balance of these two opposing effects results in a resting membrane potential in a typical neuron of –70 mV. The maintenance of the concentration differences for sodium and potassium is due to the continuous activity of the Na$^+$–K$^+$ pump.

of the membrane. Because like charges repel each other, these (+) charges would begin to repel any additional K$^+$ ions and oppose the further movement of (+) charges outward. Instead, the positively charged K$^+$ ions are now electrically attracted to the negatively charged A$^-$ ions remaining inside the cell. At this point, K$^+$ ions not only diffuse outward down their concentration gradient, but also diffuse into the cell down their *electrical gradient*. Eventually, the subsequent force that moved K$^+$ ions inward exactly balances the initial force that moved K$^+$ ions outward, so there is no further net diffusion of potassium. The membrane potential at this point has reached the *equilibrium potential for K$^+$ (E_{K^+})* and is equal to –90 mV. Therefore, when the permeability of the plasma membrane to potassium is high compared to that of sodium, the membrane potential approaches –90 mV.

Next, consider a condition in which the membrane is permeable only to sodium. Because sodium is in a greater concentration outside the cell, the Na^+ ions initially diffuse into the cell down their concentration gradient. As a result, an excess of these positively charged ions accumulates in the ICF along the internal surface of the plasma membrane; an excess of negative charges in the form of the impermeable extracellular anion, chloride (Cl^-), remains outside the cell along the external surface of the plasma membrane. This inward movement of positive charges creates a positive membrane potential because the inside of the cell is now positive relative to the outside. However, as the positively charged Na^+ ions continue to diffuse inward, once again an electrical gradient develops.

The (+) charges that have accumulated in the ICF begin to repel any additional Na^+ ions and oppose the further movement of (+) charges inward. Instead, the positively charged Na^+ ions are now attracted to the negatively charged Cl^- ions remaining outside the cell. Eventually, the initial force moving Na^+ ions inward down their concentration gradient is exactly balanced by the subsequent force moving Na^+ ions outward down their electrical gradient, so there is no further net diffusion of sodium. The membrane potential at this point has reached the *equilibrium potential for Na^+ (E_{Na}^+)* and is equal to +60 mV. Therefore, when the permeability of the plasma membrane to sodium is high compared to that of potassium, the membrane potential approaches +60 mV.

At any given time, the membrane potential is closer to the equilibrium potential of the more permeable ion. Under normal resting conditions, Na^+ ions and K^+ ions are permeable; however, potassium is significantly (50 to 75 times) more permeable than sodium. Therefore, a large number of K^+ ions diffuse outward and a very small number of Na^+ ions diffuse inward down their concentration gradients. As a result, the comparatively copious outward movement of K^+ ions exerts a powerful influence on the value of the resting membrane potential, driving it toward its equilibrium potential of –90 mV. However, the slight inward movement of Na^+ ions that would tend to drive the membrane potential toward its equilibrium potential of +60 mV renders the membrane potential slightly less negative. The balance of these two opposing effects results in a typical neuron resting membrane potential of –70 mV (see Figure 3.1).

The Na^+–K^+ pump also plays a vital role in this process. For each molecule of ATP expended, three Na^+ ions are pumped out of the cell into the ECF and two K^+ ions are pumped into the cell into the ICF. The result is the unequal transport of positively charged ions across the membrane such that the outside of the cell becomes more positive compared to its inside; in other words, the inside of the cell is more negative compared to the outside. Therefore, the activity of the pump makes a small direct contribution to generation of the resting membrane potential.

The other, even more important effect of the Na^+–K^+ pump is that it maintains the concentration differences for sodium and potassium by accumulating Na^+ ions outside the cell and K^+ ions inside the cell. As previously discussed, the passive diffusion of these ions down their concentration gradients is predominantly responsible for generating the resting membrane potential. Sodium diffuses inward and potassium diffuses outward. The continuous activity of the pump returns the Na^+ ions to the ECF and the K^+ ions to the ICF. Therefore, it can be said that the pump also makes an indirect contribution to generation of the resting membrane potential.

Bibliography

1. Lombard, J.H. and Rusch, N.J., Cells, nerves and muscles, in *Physiology Secrets*, Raff, H., Ed., Hanley and Belfus, Inc., Philadelphia, 1999, chap. 1.
2. Sherwood, L., *Human Physiology from Cells to Systems*, 4th ed., Brooks/Cole, Pacific Grove, CA, 2001.

chapter four

Electrical signals

Study objectives

- Distinguish among depolarization, hyperpolarization, and repolarization
- Compare and contrast graded potentials and action potentials
- Describe the process of local current flow
- Explain the mechanism by which action potentials are generated
- Understand the function of sodium and potassium voltage-gated channels
- Distinguish between the absolute refractory period and the relative refractory period
- Describe the process of saltatory conduction
- Explain the functional significance of myelin
- Explain why conduction of the action potential is unidirectional

4.1   Introduction

Nerve and muscle cells rely on changes in their membrane potentials in order to carry out their activities. In this chapter, the focus will be on the nerve cell, or *neuron*; however, many of the same principles also apply to muscle. The function of neurons is to convey information to other cells in the form of electrical signals. Two types of electrical signals are transmitted by neurons: graded potentials and action potentials. These signals occur due to ion flux (movement) across the plasma membrane. A given stimulus will cause its effect by altering the permeability to one or more ions. The involved ions will then diffuse into or out of the cell according to their concentration and electrical gradients, causing a change in the membrane potential.

4.2   Graded potentials

Graded potentials are short-distance signals (see Table 4.1). They are local changes in membrane potential that occur at *synapses* where one neuron

Table 4.1 Distinguishing Features of Graded Potentials and Action Potentials

Graded potentials	Action potentials
Short-distance signals	Long-distance signals
Magnitude is stimulus dependent	Magnitude is constant (all-or-none phenomenon)
Signal travels by local current flow	Signal travels by local current flow or by saltatory conduction
Magnitude of signal dissipates as it moves away from the site of stimulation	Magnitude of signal is maintained along entire length of neuron
Initiated at synapses (where one neuron comes into contract with another)	Initiated at axon hillock
Result in depolarization or hyperpolarization	Depolarization only

comes into contact with another neuron. The magnitude of these signals varies with the strength of the stimulus. As the intensity of the stimulus increases, the number of ions diffusing across the cell membrane increases and the magnitude of the change in the membrane potential increases. This change may be in either direction, so the membrane potential may become more or less negative compared to the resting membrane potential (see Figure 4.1).

Depolarization occurs when the membrane potential becomes less negative, moving toward zero. As will be discussed, depolarization makes the neuron more excitable. *Hyperpolarization* occurs when the membrane potential becomes more negative, moving away from zero. Hyperpolarization tends to make the neuron less excitable. Depolarization and hyperpolarization signals are transient or short-lived. Once the stimulus has been removed, the membrane potential returns to its resting state. Following

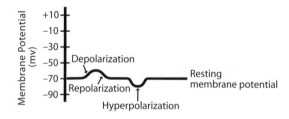

Figure 4.1 Types of changes in membrane potential. The resting membrane potential in a typical neuron is –70 mV. Movement of the membrane potential toward zero (less negative) is referred to as depolarization. The return of the membrane potential to its resting value is referred to as repolarization. Movement of the membrane potential further away from zero (more negative) is referred to as hyperpolarization.

depolarization, the membrane is said to undergo *repolarization*, returning to its resting potential.

The mechanism by which the signal is transmitted along the cell membrane is referred to as *local current flow* or the movement of positively charged ions. In the area of a stimulus causing a depolarization, the inside of the cell becomes positive (less negative) relative to the outside of the cell. Because opposite charges attract, the (+) charges in this area are attracted to and move toward the negative charges on the adjacent areas of the internal surface of the cell membrane. As a result, these adjacent areas become depolarized due to the presence of these (+) charges. This process continues and the electrical signal travels along the cell membrane away from the initial site of the stimulus; however, these graded or local potentials travel only short distances. The cell membrane is not well insulated and the current (positive charges) tends to drift away from the internal surface of the cell membrane. Consequently, as the signal travels along the membrane, the number of (+) charges causing the depolarization of the next region of membrane continually decreases and the magnitude of the depolarization therefore decreases. The further away from the initial site of stimulation, the smaller the magnitude of the signal is until it eventually dies out.

4.3   Action potentials

Action potentials are long-distance electrical signals (see Figure 4.2). These signals travel along the entire neuronal membrane. Unlike graded potentials in which the magnitude of the signal dissipates, the magnitude of the action potential is maintained throughout the length of the axon. Furthermore, in contrast to graded potentials whose magnitude is stimulus dependent, action potentials are always the same size. If a stimulus is strong enough to depolarize the membrane to a critical level referred to as *threshold*, then the membrane continues to depolarize on its own, independent of the stimulus. Typically, threshold is approximately 20 mV less negative than the resting membrane potential. Once threshold is reached, the continued depolarization takes place automatically. This is due to the diffusion of ions according to their concentration and electrical gradients and not due to the original stimulus itself.

Given that action potentials are always of a similar magnitude, how can stimuli of varied strengths be distinguished? A suprathreshold stimulus, one that is larger than necessary to depolarize the membrane simply to threshold, does not produce a larger action potential, but it does increase the *frequency* at which action potentials are generated. In other words, a stronger stimulus will trigger a greater number of action potentials per second.

The generation of an action potential involves changes in permeability to Na^+ ions and K^+ ions through *voltage-gated ion channels*. However, these permeability changes take place at slightly different times (see Figure 4.2). Voltage-gated ion channels open and close in response to changes in membrane potential. Initially, a stimulus will cause the membrane to depolarize

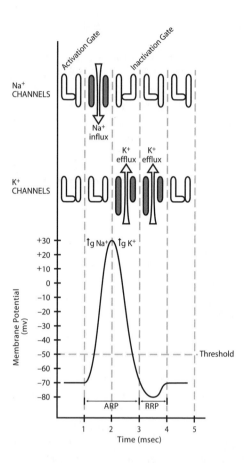

Figure 4.2 The action potential. At the resting membrane potential (–70 mV), most ion channels are in their resting state — closed but capable of opening. When the neuron is stimulated and depolarized, the activation gates of the voltage-gated Na+ channels open, permitting the influx of Na+ ions and further depolarization toward threshold. At the threshold potential, all voltage-gated Na+ channels are open, resulting in the "spike" of the action potential. Approximately 1 msec after the activation gates open, the inactivation gates of the Na+ channels close; in addition, the activation gates of the K+ channels open, resulting in the repolariza-tion of the neuron. The protracted increase in K+ ion permeability results in the after-hyperpolarization. It is during this time, when the membrane potential in the neuron is further away from threshold, that the cell is in its relative refractory period (RRP) and a larger than normal stimulus is needed to generate an action potential. The absolute refractory period (ARP) begins when the voltage-gated Na+ channels have become activated and continues through the inactivation phase. During this time, no further Na+ ion influx can take place and no new action potentials can be generated. Voltage-gated Na+ channels return to their resting state (activation gates closed, inactivation gates open) when the membrane potential approaches the resting membrane potential of the neuron.

toward threshold. When this occurs, voltage-gated Na^+ channels begin to open. As a result, Na^+ ions enter the cell down their concentration and electrical gradients. (Recall that, at this point, Na^+ is in a greater concentration outside the cell and the inside of the cell is negative relative to the outside.).

The influx of Na^+ ions causes further depolarization, resulting in the opening of more voltage-gated Na^+ channels, continued influx of Na^+ ions, and so on. This process continues until the membrane is depolarized to threshold at which point all of the Na^+ channels are open and Na^+ ion influx is rapid and abundant. At this time, the permeability to Na^+ ions is approximately 600 times greater than normal. This ion flux causes the upward swing or spike of the action potential. During this phase of the action potential, the membrane reverses polarity because of the marked influx of (+) charges; the membrane potential at the peak of the action potential is +30 mV.

Approximately 1 msec after Na^+ channels open, they close, thus preventing any further diffusion of (+) charges into the cell. At the same time, voltage-gated K^+ channels open and K^+ ions leave the cell down their concentration and electrical gradients. (At this point, K^+ is not only in a greater concentration inside the cell, but the inside is also positive relative to the outside.). During this phase of the action potential, the permeability to K^+ ions is approximately 300 times greater than normal. This efflux of (+) charges causes the membrane to repolarize back toward the resting membrane potential.

Sodium channels open more rapidly than K^+ channels because they are more voltage sensitive and a small depolarization is sufficient to open them. Larger changes in membrane potential associated with further cell excitation are required to open the less voltage-sensitive K^+ channels. Therefore, the increase in the permeability of K^+ ions occurs later than that of Na^+ ions. This is functionally significant because if both types of ion channels opened concurrently, the change in membrane potential that would occur due to Na^+ ion influx would be cancelled out by K^+ ion efflux and the action potential could not be generated.

To more fully understand the mechanism by which the action potential is generated, further explanation concerning the structure and activity of the voltage-gated ion channels is necessary. A *voltage-gated Na^+ channel* has two different gates: the *activation gate* and the *inactivation gate*. At the resting membrane potential of –70 mV in an unstimulated neuron, the activation gate is closed and the permeability to Na^+ ions is very low. In this resting state, the channel is closed but capable of opening in response to a stimulus. When stimulated by depolarization to threshold, the activation gates open very rapidly and Na^+ ions diffuse into the cell causing the upward swing of the action potential. Once these activation gates open, the inactivation gates begin to close, although these gates close more slowly. At the peak of the action potential when the inactivation gates are now closed, these channels are no longer permeable to Na^+ ions and incapable of opening regardless of further stimulation.

Therefore, Na⁺ channels cannot reopen, Na⁺ ions cannot enter the cell, and another action potential cannot be generated. In fact, these voltage-gated channels cannot return to their resting position and become capable of opening until the neuron has first repolarized to –70 mV from the existing action potential. This period of time — beginning when all the Na⁺ channels are open and lasting through their inactivation phase — is referred to as the *absolute refractory period*. Regardless of the strength of the stimulus, no new action potentials can be generated. The approximately 2-msec length of this period limits the number of action potentials that neurons can generate to up to 500 per second.

The *voltage-gated K⁺ channel* has only one gate, which is typically closed at the resting membrane potential. This gate also opens in response to depolarization of the membrane toward zero. However, unlike the activation gate of the voltage-gated Na⁺ channel that opens very quickly, this gate opens very slowly so that the permeability to K⁺ ions is delayed. In fact, it opens at approximately the same time that the inactivation gates in the Na⁺ channels close. Therefore, Na⁺ ion permeability decreases and K⁺ ion permeability increases simultaneously, resulting in the outward movement of (+) charges and rapid repolarization.

Voltage-gated K⁺ channels open and close slowly; therefore, the increase in permeability to K⁺ ions is prolonged. As a result, K⁺ ions continue to exit the cell and the membrane potential approaches the equilibrium potential for potassium. This phase of the action potential is referred to as *after-hyperpolarization*. Because the membrane potential is now further away from threshold, a larger than normal stimulus is necessary to cause depolarization to threshold. During this phase of hyperpolarization it is possible, but more difficult, for the neuron to generate another action potential. This *relative refractory period* lasts from the end of the absolute refractory period until the voltage-gated K⁺ channels have returned to their resting state and the membrane once again returns to its resting potential.

During the course of the action potential, Na⁺ ions entered the cell and K⁺ ions exited it. In order to prevent eventual dissipation of the concentration gradients for Na⁺ and K⁺ ions across the cell membrane over time, these substances must be returned to their original positions. The slow but continuous activity of the Na⁺–K⁺ pump is responsible for this function and returns Na⁺ ions to the extracellular fluid and K⁺ ions to the intracellular fluid.

4.4   Conduction of the action potential

A typical neuron consists of four functional regions:

- Cell body
- Axon hillock
- Axon
- Axon terminal

The *cell body*, with its *dendrites*, which are projections from the cell body that greatly increase the surface area, is the site of communication and input from other neurons. These inputs result in generation of graded potentials that travel a short distance to the *axon hillock*, the region of the cell body from which the axon arises. Following sufficient stimulation of the neuron, an action potential is generated at the axon hillock. This action potential must then be propagated or regenerated along the third portion of the neuron, the axon. The *axon*, or nerve fiber, is an elongated projection that transmits the action potential away from the cell body toward other cells. The final component of the neuron is the *axon terminal*, where the neuron communicates with another cell or cells by way of this action potential. Conduction of the action potential along the length of the axon is the subject of this section; communication between a neuron and another cell is discussed in the following chapter.

The action potential is initiated at the axon hillock (see Figure 4.3). This region is particularly excitable due to an abundance of voltage-gated Na^+ channels. As the axon hillock is stimulated by excitatory inputs, there is a marked influx of Na^+ ions and this region of the cell membrane becomes positive inside, resulting in an action potential. The rest of the axon is still at its resting membrane potential and is negative inside. As with graded potentials, this electrical signal also travels by local current flow (see Figure 4.3). The (+) charges in the region of the action potential are attracted to the negative charges in the immediately adjacent region of the axonal membrane.

This current flow depolarizes the new region, causing an increase in the permeability of the cell membrane to Na^+ ions through voltage-gated ion channels. The subsequent influx of Na^+ ions further depolarizes the membrane so that it reaches threshold and a *new action potential* is generated in this region. At the same time, the original site of action potential generation at the axon hillock repolarizes due to the efflux of K^+ ions. This process of generating new action potentials sequentially along the membrane enables the signal to maintain its strength as it travels the distance to the axon terminal.

Another mechanism of conduction of an action potential along the length of a neuron is the *saltatory conduction* that occurs in *myelinated* axons (see Figure 4.4). Myelin is a lipid sheath wrapped around the axon at regular intervals. The myelin is not actually part of the axon, but instead comes from other cells. In the central nervous system (brain and spinal cord), the myelin-forming cell is the *oligodendrocyte*, one of several types of support cells for centrally located neurons. In the peripheral nervous system (all neurons that lie outside the central nervous system and communicate with various body parts), myelin is formed by the *Schwann cells*. The lipid of the myelin in each case comes from multiple layers of the plasma membrane of these cells as they wrap around the axon. This lipid provides good insulation, preventing the movement of current across the cell membrane.

Without ion flux, action potentials cannot be generated in the regions covered with myelin. Instead, they occur only at breaks in the myelin sheath

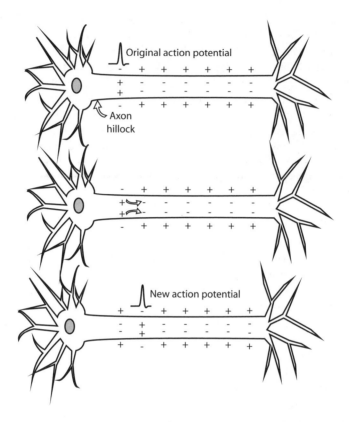

Figure 4.3 Conduction of the action potential along an axon by local current flow. Upper panel: action potentials are generated at the axon hillock. When stimulated to threshold, this region of the membrane becomes positive (+30 mV) inside relative to the outside due to the influx of Na⁺ ions. The remainder of the axon is at its resting membrane potential (−70 mV). Middle panel: because opposite charges attract, the (+) charges in the stimulated area are attracted to the (−) charges in the adjacent region of the membrane. This movement of (+) charges, or local current flow, depolarizes this adjacent region. Lower panel: the depolarization of the adjacent region causes activation of voltage-gated Na⁺ channels and generation of a new action potential. Meanwhile, the original area of stimulation has repolarized back to the resting membrane potential. This unidirectional process continues along the length of the axon.

referred to as the *nodes of Ranvier*. These nodes are located about 1 to 2 mm apart. The flow of current from an active node "skips" down the axon to the adjacent node to cause depolarization and generation of a new action potential. This transmission of the impulse from node to node is referred to as saltatory conduction, from the Latin word *saltare*, meaning "to leap."

Saltatory conduction results in a significant increase in the *velocity of conduction* of the nerve impulse down the axon compared to that of local current flow in an unmyelinated axon (see Table 4.2). The speed of conduction is

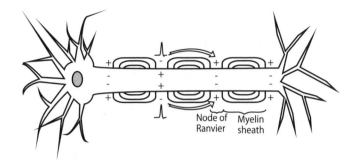

Figure 4.4 Saltatory conduction. Transmission of electrical impulses in a myelinated axon occurs by way of saltatory conduction. Composed primarily of lipid, the myelin sheath insulates the axon and prevents generation of membrane potentials. Membrane potentials occur only at gaps in the myelin sheath, referred to as the nodes of Ranvier. Therefore, transmission of the impulse, or generation of action potentials, occurs only at the nodes.

directly correlated to the urgency of the information conveyed by a given neuron. Nerve fibers carrying less important information, such as those regulating slow digestive processes, are unmyelinated. An example of a nerve fiber with myelin is one that innervates skeletal muscle so that movements can be executed rapidly.

The functional significance of myelin is revealed by the neurological deficits observed in patients with *multiple sclerosis*. This disorder is caused by the demyelination of neurons in the brain, spinal cord, and optic nerve. The loss of myelin disrupts the normal conduction of impulses along the axons of these neurons and results in weakness, numbness, loss of bladder control, and visual disturbances.

Another advantage of the presence of myelin along an axon is that impulse conduction is energetically more efficient. Because action potentials occur only at the nodes of Ranvier, fewer Na^+ and K^+ ions move in and out of the cell. Therefore, less metabolic energy is required to return these ions to their original positions along the cell membrane and to maintain the proper concentration gradients. In unmyelinated axons, action potentials, and therefore ion flux, occur along the entire length of the axon. These neurons expend more energy returning these ions to their original positions.

A second factor that influences the velocity of action potential conduction is the *diameter of the axon*. The greater the diameter is then, the lower the resistance to current flow along the axon. Therefore, the impulse is

Table 4.2 Factors Affecting Velocity of Conduction

Factor	Velocity of conduction
Myelination of axon (saltatory conduction)	↑
↑ Diameter of axon	↑

conducted along large nerve fibers more rapidly. Large myelinated nerve fibers, such as those innervating skeletal muscle, exhibit the highest conduction velocity. Small unmyelinated fibers, such as those of the autonomic nervous system innervating the heart; smooth muscle of the blood vessels and gastrointestinal tract; and glands, conduct nerve impulses more slowly.

Conduction of the action potential along the axon is *unidirectional*. In other words, the nerve impulse travels away from the cell body and the axon hillock toward the axon terminal only. As the current flows from the initial area of activity to the adjacent region of the axon, the new region becomes depolarized and generates an action potential. Simultaneously, the initial area has entered its absolute refractory period due to inactivation of voltage-gated Na^+ channels. As a result, as current flows away from the second active area, it has no effect on the original site of activity. Instead, the current continues forward and depolarizes the next adjacent region of the axon. By the time the original site has recovered from the refractory period and is capable of being restimulated, the action potential has traveled too far along the axon to affect this site by way of local current flow. This unidirectional conduction ensures that the signal reaches the axon terminal where it can influence the activity of the innervated cell as opposed to traveling back and forth along the axon ineffectively.

Pharmacy application: local anesthetics

Pain is a protective mechanism that alerts an individual to the occurrence of tissue damage. Stimulation of nociceptors (pain receptors) alters membrane permeability to ions, the predominant effect of which is the influx of Na^+ ions down their electrical and chemical gradients. Sufficient Na^+ ion influx results in generation of an action potential that is then propagated along the afferent neuron to the CNS, where the painful stimulus is perceived. Local anesthetics, such as lidocaine and procaine (also known as novocaine), prevent or relieve the perception of pain by interrupting conduction of the nervous impulse. These drugs bind to a specific receptor site on the voltage-gated Na^+ channels and block ion movement through them. Without Na^+ ion influx, an action potential cannot be generated in the afferent neuron and the signal fails to reach the CNS. In general, the action of these drugs is restricted to the site of application and becomes less effective upon diffusion of the drug away from the site of action in the nerve.

Bibliography

1. Catterall, W. and Mackie, K., Local anesthetics, in *Goodman and Gilman's: The Pharmacological Basis of Therapeutics*, 9th ed., Hardman, J.G. and Limbird, L.E., Eds., McGraw–Hill, New York, 1996, chap. 15.
2. Costanzo, L., *Physiology*, W.B. Saunders, Philadelphia, 1998.
3. Guyton, A.C. and Hall, J.E., *Textbook of Medical Physiology*, 9th ed., W.B. Saunders, Philadelphia, 1996.
4. Lombard, J.H. and Rusch, N.J., Cells, nerves and muscles, in *Physiology Secrets*, Raff, H., Ed., Hanley and Belfus, Inc., Philadelphia, 1999, chap. 1.
5. Sherwood, L., *Human Physiology from Cells to Systems*, 4th ed., Brooks/Cole, Pacific Grove, CA, 2001.
6. Silverthorn, D., *Human Physiology: An Integrated Approach*, 2nd ed., Prentice-Hall, Upper Saddle River, NJ, 2001.

chapter 5

Synaptic transmission

Study objectives

- Describe the mechanism by which chemical synapses function
- Compare and contrast excitatory synapses and inhibitory synapses
- Distinguish between an EPSP and an IPSP
- Describe how neurotransmitters are removed from the synaptic cleft
- Explain how temporal summation and spatial summation take place
- Distinguish between convergence and divergence
- Understand how pH and hypoxia affect synaptic transmission
- Describe the potential mechanisms by which drugs, toxins, and diseases affect synaptic transmission
- Distinguish between an agonist and an antagonist

5.1 Introduction

The function of a neuron is to communicate or relay information to another cell by way of an electrical impulse. A *synapse* is the site at which the impulse is transmitted from one cell to the next. A neuron may terminate on a muscle cell, glandular cell, or another neuron. The discussion in this chapter will focus on neuron-to-neuron transmission. At these types of synapses, the *presynaptic neuron* transmits the impulse *toward* the synapse and the *postsynaptic neuron* transmits the impulse *away* from the synapse. Specifically, it is the axon terminal of the presynaptic neuron that comes into contact with the cell body or the dendrites of the postsynaptic neuron. Most neurons, particularly in the CNS, receive thousands of inputs. As will become evident, the transmission of the impulse at the synapse is *unidirectional* and the presynaptic neuron influences activity of the postsynaptic neuron only.

5.2 Chemical synapses

Most of the synapses in the nervous system are *chemical synapses* in which the presynaptic neuron and the postsynaptic neuron are not in direct contact but instead are separated by a narrow (0.01 to 0.02 μm) space called the *synaptic cleft*. This space prevents the direct spread of the electrical impulse from one cell to the next. Instead, a chemical referred to as a *neurotransmitter* is released from the presynaptic neuron. The neurotransmitter diffuses across the synaptic cleft, binds to its specific receptor, and alters electrical activity of the postsynaptic neuron.

The mechanism of action of a chemical synapse is shown in Figure 5.1. The axon terminal broadens to form a swelling referred to as the *synaptic knob*. Within the synaptic knob are many *synaptic vesicles* that store the pre-formed neurotransmitter. Also found in the membrane of the synaptic knob are *voltage-gated Ca⁺⁺ channels*. When the electrical impulse, or action potential, has been transmitted along the length of the axon and reaches the axon terminal, the accompanying change in voltage causes the voltage-gated Ca^{++} channels to open. Because calcium is in greater concentration in the extra-cellular fluid compared to the intracellular fluid, Ca^{++} ions enter the cell down their concentration gradient. The Ca^{++} ions then induce the release of the neurotransmitter from synaptic vesicles into the synaptic cleft by causing the vesicles to fuse with the presynaptic membrane, thereby facilitating the process of exocytosis. The neurotransmitter molecules diffuse across the cleft and bind to specific receptors on the membrane of the postsynaptic neuron.

This binding of the neurotransmitter alters permeability of the postsyn-aptic neuron to one or more ions. As always, a change in ion permeability results in a change in the membrane potential of the cell. This change at the synapse is in the form of a *graded potential* only. At any given synapse, the change in membrane potential is not great enough to reach threshold and generate an action potential. Instead, many graded potentials generated at one or more synapses are conducted over the cell membrane toward the axon hillock. If the depolarization caused by multiple graded potentials added together is sufficient for the axon hillock to reach threshold, then an action potential is generated here.

The two types of synapses are:

- Excitatory synapses
- Inhibitory synapses

At an *excitatory synapse*, binding of the neurotransmitter to its receptor increases permeability of the membrane to Na^+ ions and K^+ ions through *chemical messenger-gated channels* closely associated with the receptor. As a result, Na^+ ions enter the cell down their concentration and electrical gradi-ents and K^+ ions leave the cell down their concentration gradient only. Because two forces cause inward diffusion of sodium and only one force causes outward diffusion of potassium, the influx of Na^+ ions is significantly greater than the efflux of K^+ ions. This greater movement of (+) charges into the cell results in a small depolarization of the neuron referred to as an *excitatory postsynaptic potential (EPSP)*, which is a graded potential only. A single action potential occurring at a single excitatory synapse opens too few

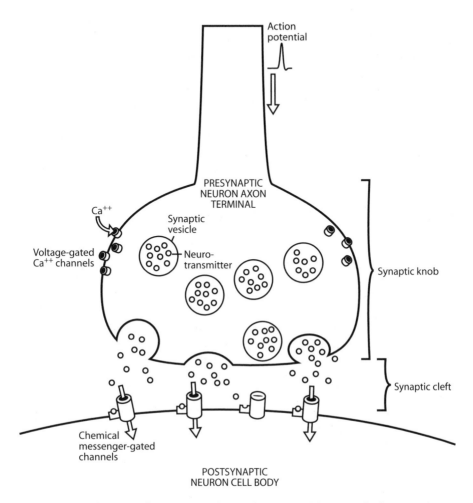

Figure 5.1 Mechanism of action at a chemical synapse. The arrival of an action potential at the axon terminal causes voltage-gated Ca^{++} channels to open. The resulting increase in concentration of Ca^{++} ions in the intracellular fluid facilitates exocytosis of the neurotransmitter into the synaptic cleft. Binding of the neurotransmitter to its specific receptor on the postsynaptic neuron alters the permeability of the membrane to one or more ions, thus causing a change in the membrane potential and generation of a graded potential in this neuron.

Na^+ channels to depolarize the membrane all the way to threshold; however, it brings the membrane potential closer toward it. This increases the likelihood that subsequent stimuli will continue depolarization to threshold and that an action potential will be generated by the postsynaptic neuron.

At an *inhibitory synapse*, binding of the neurotransmitter to its receptor increases permeability of the membrane to K^+ ions or to Cl^- ions through chemical messenger-gated channels. As a result, K^+ ions may leave the cell down their concentration gradient carrying (+) charges outward or Cl^- ions may enter the cell down their concentration gradient carrying (–) charges inward. In either case, the neuron becomes more negative inside relative to the outside and the membrane is now hyperpolarized. This small hyperpolarization is referred to as an inhibitory postsynaptic potential (IPSP). The movement of the membrane potential further away from threshold decreases the likelihood that an action potential will be generated by the postsynaptic neuron.

Almost invariably, a neuron is genetically programmed to synthesize and release only a single type of neurotransmitter. Therefore, a given synapse is either always excitatory or always inhibitory. Once a neurotransmitter has bound to its receptor on the postsynaptic neuron and has caused its effect, it is important to inactivate or remove it from the synapse in order to prevent its continuing activity indefinitely. Several mechanisms to carry this out have been identified:

- Passive diffusion of the neurotransmitter away from the synaptic cleft
- Destruction of the neurotransmitter by enzymes located in the synaptic cleft or in the plasma membranes of presynaptic or postsynaptic neurons
- Active reuptake of the neurotransmitter into the synaptic knob of the presynaptic neuron for reuse or enzymatic destruction

5.3   Summation

As previously mentioned, a single action potential at a single synapse results in a graded potential only: an EPSP or an IPSP. Therefore, generation of an action potential in the postsynaptic neuron requires the addition or *summation* of a sufficient number of excitatory inputs to depolarize this neuron to threshold. Two types of summation may occur:

- Temporal summation
- Spatial summation

Temporal summation occurs when multiple EPSPs (or IPSPs) produced by a *single* presynaptic neuron in close sequence exert their effect on membrane potential of the postsynaptic neuron. For example, an action potential in the presynaptic neuron produces an EPSP and partial depolarization of the postsynaptic neuron (see Figure 5.2). While the postsynaptic neuron is still depolarized, a second action potential in the presynaptic neuron produces another EPSP in the postsynaptic neuron that adds to the first and further depolarizes this neuron.

As more EPSPs add together, the membrane depolarizes closer to threshold until an action potential is generated. Although temporal summation is illustrated in Figure 5.2 with the summation of relatively few EPSPs, in actuality, addition of up to 50 EPSPs may be necessary to reach threshold. Because a presynaptic neuron may generate up to 500 action potentials per

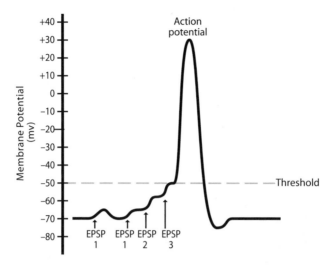

Figure 5.2 Temporal summation. Multiple excitatory postsynaptic potentials (EPSPs) produced by a single presynaptic neuron in close sequence may add together to depolarize the postsynaptic neuron to threshold and generate an action potential.

minute, temporal summation occurs quite readily. The strength of the signal to the postsynaptic neuron is therefore influenced by the *frequency of nerve impulses* generated by the presynaptic neuron.

Spatial summation occurs when multiple EPSPs (or IPSPs), produced by *many* presynaptic neurons, exert their effects on the membrane potential of the postsynaptic neuron simultaneously. For example, Figure 5.3 depicts a single postsynaptic neuron that is innervated by three presynaptic neurons. Inputs from presynaptic neurons *A* and *B* are excitatory and the input from presynaptic neuron *C* is inhibitory. Once again, single action potentials in neuron *A* or *B* produce individual EPSPs insufficient to depolarize the postsynaptic neuron to threshold. However, if EPSPs from neurons *A* and *B* are produced at the same time, the depolarizations add together and the membrane potential of the postsynaptic neuron reaches threshold, resulting in generation of an action potential. Inputs from neurons *A* (excitatory) and *C* (inhibitory) occurring simultaneously may, in effect, cancel each other out, resulting in no change in membrane potential of the postsynaptic neuron.

As with temporal summation, this example has been simplified to illustrate the concept clearly. In actuality, a large number of excitatory inputs from different presynaptic neurons are necessary to depolarize the postsynaptic neuron to threshold. Because a typical neuronal cell body receives thousands of presynaptic inputs, spatial summation also occurs quite readily. The *number of presynaptic neurons* that are active simultaneously therefore influences the strength of the signal to the postsynaptic neuron. Under normal physiological conditions, temporal summation and spatial summation may occur concurrently.

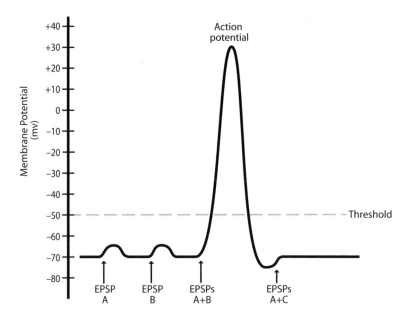

Figure 5.3 Spatial summation. Multiple excitatory postsynaptic potentials (EPSPs) or inhibitory postsynaptic potentials (IPSPs) produced by many presynaptic neurons simultaneously may add together to alter the membrane potential of the postsynaptic neuron. Sufficient excitatory input (*A* and *B*) will depolarize the membrane to threshold and generate an action potential. The simultaneous arrival of excitatory and inhibitory inputs (*A* and *C*) may cancel each other out so that the membrane potential does not change.

5.4   *Interconnections between neurons*

The interconnections or communication among neurons in humans is very extensive. Imagine the complexity of the electrical activity that may occur among 100 billion neurons in the human brain where each of these neurons provides input to and receives input from hundreds of other neurons. It is the diversity of these interconnections that accounts for the uniqueness of many abstract neurological phenomena in individuals such as intellect, personality, and memory. The two types of interconnections are:

- Convergence
- Divergence

Convergence occurs when the axon terminals of many presynaptic neurons all synapse with a single postsynaptic neuron. As discussed previously, spatial summation of nerve impulses relies on the presence of convergence. *Divergence* occurs when the axon of a single presynaptic neuron branches and synapses with multiple postsynaptic neurons. In this way, activity in a single nerve fiber can affect several regions of the nervous system, each with a different function, at the same time.

5.5   Factors affecting synaptic transmission

Several factors influence synaptic transmission of electrical impulses:

- pH of the interstitial fluid
- Hypoxia
- Drugs, toxins, and diseases

Neurons are very sensitive to changes in the *pH of the interstitial fluid* surrounding them. Normally, the pH of arterial blood is 7.4. Under conditions of *alkalosis*, in which pH increases, the excitability of neurons also increases, rendering them more likely to generate action potentials. This inappropriate stimulation of the nervous system may lead to seizures, particularly in epileptics predisposed to them. Under conditions of *acidosis*, in which pH decreases, the excitability of neurons is depressed, rendering them less likely to generate action potentials. This lack of nervous system stimulation may lead to a comatose state. Severe diabetic acidosis or acidosis associated with end-stage renal failure will often lead to coma.

Neuronal function depends on a constant supply of oxygen. *Hypoxia*, a decrease in oxygen availability, depresses neuronal activity. Interruption of blood flow to the brain for only a few seconds leads to unconsciousness. A prolonged lack of blood flow, which is characteristic of stroke, leads to permanent brain damage in the affected area.

Many *drugs, toxins*, and *diseases* exert their clinical effects by altering some phase of synaptic activity. These effects may occur by means of:

- Altered release of a neurotransmitter
- Altered interaction of a neurotransmitter with its receptor
- Altered removal of a neurotransmitter from the synaptic cleft
- Replacement of a deficient neurotransmitter

Altered release. Tetanus is an infectious disease caused by the bacterium *Clostridium tetani.* This bacterium produces a neurotoxin active on inhibitory synapses in the spinal cord. Motor neurons, which supply skeletal muscle and cause contraction, have cell bodies that lie in the spinal cord. Under normal circumstances, these motor neurons receive excitatory and inhibitory inputs from various sources. The balance of these inputs results in the appropriate degree of muscle tone or muscle contraction. Tetanus toxin prevents the release of gamma amino butyric acid (GABA), an important neurotransmitter active at these inhibitory synapses. Eliminating inhibitory inputs results in unchecked or unmodulated excitatory input to the motor neurons. The resulting uncontrolled muscle spasms initially occur in the muscles of the jaw, giving rise to the expression *lockjaw.* The muscle spasms eventually affect the respiratory muscles, thus preventing inspiration and leading to death due to asphyxiation.

Altered interaction of a neurotransmitter with its receptor. Interaction of a neurotransmitter with its receptor may be altered pharmacologically in several ways. One such mechanism involves administration of *antagonists* — drugs that bind to a given receptor and prevent the action of the neurotransmitter but, by classical definition, initiate no other effect. An interesting clinical example of this form of therapy involves schizophrenia, a severe mental disorder characterized by delusions, hallucinations, social withdrawal, and disorganized speech and behavior. Although the precise cause of schizophrenia is unknown, its pathophysiology appears to involve neuronal pathways that release excessive amounts of the neurotransmitter dopamine. Antipsychotic drugs, such as Thorazine® (chlorpromazine) and Haldol® (haloperidol), minimize symptoms of schizophrenia by blocking dopamine receptors and thus preventing excess dopamine from exerting its effects.

An *agonist* is a drug that binds to a given receptor and stimulates it. In other words, agonists mimic the effect of endogenous neurotransmitters. Albuterol, the active ingredient in medications such as Ventolin ®, is a β_2-adrenergic receptor agonist that mimics the effect of the neurotransmitter, epinephrine. Because stimulation of these receptors in the lungs causes the airways to dilate, albuterol is effective in reversing the bronchospasm and dyspnea (difficulty in breathing) associated with asthma.

Another mechanism by which neurotransmitter/receptor interaction may be altered involves administering drugs that *facilitate* binding of the neurotransmitter to its receptor. Once again, the neurotransmitter used as an example is GABA, the most prevalent inhibitory neurotransmitter in the nervous system. It not only contributes to regulation of skeletal muscle tone by inhibiting activity of motor neurons, but is also involved in the regulation of mood and emotions by acting as a CNS depressant. The benzodiazepines, antianxiety drugs that include Valium® (diazepam) and Ativan® (lorazepam), act by binding to a specific site on the GABA receptor. This binding causes a conformational change in the receptor protein that enhances the binding of GABA. As more GABA binds to the receptors, its effectiveness in the CNS is increased and anxiety is decreased.

Altered removal of a neurotransmitter from the synaptic cleft. The third mechanism by which drugs may alter synaptic activity involves changes in neurotransmitter reuptake or degradation. A very well known example of a drug in this category is Prozac® (fluoxetine), which is used to treat depression. The complete etiology is unknown, but it is widely accepted that depression involves a deficiency of monoamine neurotransmitters (e.g., norepinephrine and serotonin) in the CNS. Prozac, a selective serotonin reuptake inhibitor, prevents removal of serotonin from the synaptic cleft. As a result, the concentration and activity of serotonin are enhanced.

Replacement of a deficient neurotransmitter. Finally, synaptic activity may be altered by replacement of a deficient neurotransmitter, a form of drug therapy effective in treatment of Parkinson's disease. The pathophysiology of Parkinson's involves progressive destruction of dopaminergic (dopamine-releasing) neurons, resulting in a deficiency of dopamine in certain areas in the brain. In addition to neuronal pathways involved in regulation of mood and emotion, dopamine is released by neurons that inhibit skeletal muscle contraction. Because motor neurons normally receive excitatory and inhibitory inputs, the inhibition provided by the dopaminergic pathways results in smooth, precise muscle contractions. In the patient with Parkinson's disease, this loss of inhibition leads to increased muscle tone, or muscle rigidity, and resting tremors.

These symptoms are alleviated by administering levodopa (L-dopa), a precursor for dopamine. L-dopa is taken up by the axon terminals of dopaminergic neurons and used to form dopamine. Interestingly, in some patients, a side effect of dopamine replacement therapy is the development of symptoms characteristic of schizophrenia. (Recall that this mental disorder is caused by overactive dopaminergic neurons.) On the other hand, drugs used to treat schizophrenia — dopamine receptor antagonists — may elicit symptoms of Parkinson's disease.

Bibliography

1. Baldessarini, R., Drugs and the treatment of psychiatric disorders: psychosis and anxiety, in *Goodman and Gilman's: The Pharmacological Basis of Therapeutics*, 9th ed., Hardman, J.G. and Limbird, L.E., Eds., McGraw–Hill, New York, 1996, chap. 18.
2. Baldessarini, R., Drugs and the treatment of psychiatric disorders: depression and mania, in *Goodman and Gilman's: The Pharmacological Basis of Therapeutics*, 9th ed., Hardman, J.G. and Limbird, L.E., Eds., McGraw–Hill, New York, 1996, chap. 19.
3. Bloom, F., Neurotransmission and the central nervous system, in *Goodman and Gilman's: The Pharmacological Basis of Therapeutics*, 9th ed., Hardman, J.G. and Limbird, L.E., Eds., McGraw–Hill, New York, 1996, chap. 12.
4. Finley, P.R., Selective serotonin re-uptake inhibitors: pharmacologic profiles and potential therapeutic distinctions, *Ann. Pharmacother.*, 28(12), 1359–1369, 1994.
5. Garoutte, B., *Neuromuscular Physiology*, Mill Valley Medical Publishers, Millbrae, CA, 1996.
6. Guyton, A.C. and Hall, J.E., *Textbook of Medical Physiology*, 9th ed., W.B. Saunders, Philadelphia, 1996.
7. Hanson, M., *Pathophysiology, Foundations of Disease and Clinical Intervention*, W.B. Saunders, Philadelphia, 1998.
8. Kane, J.M., Schizophrenia, *N. Engl. J. Med.*, 334(1), 34–41, 1996.
9. Lombard, J.H. and Rusch, N.J., Cells, nerves and muscles, in *Physiology Secrets*, Raff, H., Ed., Hanley and Belfus, Inc., Philadelphia, 1999, chap. 1.
10. Ross, E.M., Pharmacodynamics: mechanisms of drug action and the relationship between drug concentration and effect, in *Goodman and Gilman's: The Pharmacological Basis of Therapeutics*, 9th ed., Hardman, J.G. and Limbird, L.E., Eds., McGraw–Hill, New York, 1996, chap. 2.

11. Sherwood, L., *Human Physiology from Cells to Systems*, 4th ed., Brooks/Cole, Pacific Grove, CA, 2001.

12. Silverthorn, D., *Human Physiology: An Integrated Approach*, 2nd ed., Prentice-Hall, Upper Saddle River, NJ, 2001.

13. *Taber's Cyclopedic Medical Dictionary*, 19th ed., F.A. Davis Co., Philadelphia, 2001.

chapter six

The nervous system

Study objectives

- Describe the organization of the nervous system including the central nervous system and the peripheral nervous system
- Distinguish among the three types of neurons: afferent neurons, efferent neurons, and interneurons
- List the three major levels of CNS function and describe their activities
- Distinguish among the three types of tracts in the CNS: projection tracts, association tracts, and commissural tracts
- Describe the activity of each of the functional areas of the cerebral cortex
- Explain how language is processed in the cerebral cortex
- Describe the functions of the basal ganglia, thalamus, hypothalamus, and brainstem
- Distinguish among the three regions of the cerebellum and their functions
- Compare and contrast the exchange of materials between the blood and peripheral tissues with that of the blood and brain
- Explain the functions of the blood–brain barrier
- Explain the functions of cerebrospinal fluid

6.1 Introduction

The nervous system is one of the two regulatory systems in the human body that influences the activity of all the other organ systems. It consists of literally billions of neurons interconnected in a highly organized manner to form circuits. The number of neurons and the manner in which they are interconnected in a given circuit distinguishes one region of the brain from another and the brain of one individual from that of another. In addition, *plasticity*, the ability to alter circuit connections and function in response to sensory input and experiences adds further complexity and distinctiveness to neurological responses and behavior. The nervous system is divided into two anatomically distinct regions:

- Central nervous system
- Peripheral nervous system

The *central nervous system* (*CNS*) consists of the brain and spinal cord. The *peripheral nervous system* (*PNS*) consists of 12 pairs of cranial nerves that arise from the brainstem and 31 pairs of spinal nerves arising from the spinal cord. These peripheral nerves carry information between the CNS and the tissues of the body. The PNS consists of two divisions:

- Afferent division
- Efferent division

The *afferent division* carries sensory information toward the CNS and the *efferent division* carries motor information away from the CNS toward the effector tissues (muscles and glands). The efferent division is further divided into two components: (1) the somatic nervous system, which consists of motor neurons that innervate skeletal muscle; and (2) the autonomic nervous system that innervates cardiac muscle, smooth muscle, and glands.

6.2   Classes of neurons

The human nervous system has three functional classes of neurons:

- Afferent neurons
- Efferent neurons
- Interneurons

Afferent neurons lie predominantly in the PNS (see Figure 6.1). Each has a sensory receptor activated by a particular type of stimulus, a cell body located adjacent to the spinal cord, and an axon. The *peripheral axon* extends from the receptor to the cell body and the *central axon* continues from the cell body into the spinal cord. *Efferent neurons* also lie predominantly in the PNS. In this case, the cell bodies are found in the CNS in the spinal cord or brainstem and the axons extend out into the periphery of the body where they innervate the effector tissues. By way of convergence, the centrally located cell bodies may receive inputs from several different regions of the brain that will influence their activity.

The third class of neurons includes the *interneurons*, which lie entirely within the CNS. Because the human brain and spinal cord contain well over 100 billion neurons, interneurons account for approximately 99% of all the neurons in the body taken together. Interneurons lie between afferent and

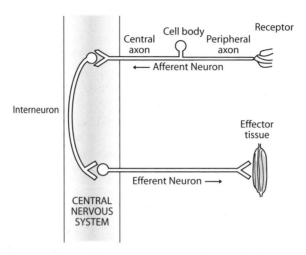

Figure 6.1 Types of neurons. Afferent neurons, which transmit impulses toward the CNS and efferent neurons, which transmit impulses away from the CNS, lie predominantly in the peripheral nervous system. Interneurons, which process sensory input and coordinate motor responses, lie entirely within the central nervous system.

efferent neurons and are responsible for integrating sensory input and coordinating a motor response. In the simplest condition, interneurons process responses at the level of the spinal cord in the form of *reflexes* that are automatic, stereotyped responses to given stimuli. For example, stimulation of pain receptors generates action potentials in their associated afferent neurons. These impulses are transmitted to the spinal cord where the afferent neurons stimulate interneurons. The interneurons then stimulate efferent neurons that cause skeletal muscle contraction in the affected area to remove the body part from the painful stimulus. This *withdrawal reflex* involves comparatively few interneurons and does not require any input from higher nervous centers in the brain. On the other hand, a response to some other stimulus may involve more sophisticated neurological phenomena such as memory, motivation, judgment, and intellect. This type of response is not automatic, is clearly far more complex and may require the activity of millions of interneurons in many regions of the brain prior to stimulation of motor neurons to carry out the desired response.

6.3   Major levels of CNS function

The three major levels of CNS function are:

- Spinal cord
- Brainstem
- Cerebrum and cerebral cortex

Table 6.1 Major Levels of CNS Function

Spinal cord	Processes reflexes
	Transmits nerve impulses to and from brain
Brainstem	Receives sensory input and initiates motor output
	Controls life-sustaining processes (e.g., respiration, circulation, digestion)
Cerebrum and cerebral cortex	Processes, integrates, and analyzes information
	Involved with highest levels of cognition, voluntary initiation of movement, sensory perception, and language

The *spinal cord* is the most anatomically inferior portion of the CNS and its functions are at the lowest level of sophistication (see Table 6.1). As mentioned earlier, the spinal cord receives sensory input from the periphery of the body and contains the cell bodies of motor neurons responsible for voluntary and involuntary movements. Once again, the involuntary and neurologically simple *reflexes* are processed entirely at the level of the spinal cord. Voluntary, deliberate movements are initiated and controlled by thought processes in the cerebrum. The second important function of the spinal cord is to *transmit nerve impulses* to and from the brain. *Ascending pathways* carry sensory input to higher levels of the CNS and *descending pathways* carry impulses from the brain to motor neurons in the spinal cord.

The *brainstem*, which consists of the medulla, pons, and midbrain, in evolutionary terms is the oldest and smallest region of the brain. Continuous with the spinal cord, the brainstem receives sensory input and initiates motor output by way of cranial nerves III through XII, which are functionally analogous to the 31 pairs of spinal nerves. Whereas the spinal cord processes sensory and motor activities in the trunk of the body and the limbs, the brainstem processes these activities primarily in the head, neck, and face. The brainstem also controls many basic life-sustaining processes, including respiration, circulation, and digestion. Even with loss of higher cognitive function, this lower level of the brain can sustain these bodily functions essential for survival.

The *cerebrum and cerebral cortex*, which account for 80% of the total brain weight in humans, constitute the highest functional level of the CNS. The more cognitively sophisticated the specie is, the larger and more highly folded the cerebral cortex is. These convolutions or folds serve to increase the surface area of the cerebral cortex, thus allowing for a greater number of neurons. Therefore, it is not unexpected that the cerebrum is most highly developed in the human. Responsible for the highest levels of processing, integration, and analysis of information, the cerebral cortex plays an important role in the most elaborate neurological functions including intellect; thought; personality; voluntary initiation of movement; final sensory perception; and language.

6.4   The brain

The brain is the integrative portion of the nervous system that serves to receive, process, and store sensory information and then plan and orchestrate the appropriate motor response. It is divided into several anatomically and functionally distinct regions (see Table 6.2). The forebrain consists of the cerebrum, basal ganglia, thalamus, and hypothalamus. The midbrain, along with the pons and the medulla of the hindbrain, composes the functional region referred to as the brainstem. The cerebellum is also considered a component of the hindbrain but is functionally distinct from the brainstem.

6.4.1   Cerebrum

The *cerebrum* is composed of two hemispheres, left and right, that are anatomically connected to ensure communication between them. Two types of tissue compose each hemisphere (see Figure 6.2):

- Gray matter
- White matter

The *gray matter*, which contains the cell bodies of neurons, is on the outer surface of the cerebrum and forms the *cerebral cortex*. The *white matter*, composed of the myelinated axons of neurons, is found underlying the cortex in the core of the cerebrum. These axons are bundled together according to function and organized into units referred to as *tracts*. The three types of tracts in the cerebrum are:

- Projection tracts
- Association tracts
- Commissural tracts

Table 6.2 Adult Brain Structures

Forebrain		
Cerebrum	→	Cerebral cortex
Basal ganglia		
Thalamus	→	Subcortical structures
Hypothalamus		(embedded within cerebrum)
Midbrain		
Hindbrain		
Pons	→	Brainstem
Medulla		
Cerebellum		

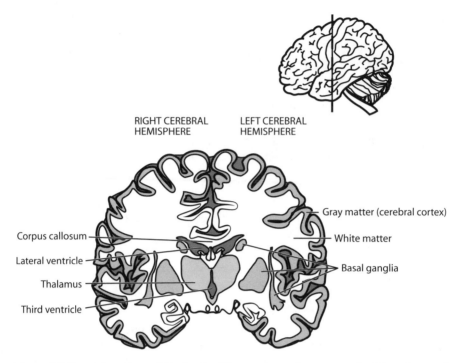

RIGHT CEREBRAL   LEFT CEREBRAL
HEMISPHERE   HEMISPHERE

Gray matter (cerebral cortex)

Corpus callosum — White matter

Lateral ventricle — Basal ganglia

Thalamus

Third ventricle

Figure 6.2 Frontal section of the brain. The cerebrum is composed of two types of tissue: internal white matter and external gray matter which forms the cerebral cortex. Embedded within the cerebral hemispheres are other masses of gray matter, basal ganglia, and thalamus. The ventricles are filled with cerebrospinal fluid (CSF).

Projection tracts may be *descending* and carry motor nerve impulses from the cerebral cortex to lower regions of the brain or spinal cord or they may be *ascending* and carry sensory impulses from lower regions of the brain or spinal cord to the cortex. *Association tracts* transmit nerve impulses from one functional region of the cerebral cortex to another within the same hemisphere. *Commissural tracts* transmit impulses from one hemisphere to the other. The primary example of this type of tract is the corpus callosum, the thick band of tissue connecting the left and right hemispheres consisting of more than 100 million neurons. The communication provided by each of these types of tracts facilitates the integration, processing, and storage of information among various regions of the brain.

The cerebral cortex is not a smooth surface, but instead is highly folded and has a furrowed appearance (see Figure 6.3). A convolution formed by these folds is referred to as a *gyrus (pl. gyri)*. Each gyrus is separated from another by a *sulcus (pl. sulci)*, which is a shallow groove, or a *fissure*, which is a deeper groove. The functional importance of gyri, sulci, and fissures is that they significantly increase the surface area of the cerebral cortex, providing space for a greater number of neurons.

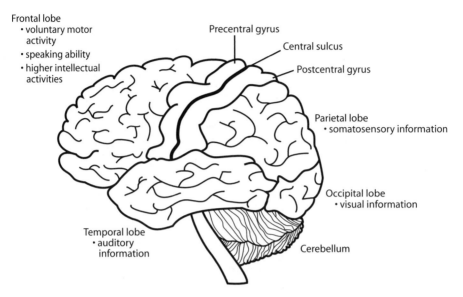

Frontal lobe
  • voluntary motor
    activity
  • speaking ability
  • higher intellectual
    activities

Precentral gyrus

Central sulcus

Postcentral gyrus

Parietal lobe
  • somatosensory information

Occipital lobe
  • visual information

Temporal lobe
  • auditory
    information

Cerebellum

Figure 6.3 Lateral view of the four lobes of the cerebral cortex.

Both hemispheres of the cerebrum consist of four lobes, including:

- Frontal lobes
- Parietal lobes
- Occipital lobes
- Temporal lobes

Named for the bones of the cranium under which they lie, the lobes are conspicuously defined by prominent sulci of the cortex, which have a relatively constant position in human brains. Each lobe is specialized for different activities (see Figure 6.3). Located in the anterior portions of the hemispheres, the *frontal lobes* are responsible for voluntary motor activity, speaking ability, and higher intellectual activities. The *parietal lobes*, which are posterior to the frontal lobes, process and integrate sensory information. The *occipital lobes*, located in the posterior-most aspects of the cerebrum, process visual information, and the *temporal lobes*, located laterally, process auditory information.

6.4.2   Functional regions of the cerebral cortex

The cerebral cortex is organized into several functionally discrete areas (see Figure 6.4). However, it is important to remember that no single area functions in isolation. The activity in each area depends on neurons in other areas for incoming and outgoing messages.

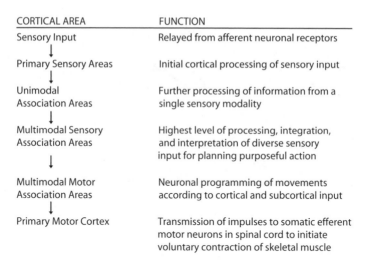

CORTICAL AREA	FUNCTION
Sensory Input ↓	Relayed from afferent neuronal receptors
Primary Sensory Areas ↓	Initial cortical processing of sensory input
Unimodal Association Areas ↓	Further processing of information from a single sensory modality
Multimodal Sensory Association Areas ↓	Highest level of processing, integration, and interpretation of diverse sensory input for planning purposeful action
Multimodal Motor Association Areas ↓	Neuronal programming of movements according to cortical and subcortical input
Primary Motor Cortex	Transmission of impulses to somatic efferent motor neurons in spinal cord to initiate voluntary contraction of skeletal muscle

Figure 6.4 Potential route of transmission of electrical impulses through association pathways of the cerebral cortex.

The *somatosensory cortex* is located in the postcentral gyrus, which is the most anterior region of the parietal lobes (see Figure 6.3). This region contains the terminations of ascending pathways that transmit nerve impulses concerning temperature, touch, pressure, pain, and proprioception. The latter is the awareness of posture, movement, changes in equilibrium, and the position of one's body parts, particularly in reference to surrounding objects. As such, the somatosensory cortex is the site for initial cerebral processing of these types of inputs.

Each section of this region of cortex receives sensory input from a specific area of the body in a highly organized and sequential manner. Interestingly, the size of the region of the cortex devoted to different areas of the body is quite disproportionate. For example, the trunk of the body and the legs are not densely innervated with sensory neurons. As a result, axonal terminations of pathways originating in these body parts are limited in number and take up only a small portion of the somatosensory cortex. Conversely, the face, tongue, and hands are very densely innervated with sensory neurons. Therefore, terminations of pathways originating in these body parts are numerous and represented in a much larger portion of the somatosensory cortex. In other words, the proportion of cortex devoted to a given body part is determined by the degree of sensory perception associated with that body part. The somatosensory cortex not only localizes the source of sensory input but it also perceives the intensity of the stimulus.

These ascending sensory pathways cross from one side of the CNS to the other so that sensory input from the left side of the body is transmitted to the somatosensory cortex of the right cerebral hemisphere and visa versa. Therefore, damage to this region of cortex in a given hemisphere results in sensory deficits such as numbness and tingling in the opposite side of the body.

In addition to the somatosensory cortex, special senses areas in the cerebral cortex are involved with the primary or initial processing of a specific type of stimulus. The *primary visual cortex* (sight) is located in the occipital lobes; the *primary auditory cortex* (hearing) and the *primary olfactory cortex* (smell) are located in the temporal lobes; and the *primary gustatory* or *taste cortex* is located at the base of the somatosensory cortex in the parietal lobes. Each of these primary areas is surrounded by a "higher order" sensory area or a *unimodal association area* that further integrates information from a single sensory modality and provides more complex aspects of the input. For example, the primary visual cortex is the first site of processing of visual information. Association tracts originating in this area then project to the surrounding unimodal association area for higher-level processing of this visual input.

The *posterior parietal cortex* is located posterior to the somatosensory cortex and serves as its unimodal association area. In addition to further processing of somatosensory input, information from the somatosensory cortex is integrated with visual inputs in this region. Association tracts from both the somatosensory cortex and the visual cortex terminate here. This activity is important for planning complex movements and for hand (proprioception)–eye (visual) coordination.

The unimodal association areas in turn project to *multimodal sensory association* areas that integrate information about more than one sensory modality. The highest level of cognitive brain function takes place in these areas. These areas process, integrate, and interpret sensory information and then link these data to the planning of movement and goal-directed action.

The *prefrontal multimodal association area* is located in the most anterior region of the frontal lobe. It is involved primarily with motor integration, including memory and planning of motor activity; long-term planning and judgment; personality traits; and behavior. Consistent with this notion, lesions to this association area result in profound cognitive deficits, impaired motor activity, and changes in personality and social behavior. These patients do not respond to environmental stimuli in a way similar to normal individuals. They tend to achieve less in life — a behavior that suggests their ability to plan and organize everyday activities is impaired. Interestingly, however, their general intelligence, perception, and long-term memory are rather intact.

The *posterior multimodal association area* is located at the junction of the parietal, temporal, and occipital lobes. It pools and integrates somatic, auditory, and visual stimuli for complex perceptual processing. As such, this area is involved primarily with visuospatial localization, language, and attention. Lesions here interfere with awareness of one's body position and of the space in which it moves as well as the ability to integrate and make sense of elements of a visual scene. In other words, these patients have normal visual acuity but cannot focus on an object of interest.

The limbic multimodal association area is partially located in each of the temporal, parietal and frontal lobes. It is concerned with emotional expression and memory storage. Although these functions appear to be unrelated, it is important to note that the emotional impact of an event is a major determinant of whether the event is remembered. Once again, it is important to remember that, although each of these multimodal association areas has its own characteristic function, all are highly interconnected and work together toward an end result.

The multimodal sensory association areas then project to the *multimodal motor association areas* located in the frontal lobes, including the *premotor cortex* and the *supplementary motor cortex*. Neurons here are active during preparation for movement. These regions receive input from the basal ganglia, cerebellum, somatosensory cortex, and posterior multimodal association cortex (all of which provide information about the ongoing movement) as well as the prefrontal multimodal association area. As such, these areas are important in programming complex sequences of movements and in orienting the body and limbs toward a specific target. Lesions in these multimodal motor association areas interfere with coordination and performance of complex integrated movements.

Following the development of the motor program, neurons originating in the multimodal motor association areas transmit impulses by way of association tracts to neurons of the primary motor cortex. The *primary motor cortex* is located in the precentral gyrus, which is the most posterior region of the frontal lobe adjacent to the multimodal motor association areas (see Figure 6.3); this area initiates voluntary contractions of specific skeletal muscles. Neurons whose cell bodies reside here transmit impulses by way of descending projection tracts to the spinal cord, where they innervate the alpha motor neurons (which innervate skeletal muscles).

As with the somatosensory cortex, neurons here are highly organized, with each section of the cortex innervating specific body parts in a sequential manner. Also like the somatosensory cortex, the size of the region of the primary motor cortex devoted to different parts of the body is quite disproportionate. Large portions of the primary motor cortex innervate the muscles of the hands, which perform complex movements, as well as muscles responsible for speech and eating. On the other hand, little cortex is devoted to motor pathways terminating in the trunk of the body or the lower extremities, which are not capable of complex movements. Therefore, the distortions in cortical representation parallel the importance of a particular part of the body in terms of complexity of motor skills. A third similarity between the primary motor cortex and the somatosensory cortex is that the projection tracts cross from one side of the CNS to the other; therefore, activity of motor neurons in the left cerebral hemisphere causes muscle contraction on the right side of the body and vice versa. Because the commands for muscle contraction originate in the primary motor cortex, lesions in this region of cortex in a given hemisphere will result in paralysis in the opposite side of the body.

The exchange of information among individuals is largely limited to species with advanced nervous systems and is found predominantly in birds and mammals. In humans, communication takes place primarily through *language* or the use of spoken or written words to convey a message. The processing of language requires a large network of interacting brain areas, both cortical and subcortical. However, the two predominant cortical areas are Wernicke's area and Broca's area. In approximately 96% of people, these cortical areas for language skills are found only in the left hemisphere. Even languages such as American sign language that rely on visuomotor abilities instead of auditory speech abilities depend primarily on the left hemisphere.

Sensory input to the language areas comes from the auditory cortex (hearing) or the visual cortex (reading). This input goes first to *Wernicke's area*, located in the left cerebral cortex near the junction of the parietal, temporal, and occipital lobes. This area is involved with language comprehension and is important for understanding spoken and written messages. It is also responsible for formulating coherent patterns of speech. In other words, this area enables an individual to attach meaning to words and to choose the appropriate words to convey his thoughts. Impulses are then transmitted to *Broca's area*, which is located in the left frontal lobe in close association with the motor areas of the cortex that control the muscles necessary for articulation. Broca's area is therefore responsible for the mechanical aspects of speaking.

A patient with a lesion in Wernicke's area is unable to understand any spoken or visual information. Furthermore, the patient's speech, while fluent, is unintelligible because of frequent errors in the choice of words. This condition is known as *receptive aphasia*. On the other hand, a patient with a lesion in Broca's area is able to understand spoken and written language but is unable to express his response in a normal manner. Speech in this patient is nonfluent and requires great effort because he cannot establish the proper motor command to articulate the desired words. This condition is known as *expressive aphasia*.

6.4.3   Basal ganglia

The *basal ganglia* consist of four nuclei or masses of gray matter embedded within the white matter of each cerebral hemisphere (see Figure 6.2). As with the cerebral cortex, this gray matter consists of functional aggregations of neuronal cell bodies. An important function of the basal ganglia is their contribution to the control of voluntary movement. The axons of neurons originating in the primary motor cortex travel through descending projection tracts to the spinal cord where they stimulate motor neurons to cause skeletal muscle contraction. At the same time, by way of divergence, these neurons transmit impulses to the basal ganglia. It is these impulses that form the primary source of input to these structures. In turn, the basal ganglia send impulses to the brainstem, which also transmits to motor neurons in the spinal cord as well as the thalamus, which transmits back to the motor areas of the cerebral cortex.

The activity of the basal ganglia tends to be inhibitory. The thalamus positively reinforces motor activity in the cerebral cortex. Impulses from the basal ganglia modulate this effect. Through their inputs to the brainstem and, ultimately the motor neurons in the spinal cord, the basal ganglia inhibit muscle tone (recall that the degree of skeletal muscle contraction and tone is determined by the summation of excitatory and inhibitory inputs to the motor neurons). They also contribute to the coordination of slow sustained contractions, especially those related to posture and body support. Motor disturbances associated with the basal ganglia include tremor and other involuntary movements; changes in posture and muscle tone; and slowness of movement without paralysis. Thus, disorders of the basal ganglia may result in diminished movement (Parkinson's disease) or excessive movement (Huntington's disease).

6.4.4 Thalamus

The *thalamus* is located between the cerebrum and the brainstem. Lying along the midline of the brain, it consists of two oval-shaped masses of gray matter, one in each cerebral hemisphere (see Figure 6.2). The thalamus is often described as a *relay station* because ascending tracts transmitting upward from the spinal cord, as well as sensory tracts from the eyes and the ears, extending ultimately to the cerebral cortex, pass through it. All sensory fiber tracts (except olfactory tracts) transmitting impulses to the cerebral cortex first synapse with neurons in the thalamus.

The thalamus acts as a *filter* for information to the cortex by preventing or enhancing the passage of specific information depending upon its significance to the individual. In fact, more than 99% of all sensory information transmitted toward the brain is discarded because it is considered irrelevant and unimportant. This selection activity is accomplished largely at the level of the thalamus. As mentioned previously in the discussion of the basal ganglia, the thalamus also plays a role in regulation of skeletal muscle contraction by positively reinforcing voluntary motor activity initiated by the cerebral cortex.

6.4.5 Hypothalamus

As its name suggests, the *hypothalamus* lies beneath the thalamus and above the pituitary gland. Although it is quite small, accounting for only about 4 g of the total 1400 g of the adult human brain, it plays a vital role in maintenance of homeostasis in the body. It is composed of numerous cell groups and fiber pathways, each with a specific function.

The hypothalamus plays a particularly important role in regulating the autonomic nervous system, which innervates cardiac muscle, smooth muscle, and glands. Many of these effects involve ascending or descending pathways of the cerebral cortex passing through the hypothalamus. Endocrine activity is also regulated by the hypothalamus by way of its control over pituitary gland secretion. Recent studies have demonstrated that the hypothalamus serves to integrate autonomic nervous system responses and endocrine function with behavior, especially behavior associated with basic homeostatic requirements. The hypothalamus provides this integrative function by regulating the following:

- Blood pressure and electrolyte composition by regulating mechanisms involved with urine output, thirst, salt appetite, maintenance of plasma osmolarity, and vascular smooth muscle tone
- Body temperature by regulating metabolic thermogenesis (e.g., shivering) and behaviors that cause an individual to seek a warmer or cooler environment
- Energy metabolism by regulating food intake, digestion, and metabolic rate
- Reproduction by way of hormonal control of sexual activity, pregnancy, and lactation
- Responses to stress by altering blood flow to skeletal muscles and other tissues as well as enhancing secretion of hormones from the adrenal cortex (glucocorticoids) whose metabolic activities enable the body to physically cope with stress

The hypothalamus regulates these physiological parameters by a three-step process involving negative feedback mechanisms (Chapter 1). First, the hypothalamus has access to and monitors sensory information from the entire body. Next, it compares this information to various biological set points that have been established for optimal cellular function. Finally, if a deviation from set point for a given parameter is detected, the hypothalamus elicits a variety of autonomic, endocrine, and behavioral responses to return the parameter to its set point and reestablish homeostasis. For example, blood glucose levels are monitored by the hypothalamus; when blood glucose is low (<50 mg glucose/100 ml blood), it mediates the sensation of hunger to drive the individual to ingest food.

6.4.6   Brainstem

The functional region known as the *brainstem* consists of the midbrain, and the pons and medulla of the hindbrain. It is continuous with the spinal cord and serves as an important connection between the brain and spinal cord because all sensory and motor pathways pass through it. The brainstem consists of numerous neuronal clusters or *centers*, each of which controls vital, life-supporting processes.

The *medulla* contains control centers for subconscious, involuntary functions, such as cardiovascular activity, respiration, swallowing, and vomiting. The primary function of the *pons* is to serve as a relay for the transfer of information between the cerebrum and the cerebellum. Along with the medulla, it also contributes to the control of breathing. The *midbrain* controls eye movement and relays signals for auditory and visual reflexes. It also provides linkages between components of the motor system including the cerebellum, basal ganglia, and cerebrum.

In addition, the brainstem contains a diffuse network of neurons known as the *reticular formation*. This network is best known for its role in cortical alertness, ability to direct attention, and sleep. It is also involved with coordination of orofacial motor activities, in particular those involved with eating and the generation of emotional facial expressions. Other functions include coordination of eating and breathing, blood pressure regulation, and response to pain.

6.4.7 Cerebellum

The *cerebellum* (Latin, little brain) is part of the hindbrain and is attached to the dorsal surface of the upper region of the brainstem. Although it constitutes only 10% of the total volume of the brain, it contains more than half of all its neurons. Its surface consists of a thin cortex of gray matter with extensive folding, a core of white matter, and three pairs of nuclei embedded within it.

The specialized function of the cerebellum is to coordinate movement by evaluating differences between intended movement and actual movement. It carries out this activity while a movement is in progress as well as during repetitions of the same movement. Three important aspects of the cerebellum's organization enable it to carry out this function. First, it receives extensive sensory input from somatic receptors in the periphery of the body and from receptors in the inner ear providing information regarding equilibrium and balance. Second, output from the cerebellum is transmitted to premotor and motor systems of the cerebral cortex and the brainstem — systems that control spinal interneurons and motor neurons. Finally, circuits within the cerebellum exhibit significant plasticity, which is necessary for motor adaptation and learning.

The cerebellum consists of three functionally distinct parts:

- Vestibulocerebellum
- Spinocerebellum
- Cerebrocerebellum

The *vestibulocerebellum* receives sensory input regarding motion of the head and its position relative to gravity as well as visual input. Outputs control axial muscles (primarily head and neck) and limb extensors, assuring balance while standing still and during movement. Outputs also control eye movements and coordinate movement of the head and eyes. Lesions here affect an individual's balance. The ability to use the incoming sensory information to control eye movements when the head is rotating and movements of the limbs and body during standing and walking is also impaired.

The *spinocerebellum* influences muscle tone and coordinates skilled voluntary movements. It receives sensory input from interneurons in the spinal cord transmitting somatic information, in particular from muscle and joint proprioceptors providing data regarding body movements and positions that are actually taking place. It also receives input from the cortical motor areas providing information regarding intended or desired movement. The spinocerebellum then compares these inputs. If the actual status of a body part differs from the intended status, the spinocerebellum transmits impulses back to the motor areas of the brain to make appropriate adjustments in activation of the associated skeletal muscles.

The *cerebrocerebellum* is involved with the planning, programming, and initiation of voluntary activity. It also participates in procedural memories or motor learning. This region of the cerebellum receives input from and provides output to the cortical motor areas directly. Lesions of the cerebrocerebellum cause delays in initiating movements and irregularities in the timing of multistep movements.

Disorders of the human cerebellum result in three types of abnormalities. The first is *hypotonia* or reduced muscle tone. Another includes abnormalities in the execution of voluntary movements or *ataxia* (defective muscular coordination). The third type of muscular malfunction is *intention tremors*. These tremors differ from the resting tremors of Parkinson's disease in that they occur *during* a movement and are most pronounced at the end of the movement when the patient attempts to terminate it.

Pharmacy application: centrally acting drugs

Combinations of centrally acting drugs are frequently used to achieve a desired therapeutic effect, particularly when the agents used have different mechanisms of action. For example, a patient with Parkinson's disease may be treated with one drug that blocks the effects of the neurotransmitter, acetylcholine, and a second drug that enhances the activity of another neurotransmitter, dopamine. However, potentially detrimental effects may occur when the agents used have additive effects. The effect of a CNS stimulant or depressant is additive with the effects of all other categories of stimulant and depressant drugs. For example, the combination of benzodiazepines (diazepam, Valium®) or barbiturates (pentobarbital, Nembutal®) with ethanol is not only additive, it may be fatal. Each of these drugs has a depressant effect on the respiratory center in the brainstem, so high doses may cause breathing to stop. The effect of a CNS drug is also additive with the physiological state of the patient. For example, anesthetics and antianxiety drugs are less effective in a hyperexcitable patient compared to a normal patient.

6.5   Blood–Brain Barrier

The movement of substances between the blood and the extracellular fluid surrounding the cells in most tissues of the body occurs very readily. This exchange takes place at the level of the capillaries, the smallest blood vessels in the cardiovascular system whose walls are formed by a single layer of endothelial cells. Lipid-soluble substances are able to move across this layer of endothelial cells at any point because they can move directly *through* the plasma membrane by passing between the phospholipid molecules of the bilayer. The movement of water-soluble substances is limited to the multiple pores found *between* the cells; however, it also takes place rapidly and efficiently.

This nonselective exchange of materials, which includes all substances except plasma proteins, does not occur in all vascular beds, however. Many substances found in the blood are potentially harmful to the CNS. Therefore, the brain and spinal cord are protected from these substances by the *blood–brain barrier*. In the capillaries of the brain and spinal cord, there are no pores between the endothelial cells; instead, *tight junctions* fuse the cells together. As a result, exchange between blood and the extracellular fluid of the brain is altered. Lipid-soluble substances, such as oxygen; carbon dioxide; steroid hormones; most anesthetics; and alcohol, continue to move directly through the plasma membrane and therefore remain very permeable. Because the blood–brain barrier anatomically prevents movement of materials between the cells, it is impermeable to water-soluble substances such as glucose, amino acids, and ions. These substances are exchanged between the blood and extracellular fluid of the brain by way of highly selective membrane-bound protein carriers.

There are several benefits to the presence of this barrier. It protects the neurons of the CNS from fluctuations in plasma components. For example, a change in the potassium ion concentration could alter neuronal function due to its effect on membrane potential. Second, the barrier minimizes the possibility that harmful blood-borne substances reach the CNS. Finally, it prevents any blood-borne substances that could function as neurotransmitters from reaching the brain and causing inappropriate neuronal stimulation.

The blood–brain barrier exists in capillaries in all areas of the brain and spinal cord except the hypothalamus and some regions of the brainstem. The absence of the barrier in a given region coincides with the function of that area. For example, the hypothalamus contributes to homeostasis by monitoring concentration of various blood-borne substances such as glucose and hormones. Glucose and amino acid-derived hormones are hydrophilic and would be unable to come into contact with hypothalamic neurons if the barrier were present. Another instance includes the vomit center of the medulla whose neurons detect the presence of potentially toxic substances in the blood. This center prevents the further absorption of these substances from the gastrointestinal tract by inducing vomiting. Once again, neurons in this region need to be exposed to any hydrophilic toxins in order to carry out this function.

Pharmacy application: antihistamines and the blood–brain barrier

Antihistamine drugs have long been used to treat symptoms of allergy such as sneezing, itching, watery discharge from the eyes and nose, and possibly wheezing. The older or first-generation histamine H_1 receptor antagonists such as Benadryl® and Tavist® effectively relieve these peripheral symptoms. However, these medications, of the drug class ethanolamines, are very lipophilic and readily cross the blood–brain barrier to interact with histamine H_1 receptors in the CNS as well. As a result, they also cause central effects such as diminished alertness, slowed reaction times, and sedation. The newer or second-generation histamine H_1 receptor antagonists such as Claritin® and Hismanal® have been chemically designed to be less lipophilic and not cross the blood–brain barrier at therapeutic doses. Therefore, these medications which are of the drug class piperidines, eliminate the peripheral symptoms of allergy without this depression of CNS activity.

6.6   Cerebrospinal fluid

Embedded within the brain are four *ventricles* or chambers that form a continuous fluid-filled system. In the roof of each of these ventricles is a network of capillaries referred to as the *choroid plexus*. It is from the choroid plexuses of the two lateral ventricles (one in each cerebral hemisphere) that *cerebrospinal fluid (CSF)* is primarily derived. Due to the presence of the blood–brain barrier, the selective transport processes of the choroid plexus determine the composition of the CSF. Therefore, the composition of the CSF is markedly different from the composition of the plasma. However, the CSF is in equilibrium with the interstitial fluid of the brain and contributes to the maintenance of a consistent chemical environment for neurons, which serves to optimize their function.

The CSF flows through the ventricles, downward through the central canal of the spinal cord, and then upward toward the brain through the subarachnoid space that completely surrounds the brain and spinal cord. As the CSF flows over the superior surface of the brain, it leaves the subarachnoid space and is absorbed into the venous system. Although CSF is actively secreted at a rate of 500 ml/day, the volume of this fluid in the system is approximately 140 ml. Therefore, the entire volume of CSF is turned over three to four times per day.

The one-way flow of the CSF and the constant turnover facilitate its important function of *removing potentially harmful brain metabolites*. The CSF also protects the brain from impact by serving as a *shock-absorbing system* that lies between the brain and its bony capsule. Finally, because the brain and the CSF have about the same specific gravity, the brain floats in this fluid. This *reduces the effective weight of the brain* from 1400 g to less than 50 g and prevents compression of neurons on the inferior surface of the brain.

Bibliography

1. Amaral, D.G., The anatomical organization of the nervous system, in *Principles of Neuroscience*, 4th ed., Kandel, E.R., Schwartz, J.H., and Jessell, T.M., Eds., McGraw–Hill, New York, 2000, chap. 17.
2. Babe, K.S., Jr. and Serafin, W.E., Histamine, bradykinin and their antagonists, in *Goodman and Gilman's, The Pharmacological Basis of Therapeutics*, 9th ed., Hardman, J.G. and Limbird, L.E., Eds., McGraw–Hill, New York, 1996, chap. 25.
3. Bloom, F.E., Neurotransmission and the central nervous system, in *Goodman and Gilman's, The Pharmacological Basis of Therapeutics*, 9th ed., Hardman, J.G. and Limbird, L.E., Eds., McGraw–Hill, New York, 1996, chap. 12.
4. Garoutte, B., *Neuromuscular Physiology*, 4th ed., Mill Valley Medical Publishers, Millbrae, CA, 1996.
5. Ghez, C. and Thach, W.T., The cerebellum, in *Principles of Neuroscience*, 4th ed., Kandel, E.R., Schwartz, J.H., and Jessell, T.M., Eds., McGraw–Hill, New York, 2000, chap. 42.
6. Laterra, L. and Goldstein, G.W., Ventricular organization of cerebral spinal fluid: blood–brain barrier, brain edema, and hydrocephalus, in *Principles of Neuroscience*, 4th ed., Kandel, E.R., Schwartz, J.H., and Jessell, T.M., Eds., McGraw–Hill, New York, 2000, appendix B.
7. Rechtschaffen, A. and Siegel, J., Sleep and dreaming, in *Principles of Neuroscience*, 4th ed., Kandel, E.R., Schwartz, J.H., and Jessell, T.M., Eds., McGraw–Hill, New York, 2000, chap. 47.
8. Saper, C.B., Iversen, S., and Frackowiak, R., Integration of sensory and motor function: the association areas of the cerebral cortex and the cognitive capabilities of the brain, in *Principles of Neuroscience*, 4th ed., Kandel, E.R., Schwartz, J.H., and Jessell, T.M., Eds., McGraw–Hill, New York, 2000, chap. 19.
9. Sherwood, L., *Human Physiology from Cells to Systems*, 4th ed., Brooks/Cole, Pacific Grove, CA, 2001.
10. Silverthorn, D.U., *Human Physiology: An Integrated Approach*, 2nd ed., Prentice-Hall, Upper Saddle River, NJ, 2001.

chapter seven

The spinal cord

Study objectives

- Define "cauda equina" and explain how it is formed
- Distinguish between a nerve and a tract
- Explain the function of the gray matter of the spinal cord
- Describe the location and function of each of the four types of neurons found in the gray matter of the spinal cord
- Explain the function of the white matter of the spinal cord
- Describe the composition of the ascending tracts including the origin and termination of each of the neurons
- Distinguish between corticospinal tracts and multineuronal tracts
- Discuss the mechanisms by which spinal anesthesia and epidural anesthesia exert their effects
- Define the various categories of reflexes
- List the components of the reflex arc
- Explain the mechanism of the withdrawal reflex
- Explain the mechanism of the crossed-extensor reflex

7.1 Introduction

The lowest level of the central nervous system (CNS), anatomically and functionally, is the *spinal cord*. Continuous with the brainstem, it exits the skull through the *foramen magnum*. The spinal cord then passes through the *vertebral canal* of the vertebral column to the level of the first or second lumbar vertebrae. The spinal cord is divided into four anatomical regions: cervical, thoracic, lumbar, and sacral. These regions are named according to the vertebrae adjacent to them during embryonic development. Each region is subdivided into functional segments. A pair of spinal nerves extends from each segment (one nerve from the left side of the spinal cord and one nerve from the right) and exits the CNS through the *intervertebral foramina*, or openings between adjacent vertebrae. There are a total of 31 pairs of spinal nerves:

- 8 Cervical
- 12 Thoracic
- 5 Lumbar
- 5 Sacral
- 1 Coccygeal

Spinal nerves arising from the *cervical level* of the cord are involved with sensory perception and motor function of the back of the head, neck, and arms. Nerves arising from the *thoracic level* innervate the upper trunk. Spinal nerves from the *lumbar* and *sacral regions* of the cord innervate the lower trunk, back, and legs. Lesions of the spinal cord interrupt sensation and motor function. The affected regions of the body are those innervated by spinal nerves below the level of the lesion. Interestingly, the phrenic nerves that innervate the diaphragm, the major muscle of inspiration, arise from spinal cord segments C_3 through C_5. Therefore, only lesions high in the cervical region will affect breathing.

The human spinal cord and the vertebral column initially grow at the same rate during embryonic development. In this way, spinal segments and the vertebral bones for which they are named are aligned. Therefore, the spinal nerves emerge from the vertebral column at the same level as the spinal cord segment from which they arise. However, after the third month of gestation, each vertebral bone becomes larger compared to the associated spinal segment; therefore, the vertebral column grows approximately 25 cm longer than the spinal cord. (This explains why the spinal cord extends only as far as the upper lumbar vertebrae.) As a result, the spinal cord segment from which each pair of spinal nerves arises is no longer aligned with its associated vertebral bone.

Because the vertebral column is now longer than the spinal cord, the intervertebral foramina have shifted downward relative to their corresponding spinal cord segment. Therefore, the spinal nerve roots arising from each segment must extend downward through the vertebral canal to reach their points of exit. This is the case especially for spinal nerves arising from the lumbar and sacral regions of the cord. As a result, only spinal nerve roots are found in the vertebral canal below the level of the first or second lumbar vertebrae. Because of its appearance, this bundle of nerve roots is collectively referred to as the *cauda equina*, or "horse's tail." A sample of cerebrospinal fluid may be obtained from this region by way of a *lumbar puncture* or "spinal tap." A needle may be safely inserted into the vertebral canal without the possibility of penetrating the spinal cord. The spinal nerve roots are easily pushed aside by the needle, significantly reducing the possibility of puncturing one of these nerves.

The spinal nerves associate with the spinal cord by way of two branches, or roots:

- Dorsal root
- Ventral root

The *dorsal root* contains afferent, or sensory, neurons. Impulses in these neurons travel from peripheral tissues toward the spinal cord. The *ventral root* contains efferent, or motor, neurons. Impulses in these neurons travel away from the spinal cord toward the peripheral tissues.

At this point, it is important to note that a *nerve* is defined as a bundle of neuronal axons; some are afferent and some are efferent. A nerve does not consist of entire neurons, only their axons. Furthermore, nerves are found only in the peripheral nervous system. Bundles of neurons with similar functions located within the CNS are referred to as *tracts*. Therefore, technically speaking, no nerves are within the brain or the spinal cord.

7.2 Functions of the spinal cord

The spinal cord is responsible for two vital CNS functions. The cord:

- Conducts nerve impulses to and from the brain
- Processes sensory input from the skin, joints, and muscles of the trunk and limbs and initiates reflex responses to this input

7.3 Composition of the cord

The spinal cord consists of:

- Gray matter
- White matter

The *gray matter* is composed of nerve cell bodies and unmyelinated interneuron fibers. The location of the gray matter in the spinal cord is opposite to that of the brain. In the brain, the gray matter of the cerebrum and the cerebellum is found externally forming a cortex, or covering, over the internally located white matter. In the spinal cord, the gray matter is found internally and is surrounded by the white matter.

The *white matter* is composed of myelinated axons of neurons. These axons are grouped together according to function to form tracts. Neurons transmitting impulses toward the brain in the *ascending tracts* carry sensory information. Those transmitting impulses away from the brain in the *descending tracts* carry motor information.

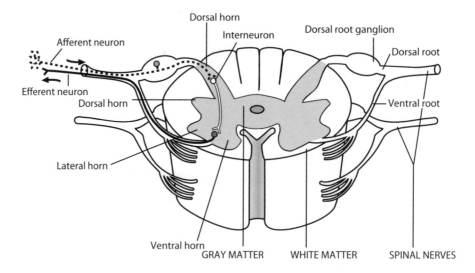

Figure 7.1 Cross-sectional view of the spinal cord. In contrast to the brain, the gray matter of the spinal cord is located internally, surrounded by the white matter. The gray matter consists of nerve cell bodies and unmyelinated interneuron fibers. This component of the spinal cord is divided into three regions: the dorsal, lateral, and ventral horns. The white matter consists of bundles of myelinated axons of neurons, or tracts. Each segment of the spinal cord gives rise to a pair of spinal nerves containing afferent and efferent neurons. Afferent neurons enter the spinal cord through the dorsal root and efferent neurons exit it through the ventral root.

7.3.1 Gray matter

A cross-sectional view of the spinal cord reveals that the gray matter has a butterfly or "H" shape (see Figure 7.1). As such, on each side of the spinal cord the gray matter is divided into three regions:

- Dorsal horn (posterior, toward the back)
- Ventral horn (anterior)
- Lateral horn

Each spinal segment contains millions of neurons within the gray matter. Functionally, four types of neurons exist:

- Second-order sensory neurons
- Somatic motor neurons
- Visceral motor neurons
- Interneurons

The cell bodies of *second-order sensory neurons* are found in the dorsal horn. These neurons receive input from afferent neurons (first-order sensory neurons) entering the CNS from the periphery of the body through the dorsal root of the spinal nerve. The function of the second-order sensory neuron is to transmit nerve impulses to higher levels in the CNS. The axons of these neurons leave the gray matter and travel upward in the appropriate ascending tracts of the white matter.

The cell bodies of *somatic motor neurons* are found in the ventral horn. The axons of these neurons exit the CNS through the ventral root of the spinal nerve and innervate skeletal muscles. The two types of motor neurons located in the ventral horn are:

- *Alpha motor neurons* innervate skeletal muscle fibers to cause contraction.
- *Gamma motor neurons* innervate intrafusal fibers of the muscle spindle, which monitors muscle length.

The spatial organization of the cell bodies of the motor neurons follows a *proximal–distal rule*. Motor neurons that innervate the most proximal muscles (axial muscles of the neck and trunk) lie most medially in the gray matter. Motor neurons innervating the most distal muscles (wrists, ankles, digits) lie most laterally in the gray matter.

The cell bodies of *visceral motor neurons* are found in the lateral horn. The axons of these neurons form efferent nerve fibers of the autonomic nervous system (ANS). The ANS innervates cardiac muscle, smooth muscle and glands (see Chapter 9). The axons of these neurons exit the spinal cord by way of the ventral root.

Interneurons are found in all areas of the spinal cord gray matter. These neurons are quite numerous, small, and highly excitable; they have many interconnections. They receive input from higher levels of the CNS as well as from sensory neurons entering the CNS through the spinal nerves. Many interneurons in the spinal cord synapse with motor neurons in the ventral horn. These interconnections are responsible for the integrative functions of the spinal cord including reflexes.

Afferent neurons that transmit sensory information toward the spinal cord are referred to as *first-order sensory neurons*. The cell bodies of these neurons are found in the *dorsal root ganglia*. These ganglia form a swelling in each of the dorsal roots just outside the spinal cord. The portion of the axon between the distal receptor and the cell body is referred to as the *peripheral axon* and the portion of the axon between the cell body and the axon terminal within the CNS is referred to as the *central axon*.

Upon entering the spinal cord, the first-order sensory neurons may enter the gray matter and may then synapse with one or more of the following neurons:

- Second-order sensory neuron that transmits impulses to higher levels of the CNS
- Alpha motor neuron that transmits impulses to skeletal muscles
- Interneurons that transmit impulses to motor neurons

Synapses between first-order sensory neurons and alpha motor neurons, either directly or by way of interneurons, result in spinal cord reflexes. Reflexes are discussed in more detail in a subsequent section in this chapter.

Alternatively, the first-order sensory neurons may initially enter the white matter of the spinal cord. In this case, the axons of these neurons may ascend the cord to the medulla or travel up or down the cord to a different spinal segment. Upon reaching its destination, the axon then enters the gray matter of the spinal cord and synapses with one or more of the neurons discussed previously.

7.3.2   White matter

The white matter of the spinal cord consists of myelinated axons of neurons. These axons may travel up the spinal cord to a higher spinal segment or to the brain. On the other hand, they may travel down the spinal cord to a lower spinal segment. The axons of neurons that carry similar types of impulses are bundled together to form tracts. *Ascending tracts* carry sensory information from the spinal cord toward the brain. *Descending tracts* carry motor impulses from the brain toward the motor neurons in the lateral or ventral horns of the spinal cord gray matter. In general, these tracts are named according to their origin and termination. For example, the ventral spinocerebellar tract is an ascending tract carrying information regarding unconscious muscle sense (proprioception) from the spinal cord to the cerebellum. On the other hand, the ventral corticospinal tract is a descending tract carrying information regarding voluntary muscle control from the cerebral cortex to the spinal cord.

Ascending tracts. These tracts contain three successive neurons:

- First-order neurons
- Second-order neurons
- Third-order neurons

As discussed, the *first-order neuron* is the afferent neuron that transmits impulses from a peripheral receptor toward the CNS. Its cell body is located in the dorsal root ganglion. This neuron synapses with the *second-order neuron* whose cell body is located in the dorsal horn of the spinal cord or in the medulla of the brainstem. The second-order neuron travels upward and synapses with the *third-order neuron,* whose cell body is located in the thalamus. Limited processing of sensory information takes place in the thalamus. Finally, the third-order neuron travels upward and terminates in the somatosensory cortex where more complex, cortical processing begins.

All ascending tracts cross to the opposite side of the CNS. For example, sensory input entering the left side of the spinal cord ultimately terminates on the right side of the cerebral cortex. These tracts may cross — at the level of entry into the spinal cord; a few segments above the level of entry; or within the medulla of the brainstem. The locations of specific ascending tracts are illustrated in Figure 7.2 and a summary of their functions is found in Table 7.1.

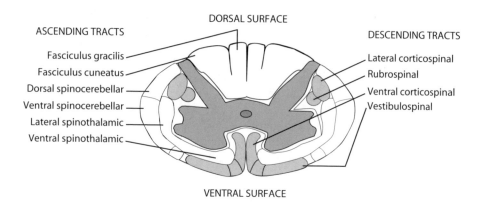

Figure 7.2 Ascending and descending tracts in white matter of the spinal cord. Tracts are formed of bundles of neuronal axons that transmit similar types of information.

Table 7.1 Ascending and Descending Tracts in White Matter of the Spinal Cord

Ascending pathway	Function
Fasciculus gracilis	Fine touch discrimination (ability to recognize size, shape, and texture of objects and their movement across the skin); proprioception; vibration from legs and lower trunk; crossed
Fasciculus cuneatus	Fine touch discrimination; proprioception; vibration from neck, arms, upper trunk; crossed
Dorsal spinocerebellar	Proprioception (important for muscle tone and posture); uncrossed
Ventral spinocerebellar	Proprioception; crossed
Lateral spinothalamic	Pain; temperature; crossed
Ventral spinothalamic	Light touch; pressure; crossed

Descending pathway	Function
Lateral corticospinal	Voluntary control of skeletal muscles; crossed
Rubrospinal	Originates in brainstem; subconscious control of skeletal muscle (muscle tone, posture); crossed
Ventral corticospinal	Voluntary control of skeletal muscles; uncrossed
Vestibulospinal	Originates in brainstem; subconscious control of skeletal muscle (muscle tone, balance, equilibrium); uncrossed

Pharmacy application: spinal anesthesia

Injecting a local form of anesthetic into the cerebrospinal fluid surrounding the spinal cord causes spinal anesthesia. This injection is made below the level of the second lumbar vertebra in order to minimize direct nerve trauma. Spinal anesthesia is effective in the control of pain during lower body surgical procedures, such as knee surgery. Currently, the drugs most commonly used in the U.S. include lidocaine, bupivacaine, and tetracaine. The choice of anesthetic is determined by the duration of anesthesia required: lidocaine is used for short procedures; bupivacaine is chosen for procedures of intermediate length; and tetracaine is used for long-duration procedures.

The mechanism of action of these anesthetics involves the blockade of sodium channels in the membrane of the second-order sensory neuron. The binding site for these anesthetics is on a subunit of the sodium channel located near the internal surface of the cell membrane. Therefore, the agent must enter the neuron in order to block the sodium channel effectively. Without the influx of sodium, neurons cannot depolarize and generate an action potential, so the second-order sensory neuron cannot be stimulated by impulses elicited by pain receptors associated with the first-order sensory neuron. In other words, the pain signal is effectively interrupted at the level of the spinal cord and does not travel any higher in the CNS. In this way, the brain does not perceive pain.

Interestingly, second-order sensory neurons are neurons of the spinal cord gray matter most susceptible to the effects of spinal anesthesia. These neurons have a small diameter and are unmyelinated. The small diameter allows the drug to locate its binding site on the sodium channel more readily due to a smaller volume of distribution of drug within the neuron. Furthermore, unmyelinated neurons have a greater number of sodium channels located over a larger surface area. Alpha motor neurons in the ventral horn are susceptible to these anesthetics only at high doses because alpha motor neurons have a large diameter and are myelinated. The larger diameter results in a larger volume of distribution of the drug within the neuron. Myelination limits the number and availability of sodium channels upon which the anesthetic can exert its effect.

Descending tracts. Voluntary movement of skeletal muscles is controlled by two types of descending tracts. Neurons in these tracts terminate on and influence activity of alpha motor neurons in the ventral horn. The two types of tracts include:

- Corticospinal (pyramidal) tracts
- Multineuronal (extrapyramidal) tracts

The *corticospinal tracts* originate in the cerebral cortex. Neurons of the primary motor cortex are referred to as *pyramidal cells*. Most of these neurons' axons descend directly to the alpha motor neurons in the spinal cord. In other words, these are primarily monosynaptic pathways. This type of synaptic connection is particularly important for the movement of individual fingers. A primary function of these tracts is to regulate fine, discrete, voluntary movements of the hands and fingers. The *multineuronal tracts* originate in many regions of the brain, including the motor regions of the cerebral cortex, the cerebellum, and the basal ganglia. Impulses from these various regions are transmitted to nuclei in the brainstem, in particular the reticular formation and vestibular nuclei. The axons of neurons in these nuclei descend to the alpha motor neurons in the spinal cord. The multineuronal tracts regulate overall body posture. Specifically, these tracts control subconscious movements of large muscle groups in the trunk and limbs.

These two types of descending motor tracts do not function in isolation. They are extensively interconnected and cooperate in the control of movement. For example, in order to grasp a doorknob to open a door, there is subconscious positioning of the body to face the door and extend an arm toward the doorknob.

As with the ascending tracts, descending tracts cross from one side of the CNS to the other. Most of the tracts cross over in the medulla of the brainstem. Therefore, the right side of the brain influences the activity of the alpha motor neurons and thus the skeletal muscles on the left side of the body. The locations of specific descending tracts are illustrated in Figure 7.2 and a summary of their functions is found in Table 7.1.

Pharmacy application: epidural anesthesia

Epidural anesthesia is administered by injecting local anesthetic into the epidural space. Located outside the spinal cord on its dorsal surface, the epidural space contains fat and is highly vascular. Therefore, this form of anesthesia can be performed safely at any level of the spinal cord. Furthermore, a catheter may be placed into the epidural space, allowing for continuous infusions or repeated bolus administrations of anesthetic.

The primary site of action of epidurally administered agents is on the spinal nerve roots. As with spinal anesthesia, the choice of drug to be used is determined primarily by the duration of anesthesia desired. However, when a catheter has been placed, short-acting drugs can be administered repeatedly. Bupivacaine is typically used when a long duration of surgical block is needed. Lidocaine is used most often for intermediate length procedures; chloroprocaine is used when only a very short duration of anesthesia is required.

An important difference between epidural anesthesia and spinal anesthesia is that agents injected into the epidural space may readily enter the blood due to the presence of a rich venous plexus in this area. This is an important consideration when epidural anesthesia is used to control pain during labor and delivery. The agents used are able to cross the placenta, enter the fetal circulation, and exert a depressant effect on the neonate.

7.4 Spinal reflexes

Reflexes may be classified in several ways. They may be named according to the effector tissues that carry out the reflex response:

- *Skeletal muscle reflexes* control skeletal muscles.
- *Autonomic reflexes* control cardiac muscle, smooth muscle and glands.

They may be named according to the region of the CNS that integrates incoming sensory information and elicits the reflex response:

- *Cranial reflexes* are processed within the brain.
- *Spinal reflexes* are processed at the level of the spinal cord.

Finally, reflexes may be innate or learned:

- *Simple*, or *basic*, *reflexes* are preprogrammed (built-in), unlearned responses.
- *Acquired*, or *conditioned*, *reflexes* are learned responses that require experience or training.

This section will examine the mechanism of simple or basic spinal reflexes that control skeletal muscles.

A reflex occurs when a particular stimulus always elicits a particular response. This response is automatic and involuntary; in other words, it occurs without conscious effort. Therefore, reflexes are specific, predictable, and, furthermore, often purposeful. For example, the withdrawal reflex causes a body part to be pulled away from a painful stimulus so that tissue injury is avoided. Spinal reflexes require no input from the brain because they are elicited entirely at the level of the spinal cord. However, while the reflex is underway, nervous impulses are also transmitted to the brain for further processing. In fact, input from the brain may modulate a reflex or alter the response to a stimulus through conscious effort.

A reflex response requires an intact neural pathway between the stimulated area and the responding muscle. This pathway is referred to as a *reflex arc* and includes the following components (see Figure 7.3):

- Sensory receptor
- Afferent or first-order sensory neuron
- Integrating center in the spinal cord (synapses)

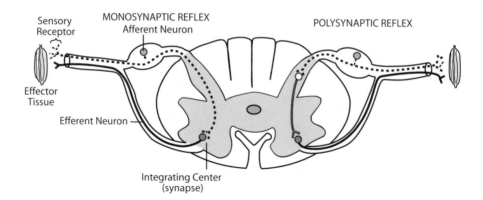

Figure 7.3 Components of a reflex arc. As illustrated by the components of the reflex arc, reflexes may be processed entirely at the level of the spinal cord with no need for input from the brain. A monosynaptic reflex has a single synapse between afferent and efferent neurons; a polysynaptic reflex has two or more synapses between these neurons. In this case, interneurons lie between the sensory and motor neurons. The more interneurons involved, the more complex the response is.

- Efferent or motor neuron
- Effector tissue (skeletal muscle)

A reflex is initiated by stimulation of a *sensory receptor* located at the peripheral ending of an afferent or first-order sensory neuron. This *afferent neuron* transmits impulses to the spinal cord. Within the gray matter of the spinal cord, the afferent neuron synapses with other neurons. As such, the spinal cord serves as an *integrating center* for the sensory input. The afferent neuron must ultimately synapse with an efferent or *motor neuron*. When the afferent neuron synapses directly with the motor neuron, it forms a *monosynaptic reflex*. An example of this type of reflex is the stretch reflex. When the afferent neuron synapses with an interneuron that then synapses with the motor neuron, it forms a *polysynaptic reflex*, e.g., the withdrawal reflex. Most reflexes are polysynaptic. The motor neuron then exits the spinal cord to innervate an *effector tissue*, which carries out the reflex response.

Withdrawal reflex. The *withdrawal reflex* is elicited by a painful or tissue-damaging stimulus. The response is to move the body part away from the source of the stimulus quickly, usually by flexing a limb. Any of the major joints, and therefore muscle groups, may be involved in a reflex, depending upon the point of stimulation. For example, all of the joints of a limb are involved when a digit, such as a finger, is stimulated (e.g., finger, wrist, elbow, shoulder). Furthermore, the withdrawal reflex is a very powerful reflex and may override other nervous impulses, such as those regarding locomotion, or walking.

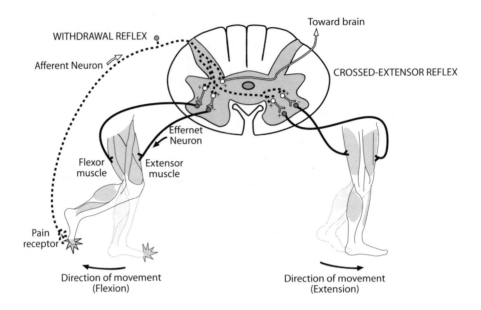

WITHDRAWAL REFLEX

Afferent Neuron

Toward brain

CROSSED-EXTENSOR REFLEX

Effernet Neuron

Flexor muscle   Extensor muscle

Pain receptor

Direction of movement
(Flexion)

Direction of movement
(Extension)

Figure 7.4 The withdrawal reflex coupled with the crossed-extensor reflex. A painful stimulus will elicit the withdrawal reflex, which causes flexor muscles to contract and move the affected body part away from the stimulus. At the same time, the crossed-extensor reflex causes extensor muscles in the opposite limb to contract. The straightening of the opposite limb provides support for the body.

An example of the mechanism of the withdrawal reflex is illustrated in Figure 7.4. When a painful stimulus activates a sensory receptor on the right foot, action potentials are transmitted along the afferent neuron to the spinal cord. By way of divergence, this neuron synapses with several other neurons within the gray matter of the spinal cord:

- Excitatory interneuron
- Inhibitory interneuron
- Second-order sensory neuron

The *excitatory interneuron* then synapses with the alpha motor neuron that innervates the *flexor muscles* of the right leg. Consequently, stimulation of the excitatory interneuron leads to stimulation of the alpha motor neuron, which then stimulates the flexor muscles to contract and pick up or withdraw the foot from the painful stimulus. The *inhibitory interneuron* synapses with the alpha motor neuron that innervates the *extensor muscles* of the right leg. Therefore, stimulation of the inhibitory interneuron leads to inhibition of the alpha motor neuron. As a result, the extensor muscles relax.

The flexor muscles and the extensor muscles are *antagonistic* — they cause opposite effects. Therefore, when one of these groups of muscles is activated, the other group must be inhibited. This is referred to as *reciprocal inhibition*. In this way, activation of the withdrawal reflex leads to unimpeded flexion.

The *second-order sensory neuron* transmits impulses ultimately to the left side of the brain. This permits the awareness of pain, identification of its source, and, if necessary, postural adjustment. As discussed, impulses in this pathway do not play a role in the reflex per se.

Crossed-extensor reflex. Where appropriate, the withdrawal reflex may be accompanied by the *crossed-extensor reflex*. In the example discussed, when the right leg is flexed or lifted, the left leg must be extended or straightened in order to support the body. In addition to stimulating interneurons on the right side of the spinal cord to influence skeletal muscle activity on the right side of the body, the afferent neuron may also stimulate interneurons on the left side of the spinal cord to influence skeletal muscle activity on the left side of the body. Once again, excitatory and inhibitory interneurons are involved; however, in this case these interneurons influence the activity of the opposite muscle groups. Stimulation of the excitatory interneuron on the left side of the spinal cord leads to stimulation of the alpha motor neuron that innervates the extensor muscles, causing the left leg to straighten. Stimulation of the inhibitory interneuron on the left side of the spinal cord leads to inhibition of the alpha motor neuron that innervates the flexor muscles. This results in unimpeded extension of the left leg and support of the body during withdrawal of the right leg.

Bibliography

1. Amaral, D.G., The anatomical organization of the nervous system, in *Principles of Neuroscience*, 4th ed., Kandel, E.R., Schwartz, J.H., and Jessell, T.M., Eds., McGraw–Hill, New York, 2000, chap. 17.
2. Amaral, D.G., The functional organization of perception and movement, in *Principles of Neuroscience*, 4th ed., Kandel, E.R., Schwartz, J.H., and Jessell, T.M., Eds., McGraw–Hill, New York, 2000, chap. 18.
3. Carroll, E.W. and Curtis, R.L., Organization and control of neural function, in *Pathophysiology, Concepts of Altered Health States*, 5th ed., Porth, C.M., Ed., Lippincott–Raven Publishers, Philadelphia, 1998, chap. 37.
4. Catterall, W.A. and Mackie, K., Local anesthetics, in *Goodman and Gilman's: The Pharmacological Basis of Therapeutics*, 9th ed., Hardman, J.G. and Limbird, L.E., Eds., McGraw–Hill, New York, 1996, chap. 15.
5. DeLong, M.R., The basal ganglia, in *Principles of Neuroscience*, 4th ed., Kandel, E.R., Schwartz, J.H., and Jessell, T.M., Eds., McGraw–Hill, New York, 2000, chap. 43.
6. Ghez, C. and Krakauer, J., The organization of movement, in *Principles of Neuroscience*, 4th ed., Kandel, E.R., Schwartz, J.H., and Jessell, T.M., Eds., McGraw–Hill, New York, 2000, chap. 33.
7. Krakauer, J. and Ghez, C., Voluntary movement, in *Principles of Neuroscience*, 4th ed., Kandel, E.R., Schwartz, J.H., and Jessell, T.M., Eds., McGraw–Hill, New York, 2000, chap. 38.
8. Sherwood, L., *Human Physiology from Cells to Systems*, 4th ed., Brooks/Cole, Pacific Grove, CA, 2001.

9. Silverthorn, D.U., *Human Physiology: An Integrated Approach,* 2nd ed., Prentice-Hall, Upper Saddle River, NJ, 2001.

10. *Taber's Cyclopedic Medical Dictionary,* 19th ed., F.A. Davis Co., Philadelphia, PA, 2001.

chapter eight

Pain

Study objectives

- Describe the three types of nociceptors and the stimuli that activate them
- Distinguish between A-delta fibers and C fibers
- Compare and contrast fast pain and slow pain
- Distinguish between primary hyperalgesia and centrally mediated hyperalgesia
- Discuss functions of the neurotransmitters, glutamate, and substance P
- Describe the pain pathway and the role that each stimulated region of the brain plays in the response to pain
- Explain how the endogenous analgesic system suppresses pain
- Distinguish between cutaneous pain and deep visceral pain
- Describe the mechanisms by which tissue ischemia and muscle spasm lead to pain
- Discuss potential causes of visceral pain
- Describe the mechanism of referred pain
- Explain how phantom pain occurs
- List properties of an ideal analgesic medication
- List and discuss effects of nonnarcotic analgesic medications
- Discuss effects of opioid analgesic medications
- Discuss effects of adjuvant medications

8.1 Introduction

Sensations interpreted as *pain*, including burning, aching, stinging, and soreness, are the most distinctive forms of sensory input to the central nervous system. Pain serves an important protective function because it causes awareness of actual or potential tissue damage. Furthermore, it stimulates an individual to react to remove or withdraw from the source of the pain. Unlike other forms of sensory input, such as vision, hearing, and smell, pain has an urgent, primitive quality. This quality is responsible for the behavioral and emotional aspect of pain perception.

8.2   Nociceptors

Nociceptors are bare or free nerve endings; therefore, they do not adapt, or stop responding, to sustained or repeated stimulation. This is beneficial in that it keeps the individual aware of the damaging stimulus for as long as it persists. Nociceptors are widely distributed in the skin, dental pulp, periosteum, joints, meninges, and some internal organs. The three major classes of nociceptors are:

- Thermal nociceptors
- Mechanical nociceptors
- Polymodal nociceptors

Thermal nociceptors are activated by extreme temperatures, especially heat. One group of these receptors is stimulated by noxious heat (>45°C) and a second group is stimulated by noxious cold (<5°C). These are the temperatures at which the tissues begin to be damaged. *Mechanical nociceptors* are activated by mechanical damage, such as cutting, pinching, or tissue distortion, as well as by intensive pressure applied to the skin. Their firing rates increase with the destructiveness of the mechanical stimulus. *Polymodal nociceptors* are activated by all types of damaging stimuli (thermal, mechanical, chemical), including irritating exogenous substances that may penetrate the skin. Endogenous substances that may stimulate these receptors to elicit pain include potassium released from damaged cells; bradykinin; histamine; substance P; acids; and proteolytic enzymes (see Table 8.1). Stimulation of polymodal nociceptors elicits sensations of slow, burning pain.

Two types of afferent neurons are associated with nociceptors:

- A-delta fibers
- C fibers

Thermal nociceptors and mechanical nociceptors are associated with *A-delta fibers*. These are small myelinated fibers that transmit impulses at a rate of 5 to 30 m/sec. Polymodal nociceptors are associated with *C fibers*. These are small unmyelinated fibers that transmit impulses at a rate generally less than 1.0 m/sec (range of 0.5 to 2.0 m/sec).

The two types of pain are:

- Fast pain
- Slow pain

Fast pain may be described as sharp or prickling pain (see Table 8.2). This pain is perceived first (within 0.1 sec) as it is carried by the more rapidly

Table 8.1 Endogenous Chemicals Activating or Sensitizing Nociceptors

Chemical	Source	Enzyme involved in synthesis	Effect on first-order sensory neuron	Pharmacological intervention
Potassium	Damaged cells		Activation	
Serotonin	Platelets	Tryptophan hydroxylase	Activation	
Bradykinin	Plasma kininogen	Kallikrein	Activation	
Histamine	Mast cells		Activation	H_1 receptor antagonists (e.g., diphenhydramine chloride, Benadryl®)
Prostaglandins	Arachidonic acid/damaged cells	Cyclooxygenase	Sensitization	Non-steroidal anti-inflammatory drugs (e.g. aspirin, ibuprofen)
Leukotrienes	Arachidonic acid/damaged cells	Lipoxygenase	Sensitization	
Substance P	First order sensory neuron		Sensitization	Opioid receptor agonists (e.g., morphine)

Table 8.2 Characteristics of Fast and Slow Pain

Fast pain	Slow pain
Occurs first	Occurs second, persists longer
Sharp, prickling sensation	Dull, aching, throbbing sensation; more unpleasant
A-delta fibers	C fibers
Thermal or mechanical nociceptors	Polymodal nociceptors
Easily localized	Poorly localized

conducting A-delta fibers. Because fast pain is elicited by stimulation of specific thermal or mechanical nociceptors, it is easily localized. This type of pain is not felt in most of the deeper tissues of the body. *Slow pain* may be described as dull, aching, or throbbing pain. This pain is perceived second (only after 1 sec or more) because it is carried by C fibers. Slow pain persists longer and is typically more unpleasant; in fact, it tends to become greater over time. Slow pain is typically associated with tissue destruction. Noxious chemicals released from damaged cells or activated in the interstitial fluid can spread in the tissue, causing a relatively diffuse stimulation of polymodal receptors. As a result, slow pain is poorly localized; it may occur in the skin as well as almost any deep tissue or organ.

8.3   Hyperalgesia

An injured area is typically more sensitive to subsequent stimuli. As a result, painful stimuli, or even normally nonpainful stimuli, may cause an excessive pain response. An increase in the sensitivity of nociceptors is referred to as *primary hyperalgesia*. A classic example of hyperalgesia is a burn. Even light touch of a burned area may be painful.

The sensitization of nociceptors following tissue damage or inflammation results from a variety of chemicals released or activated in the injured area (see Table 8.1). These substances decrease the threshold for activation of the nociceptors. One such substance that seems to be more painful than the others is *bradykinin*. Activated by enzymes released from damaged cells, bradykinin causes pain by several mechanisms. First, it activates A-delta and C fibers directly. Second, along with histamine, it contributes to the inflammatory response to tissue injury. Third, it promotes synthesis and release of prostaglandins from nearby cells. The *prostaglandins* sensitize all three types of pain receptors, thus enhancing the response to a noxious stimulus. In other words, it hurts more when prostaglandins are present. Aspirin and nonsteroidal anti-inflammatory drugs (NSAIDs) inhibit the synthesis of prostaglandins, which accounts, in part, for their analgesic effects.

Centrally mediated hyperalgesia involves the hyperexcitability of second-order sensory neurons in the dorsal horn of the spinal cord. In the case of severe or persistent tissue injury, C fibers fire action potentials repetitively. As a result, response of the second-order sensory neurons increases progressively. The mechanism of this enhanced response, also referred to as *"wind-up,"* depends on the release of the neurotransmitter *glutamate* from the C fibers. An excitatory neurotransmitter, glutamate stimulates the opening of calcium channels gated by the N-methyl-D-aspartate (NMDA)-type glutamate receptor. Calcium influx ultimately leads to long-term biochemical changes and hyperexcitability of the second-order neuron.

8.4   Neurotransmitters of nociceptive afferent fibers

Two neurotransmitters are released by the nociceptive afferent fibers in the dorsal horn of the spinal cord. These neurotransmitters, which stimulate the second-order sensory neurons, include:

- Glutamate
- Substance P

The amino acid *glutamate* is the major neurotransmitter released by A-delta fibers and C fibers. Glutamate binds to the AMPA-type glutamate receptor on the second-order sensory neuron to elicit action potentials and continue transmission of the signal to higher levels of the CNS. *Substance P* is released primarily from C fibers. Levels of this neurotransmitter increase significantly under conditions of persistent pain. This neurotransmitter also stimulates ascending pathways in the spinal cord and appears to enhance and prolong the actions of glutamate.

8.5   Pain pathway

Stimulation of a nociceptor in the periphery of the body elicits action potentials in the *first-order neuron*, which transmits the signal to the *second-order neuron* in the dorsal horn of the spinal cord. From the spinal cord, the signal is transmitted to several regions of the brain. The most prominent ascending nociceptive pathway is the *spinothalamic tract*. Axons of the second-order sensory neurons project to the contralateral (opposite) side of the spinal cord and ascend in the white matter, terminating in the *thalamus* (see Figure 8.1). The thalamus contributes to the basic sensation or awareness of pain only; it cannot determine the source of the painful stimulus.

Signals are also transmitted to the *reticular formation* of the brainstem by way of the *spinoreticular tract*. The reticular formation plays an important role in the response to pain. First, it facilitates avoidance reflexes at all levels of the spinal cord and, second, it is responsible for the significant arousal effects of pain. Signals from the reticular formation cause an increase in the electrical activity of the cerebral cortex associated with increased alertness. Furthermore, it sends nerve impulses to the *hypothalamus* to influence its functions associated with sudden alertness, such as increased heart rate and

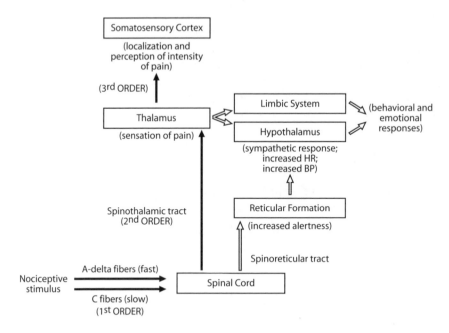

Figure 8.1 The pain pathway. The pain signal is transmitted to several regions of the brain, including the thalamus; reticular formation; hypothalamus; limbic system; and somatosensory cortex. Each region carries out a specific aspect of the response to pain.

blood pressure. These responses are mediated by the sympathetic nervous system.

Nerve signals from the thalamus and the reticular formation are transmitted to the *limbic system* as well as the hypothalamus. Together, these regions of the brain are responsible for behavioral and emotional responses to pain. The limbic system, in particular, may be involved with the mood-altering and attention-narrowing effect of pain.

The cell bodies of *third-order sensory* neurons are located in the thalamus. These neurons transmit the pain signal to the *somatosensory cortex*. The function of this region of the brain is to localize and perceive the intensity of the painful stimulus. Further transmission of the signal to the *association areas* of the cerebral cortex is important for the perception and meaningfulness of the painful stimulus.

8.6   *Endogenous analgesic system*

The *endogenous analgesic system* is a built-in neuronal system that suppresses transmission of nervous impulses in the pain pathway. It functions by way of the following neurotransmitters produced in the CNS:

- Endorphins
- Enkephalins
- Dynorphin

Endorphins are found primarily in the limbic system, hypothalamus, and brainstem. *Enkephalins* and *dynorphin* (in smaller quantities) are found primarily in the *periaqueductal gray matter* (*PAG*) of the midbrain, the limbic system, and the hypothalamus. These endogenous substances mimic the effects of morphine and other opiate drugs at many points in the analgesic system, including in the dorsal horns of the spinal cord.

Opioid receptors are highly concentrated in the PAG area of the midbrain. Stimulation of this region produces long-lasting analgesia with no effect on the level of consciousness. For these reasons, the PAG area is often referred to as the *endogenous analgesia center*. This area receives input from many regions of the CNS, including the cerebral cortex; hypothalamus; reticular formation of the brainstem; and spinal cord by way of the spinothalamic tracts. This region is also interconnected with the limbic system, which is responsible for the emotional response to pain.

The endogenous analgesic pathway has three major components:

- Periaqueductal gray area
- Nucleus raphe magnus
- Pain inhibitory complex in the dorsal horns of the spinal cord

The endogenous analgesic pathway begins in the PAG area, in which neurons descend to the *nucleus raphe magnus* (*NRM*) in the medulla (see Figure 8.2). Neurons of the NRM then descend to the dorsal horn of the spinal cord where they synapse with local spinal interneurons. The interneurons then synapse with incoming pain fibers. Many of the neurons derived from the PAG area secrete enkephalin from their axon terminals in the NRM. The neurons derived from the NRM secrete serotonin from their axon terminals in the spinal cord. The serotonin stimulates the local cord interneurons to secrete enkephalin. The enkephalin then causes presynaptic inhibition of the incoming pain fibers. Binding of enkephalin to opioid receptors on these pain fibers blocks calcium channels in the axon terminals. Because the influx of calcium is necessary for the exocytosis of neurotransmitter, blocking these channels prevents release of substance P. As a result, this system interrupts the pain signal at the level of the spinal cord.

The endogenous analgesic system is normally inactive. It remains unclear how this system becomes activated. Potential activating factors include exercise, stress, acupuncture, and hypnosis.

8.7   *Cutaneous pain*

Cutaneous pain is felt in superficial structures such as the skin and subcutaneous tissues. A pin prick and a paper cut are examples of cutaneous pain.

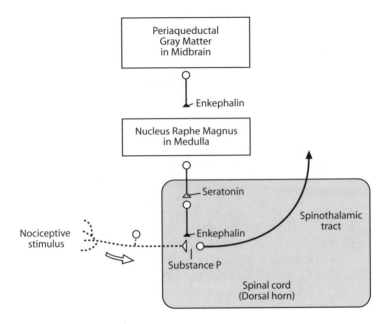

Figure 8.2 The endogenous analgesic system. The three major components of the endogenous analgesic system include the periaqueductal gray matter in the mid-brain; nucleus raphe magnus in the medulla; and pain inhibitory complex in the dorsal horns of the spinal cord. This system causes presynaptic inhibition of pain fibers entering the spinal cord. The binding of enkephalin to opioid receptors on the pain fibers prevents release of the neurotransmitter, substance P. As a result, the pain signal is terminated in the spinal cord and does not ascend to higher centers in the CNS.

It is a sharp pain with a burning quality that may be easily localized. This pain may be abrupt or slow in onset.

8.8 Deep somatic pain

As its name implies, *deep somatic pain* is generated in deep body structures, such as the periosteum, muscles, tendons, joints, and blood vessels. This type of pain is more diffuse than cutaneous pain. It may be elicited by strong pressure, ischemia, and tissue damage.

Tissue ischemia. When blood flow to a tissue is decreased or interrupted, the tissue becomes painful within a few minutes. In fact, the greater the rate of metabolism in the tissue, the more rapid is the onset of pain. The causes of pain due to *tissue ischemia* include:

- Accumulation of *lactic acid* due to the anaerobic metabolism that occurs during ischemia
- *Release and activation of noxious chemicals* in the area of tissue ischemia due to tissue damage (see Table 8.1)

The lactic acid and other noxious chemicals stimulate polymodal nociceptors.

Muscle spasm. The pain induced by *muscle spasm* results partially from the direct effect of tissue distortion on mechanical nociceptors. Muscle spasm also causes tissue ischemia. The increased muscle tension compresses blood vessels and decreases blood flow. Furthermore, the increased rate of metabolism associated with the spasm exacerbates the ischemia. As discussed earlier, ischemia leads to stimulation of polymodal nociceptors.

8.9 Visceral pain

Visceral pain occurs in organs and tissues of the thoracic and abdominal cavities. It may be caused by several factors, including:

- Inflammation
- Chemical stimuli
- Spasm of a hollow organ
- Overdistension of a hollow organ

Inflammation of the appendix (appendicitis) and gallbladder (cholecystitis) are common examples of visceral pain. *Chemical stimuli* may include gastric acid (gastroesophageal reflux disease (GERD), gastric ulcer, duodenal ulcer) or those substances associated with tissue ischemia and tissue damage. *Spasm* of the smooth muscle in the wall of a hollow organ causes pain due to the direct stimulation of mechanical nociceptors as well as ischemia-induced stimulation of polymodal nociceptors. This type of pain often occurs in the form of *cramps*. In other words, the pain increases to a high intensity and then subsides. This process occurs rhythmically, once every few minutes. Cramping pain frequently occurs in gastroenteritis, menstruation, and parturition (labor). *Overdistension* of a hollow organ causes pain by excessive stretch of the tissue and stimulation of mechanical nociceptors. Overdistension may also cause collapse of the blood vessels, resulting in development of ischemic pain. Severe visceral pain is typically accompanied by autonomic nervous system responses, such as nausea, vomiting, sweating, and pallor. This type of pain is poorly localized.

8.10 Referred pain

Referred pain is felt in a part of the body different from the actual tissue causing the pain. Typically, the pain is initiated in a visceral organ or tissue and referred to an area of the body surface. Classic examples of referred pain include *headache* and *angina*. Interestingly, the brain does not contain nociceptors; therefore, pain perceived as a headache originates in other tissues, such as the eyes; sinuses; muscles of the head and neck; and meninges. Angina, or chest pain, is caused by coronary ischemia. It may be accompanied by pain referred to the neck, left shoulder, and left arm.

Referred pain most likely results from the convergence of visceral and somatic afferent fibers on the same second-order neurons in the dorsal horn of the spinal cord (see Figure 8.3). Therefore, the brain has no way of identifying the original source of the pain. Because superficial inputs normally predominate over visceral inputs, higher centers may incorrectly attribute the pain to the skin instead of the deeper tissue.

8.11 Phantom pain

Phantom pain is pain that appears to arise from an amputated limb or body part; as many as 70% of amputees experience phantom pain. This pain may begin with sensations of tingling, heat and cold, or heaviness, followed by burning, cramping, or shooting pain. Phantom pain may disappear spontaneously or persist for many years.

The exact cause of phantom pain is not clearly understood. One proposed mechanism involves stimulation of the sensory pathway that had once originated in the amputated body part. An important point is that the sensory pathway originating in a given body part transmits impulses to the region of the somatosensory cortex devoted to that body part regardless of amputation. Stimulation at any point along this pathway results in the same sensation that would be produced by stimulation of the nociceptor in the body part itself. Following amputation of a body part, the ends of the afferent nerves arising from that body part become trapped in the scar tissue of the

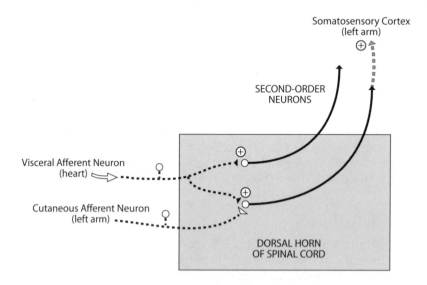

Figure 8.3 Referred pain. The mechanism of referred pain involves convergence of visceral afferent neurons and cutaneous afferent neurons with the same second-order neurons in the dorsal horn of the spinal cord. In this example, the pain of angina that originates in the heart is referred to the left arm.

stump. These afferent nerve endings exhibit increased sensitivity and are easily stimulated. Therefore, action potentials are generated at these nerve endings and transmitted to the area of the somatosensory cortex devoted to the amputated body part. This results in the perception of pain arising from the amputated portion of the body.

A second theory of phantom pain suggests that second-order neurons in the dorsal horn of the spinal cord become hyperactive. Spontaneous firing of these neurons causes transmission of nerve impulses to the brain and the perception of pain.

8.12 Pharmacologic treatment of pain

An *analgesic drug* acts on the nervous system to suppress or eliminate pain without causing loss of consciousness. As such, an ideal analgesic would exhibit the following qualities:

- Potent
- Nonaddictive
- Minimal adverse effects
- Effective without altering the patient's state of awareness
- Does not cause tolerance
- Inexpensive

Pain medications may be divided into three categories:

- Nonnarcotic analgesics
- Opioid analgesics
- Adjuvant analgesics

Nonnarcotic analgesics. The *nonnarcotic analgesics* include aspirin, NSAIDs, and acetaminophen. *Aspirin* acts centrally and peripherally to block the transmission of pain impulses. Furthermore, it reduces fever and inflammation and inhibits synthesis of the prostaglandins that increase the sensitivity of nociceptors.

The *NSAIDs* exert their analgesic effects primarily through inhibition of cyclooxygenase, the rate-limiting enzyme for prostaglandin synthesis. Typical NSAIDs inhibit cyclooxygenase 1 (COX-1; constitutive) and cyclooxygenase 2 (COX-2; induced in areas of inflammation). More recently, medications specific for COX-2 (rofecoxib, Vioxx®) have been developed. The advantage of these agents is that they reduce pain, fever, and inflammation without the unwanted side effects accompanying COX-1 inhibition, particularly those leading to gastric ulcers. NSAIDs inhibit the inflammatory response by decreasing the sensitivity of blood vessels to bradykinin and histamine, reversing vasodilation, and reducing the release of inflammatory mediators from mast cells, basophils, and granulocytes.

Acetaminophen, another alternative to aspirin, is an effective analgesic and fever-reducing agent. However, this medication has no effect on inflammation.

Opioid analgesics. Medications with morphine-like actions are referred to as *opioid* or *narcotic agents*. Opioid drugs exert their effects through three major categories of opioid receptors: mu (μ), kappa (κ) and delta (Δ). Analgesia appears to involve μ-receptors (largely at supraspinal sites) and κ-receptors (principally within the spinal cord). *Morphine* produces analgesia through interaction with μ-receptors. In fact, most clinically used opioids are relatively selective for μ-receptors. Morphine can stimulate μ_2-receptors spinally or μ_1-receptors supraspinally. When given systemically, it acts predominantly through supraspinal μ_1-receptors. Other effects of μ-receptor activation include respiratory depression; reduced gastrointestinal motility (leading to constipation); and feelings of well-being or euphoria.

Morphine may be administered orally, intravenously, or epidurally. An advantage of epidural administration is that it provides effective analgesia while minimizing the central depressant effects associated with systemic administration. The mechanism of action with the epidural route of administration involves opioid receptors on the cell bodies of first-order sensory neurons in the dorsal root ganglia as well as their axon terminals in the dorsal horn. Stimulation of these receptors inhibits release of substance P and interrupts transmission of the pain signal to the second-order sensory neuron.

Adjuvant analgesics. *Adjuvant analgesics* include medications such as *antidepressants* and *antiseizure medications*. The effectiveness of these agents may be due to the existence of nonendorphin synapses in the endogenous analgesic pathway. For example, the neurotransmitter serotonin has been shown to play a role in producing analgesia. Tricyclic antidepressant medications, such as imipramine, that block the removal of serotonin from the synapse suppress pain in some individuals. Certain antiseizure medications, such as carbamazepine and phenytoin, have specific analgesic effects that are effective under certain conditions. For example, these medications, which suppress spontaneous neuronal firing, are particularly effective in management of pain that occurs following nerve injury. Other agents, such as the *corticosteroids*, reduce pain by decreasing inflammation and the nociceptive stimuli responsible for the pain.

Bibliography

1. Basbaum, A.I. and Jessell, T.M., The perception of pain, in   *Principles of Neuroscience*, 4th ed., Kandel, E.R., Schwartz, J.H., and Jessell, T.M., Eds., McGraw–Hill, New York, 2000, chap. 24.
2. Curtis, S., Kolotylo, C., and Broome, M.E., Somatosensory function and pain, in *Pathophysiology, Concepts of Altered Health States*, 5th ed., Porth, C.M., Ed., Lippincott–Raven Publications, Philadelphia, 1998, chap. 40.

3. Gardner, E.P., Martin, J.H., and Jessell, T.M., The bodily senses, in *Principles of Neuroscience,* 4th ed., Kandel, E.R., Schwartz, J.H., and Jessell, T.M., Eds., McGraw–Hill, New York, 2000, chap. 22.

4. Guyton, A.C. and Hall, J.E., *Textbook of Medical Physiology,* 10th ed., W.B. Saunders, Philadelphia, 2000.

5. Rhoades, R. and Pflanzer, R., *Human Physiology,* 4th ed., Brooks/Cole, Pacific Grove, CA, 2003.

6. Sherwood, L., *Human Physiology from Cells to Systems,* 4th ed., Brooks/Cole, Pacific Grove, CA, 2001.

7. Silverthorn, D.U., *Human Physiology: An Integrated Approach,* 2nd ed., Prentice- Hall, Upper Saddle River, NJ, 2001.

chapter nine

The autonomic nervous system

Study objectives

- Explain how various regions of the central nervous system regulate autonomic nervous system function
- Explain how autonomic reflexes contribute to homeostasis
- Describe how the neuroeffector junction in the autonomic nervous system differs from that of a neuron-to-neuron synapse
- Compare and contrast anatomical features of the sympathetic and parasympathetic systems
- For each neurotransmitter in the autonomic nervous system, list the neurons that release it and the type and location of receptors that bind with it
- Describe the mechanisms by which neurotransmitters are removed
- Distinguish between cholinergic and adrenergic receptors
- Describe the overall and specific functions of the sympathetic system
- Describe the overall and specific functions of the parasympathetic system
- Explain how effects of the catecholamines differ from those of direct sympathetic stimulation

9.1 Introduction

The *autonomic nervous system (ANS)*, also known as the visceral or involuntary nervous system, functions below the level of consciousness. Because it innervates cardiac muscle, smooth muscle, and various endocrine and exocrine glands, this nervous system influences the activity of most of the organ systems in the body. Therefore, it is evident that the ANS makes an important contribution to the maintenance of homeostasis. Regulation of blood pressure; gastrointestinal responses to food; contraction of the urinary bladder; focusing of the eyes; and thermoregulation are just a few of the many

Table 9.1 Distinguishing Features of Autonomic and Somatic Nervous Systems

Autonomic nervous system	Somatic nervous system
Unconscious control; involuntary	Conscious control; voluntary
All innervated structures except skeletal muscle (e.g., cardiac and smooth muscles; glands)	Skeletal muscle
Visceral functions (e.g., cardiac activity, blood flow, digestion, etc.)	Movement; respiration; posture
Peripheral ganglia located outside cerebrospinal axis	No peripheral ganglia; synapses located entirely within cerebrospinal axis
Preganglionic and postganglionic neurons	Alpha motor neuron
Nonmyelinated	Myelinated
Neurotransmitters: acetylcholine, norepinephrine	Neurotransmitter: acetylcholine only
Cell bodies in brainstem, lateral horn of spinal cord	Cell bodies in ventral horn of spinal cord
No discrete innervation of individual effector cells	Axon divides; each axon terminal innervates single muscle fiber directly
Axon terminal with multiple varicosities releases neurotransmitter over wide surface area affecting many tissue cells	Motor end-plate or neuromuscular junction = axon terminal in apposition to specialized surface of muscle cell membrane
Gap junctions allow spread of nervous stimulation throughout tissue	No gap junctions between effector cells; no spread of electrical activity from one muscle fiber to another

homeostatic functions regulated by the ANS. Several distinguishing features of the ANS and the somatic nervous system, which innervates skeletal muscle, are summarized in Table 9.1.

9.2   *Regulation of autonomic nervous system activity*

The efferent nervous activity of the ANS is regulated by several regions in the central nervous system (CNS):

- Hypothalamus and brainstem
- Cerebral cortex and limbic system
- Spinal cord

Many homeostatic control centers are located in the *hypothalamus* and the *brainstem*. Through their effects on the ANS, these regions of the brain work together to control cardiovascular, respiratory, and digestive activity. The *cerebral cortex* and the *limbic system* also influence ANS activities associated with emotional responses by way of hypothalamic–brainstem pathways. For example, blushing during an embarrassing moment, a response most likely originating in the frontal association cortex, involves vasodilation of blood vessels to the face. Finally, many autonomic reflexes, such as the micturition reflex (urination), are mediated at the level of the *spinal cord*. Although these reflexes are subject to influence from higher nervous centers, they may occur without input from the brain.

The significance of the contribution to homeostasis by *autonomic reflexes* warrants further discussion. As described in Chapter 1, maintenance of homeostasis requires continuous sensory input through afferent pathways to the CNS regarding the internal state of the body. The CNS then integrates this information and initiates various negative feedback responses through motor pathways that alter organ activity. The result is the maintenance of the appropriate balance or equilibrium of variables in the internal environment needed for optimal body function. When considering the ANS, much of this sensory input from the thoracic and abdominal viscera is transmitted by afferent fibers of cranial nerve X, the vagus nerve. Other cranial nerves also contribute sensory input to the brain. The sensory signals are transmitted to control centers in the hypothalamus and brainstem. These centers then initiate the proper reflex responses from the visceral organs and tissues by way of the ANS.

An example of this type of reflex is the baroreceptor reflex (see Figure 1.2). Baroreceptors located in some of the major systemic arteries are sensory receptors that monitor blood pressure. If blood pressure decreases, the number of sensory impulses sent from the baroreceptors to the cardiovascular control center in the brainstem also decreases. As a result of this change in baroreceptor stimulation and sensory input to the brainstem, ANS discharge to the heart and blood vessels is adjusted to increase heart rate and vascular resistance so that blood pressure increases to its normal value.

9.3   Efferent pathways of autonomic nervous system

The efferent pathways of the ANS consist of two neurons that transmit impulses from the CNS to the effector tissue. The *preganglionic neuron* originates in the CNS with its cell body in the lateral horn of the gray matter of the spinal cord or in the brainstem. The axon of this neuron travels to an autonomic ganglion located outside the CNS, where it synapses with a *postganglionic neuron*. This neuron innervates the effector tissue.

Synapses between the autonomic postganglionic neuron and effector tissue — the *neuroeffector junction* — differ greatly from the neuron-to-neuron synapses discussed previously in Chapter 5 (see Table 9.1). The postganglionic fibers in the ANS do not terminate in a single swelling like the synaptic knob, nor do they synapse directly with the cells of a tissue. Instead, the axon terminals branch and contain multiple swellings called *varicosities* that lie across the surface of the tissue. When the neuron is stimulated, these varicosities release neurotransmitter over a large surface area of the effector tissue. This diffuse release of the neurotransmitter affects many tissue cells simultaneously. Furthermore, cardiac muscle and most smooth muscle have *gap junctions* between cells. These specialized intercellular communications allow for spread of electrical activity from one cell to the next. As a result, the discharge of a single autonomic nerve fiber to an effector tissue may alter activity of the entire tissue.

9.4   *Divisions of autonomic nervous system*

The ANS is composed of two anatomically and functionally distinct divisions: the *sympathetic system* and the *parasympathetic system*. Two important features of these divisions include:

- Tonic activity
- Dual innervation

Both systems are *tonically active*. In other words, they provide some degree of nervous input to a given tissue at all times. Therefore, the frequency of discharge of neurons in both systems can increase or decrease and, as a result, tissue activity may be enhanced or inhibited. This characteristic of the ANS improves its ability to regulate a tissue's function more precisely. Without tonic activity, nervous input to a tissue could only increase.

Many tissues are *innervated by both systems*. Because the sympathetic and parasympathetic systems typically have opposing effects on a given tissue, increasing the activity of one system while simultaneously decreasing the activity of the other results in very rapid and precise control of a tissue's function. Several distinguishing features of these two divisions of the ANS are summarized in Table 9.2.

Each system is dominant under certain conditions. The sympathetic system predominates during emergency *"fight-or-flight"* reactions and during exercise. The overall effect of the sympathetic system under these conditions is to prepare the body for strenuous physical activity. More specifically, sympathetic nervous activity will increase the flow of blood that is well-oxygenated and rich in nutrients to tissues that need it, in particular, the working skeletal muscles. The parasympathetic system predominates during quiet, resting conditions. The overall effect of the parasympathetic system under these conditions is to *conserve and store energy* and to regulate basic body functions such as digestion and urination.

9.5   *Sympathetic division*

The preganglionic neurons of the sympathetic system arise from the thoracic and lumbar regions of the spinal cord (segments T_1 through L_2; see Figure 9.1). Most of these preganglionic axons are short and synapse with postganglionic neurons within ganglia found in *sympathetic ganglion chains*. Running parallel immediately along either side of the spinal cord, each of these chains consists of 22 ganglia. The preganglionic neuron may exit the spinal cord and synapse with a postganglionic neuron in a ganglion at the same spinal cord level from which it arises. This neuron may also travel more rostrally

Table 9.2 Distinguishing Features of Sympathetic and Parasympathetic Systems

Sympathetic system	Parasympathetic system
Originates in thoracic and lumbar regions of the spinal cord (T_1–L_2)	Originates in brainstem (cranial nerves III, VII, IX, and X) and sacral region of spinal cord (S_2–S_4)
Ganglia located in paravertebral sympathetic ganglion chain or collateral ganglia	Terminal ganglia located near or embedded within target tissue
Short cholinergic preganglionic fibers; long adrenergic postganglionic fibers	Long cholinergic preganglionic fibers; short cholinergic postganglionic fibers
Ratio of preganglionic fibers to postganglionic fibers is 1:20	Ratio of preganglionic fibers to postganglionic fibers is 1:3
Divergence coordinates activity of neurons at multiple levels of spinal cord	Limited divergence
Activity often involves mass discharge of entire system	Activity normally to discrete organs
Predominates during emergency "fight-or-flight" reactions and exercise	Predominates during quiet resting conditions

or caudally (upward or downward) in the ganglion chain to synapse with postganglionic neurons in ganglia at other levels. In fact, a single preganglionic neuron may synapse with several postganglionic neurons in many different ganglia. Overall, the ratio of preganglionic fibers to postganglionic fibers is about 1:20. The long postganglionic neurons originating in the ganglion chain then travel outward and terminate on the effector tissues. This divergence of the preganglionic neuron results in coordinated sympathetic stimulation to tissues throughout the body. The concurrent stimulation of many organs and tissues in the body is referred to as *mass sympathetic discharge*.

Other preganglionic neurons exit the spinal cord and pass through the ganglion chain without synapsing with a postganglionic neuron. Instead, the axons of these neurons travel more peripherally and synapse with postganglionic neurons in one of the *sympathetic collateral ganglia* (see Figure 9.1). These ganglia are located about halfway between the CNS and effector tissue.

Finally, the preganglionic neuron may travel to the *adrenal medulla* and synapse directly with this glandular tissue. The cells of the adrenal medulla have the same embryonic origin as neural tissue and, in fact, function as *modified postganglionic neurons*. Instead of the release of neurotransmitter directly at the synapse with an effector tissue, the secretory products of the adrenal medulla are picked up by the blood and travel throughout the body to all of the effector tissues of the sympathetic system.

An important feature of this system, which is quite distinct from the parasympathetic system, is that the postganglionic neurons of the sympathetic

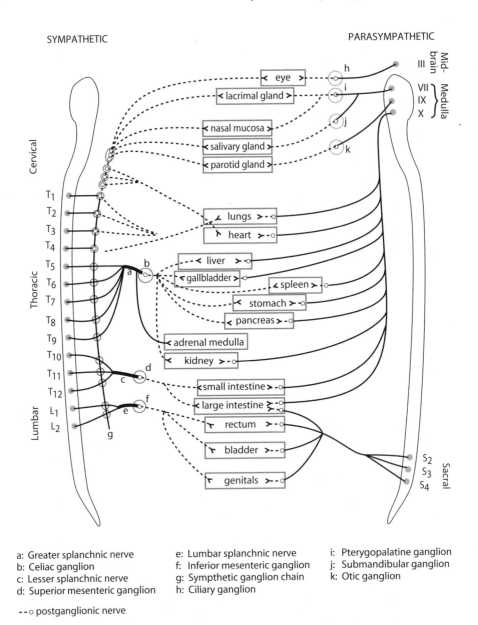

SYMPATHETIC   PARASYMPATHETIC

Figure 9.1 The autonomic nervous system and its effector organs. The efferent pathways of this system consist of two neurons that transmit impulses from the CNS to the effector tissue, preganglionic neuron (solid line), and postganglionic neuron (dashed line). As illustrated, most tissues receive nervous input from both divisions of the ANS: the sympathetic and the parasympathetic.

a: Greater splanchnic nerve   e: Lumbar splanchnic nerve   i: Pterygopalatine ganglion
b: Celiac ganglion   f: Inferior mesenteric ganglion   j: Submandibular ganglion
c: Lesser splanchnic nerve   g: Sympthetic ganglion chain   k: Otic ganglion
d: Superior mesenteric ganglion   h: Ciliary ganglion

- - o postganglionic nerve

system travel within each of the 31 pairs of spinal nerves (see Chapter 7). Interestingly, 8% of the fibers that constitute a spinal nerve are sympathetic fibers. This allows for distribution of sympathetic nerve fibers to the effectors of the skin, including blood vessels and sweat glands. In fact, because most innervated blood vessels in the entire body, primarily arterioles and veins, receive only sympathetic nerve fibers, vascular smooth muscle tone and sweating are regulated by the sympathetic system only. In addition, the sympathetic system innervates structures of the head (eye, salivary glands, mucus membranes of the nasal cavity), thoracic viscera (heart, lungs) and viscera of the abdominal and pelvic cavities (e.g., stomach, intestines, pancreas, spleen, adrenal medulla, urinary bladder; see Figure 9.1).

9.6 Parasympathetic division

Preganglionic neurons of the parasympathetic system arise from several nuclei of the brainstem and from the sacral region of the spinal cord (segments S_2 to S_4; see Figure 9.1). The axons of the preganglionic neurons are quite long compared to those of the sympathetic system and synapse with postganglionic neurons within *terminal ganglia* that are close to or embedded within the effector tissues. The very short axons of the postganglionic neurons then provide input to the cells of that effector tissue.

The preganglionic neurons that arise from the brainstem exit the CNS through cranial nerves. The occulomotor nerve (III) innervates the eyes; the facial nerve (VII) innervates the lacrimal gland, salivary glands, and mucus membranes of the nasal cavity; the glossopharyngeal nerve (IX) innervates the parotid (salivary) gland; and the vagus nerve (X) innervates the viscera of the thorax and abdomen (e.g., heart, lungs, stomach, intestines, and pancreas). The physiological significance of this latter nerve in terms of influence of the parasympathetic system is clearly illustrated by its widespread distribution and the fact that 75% of all parasympathetic fibers are in the vagus nerve. Preganglionic neurons that arise from the sacral region of the spinal cord exit the CNS and join together to form the pelvic nerves. These nerves innervate the viscera of the pelvic cavity (e.g., urinary bladder, colon).

Because the terminal ganglia are located within the innervated tissue, there is typically little divergence in the parasympathetic system compared to the sympathetic system. In many organs, the ratio of preganglionic fibers to postganglionic fibers is 1:1. Therefore, the effects of the parasympathetic system tend to be more discrete and localized, with only specific tissues stimulated at any given moment, compared to the sympathetic system in which a more diffuse discharge is possible.

9.7 Neurotransmitters of autonomic nervous system

The two most common neurotransmitters released by neurons of the ANS are *acetylcholine (Ach)* and *norepinephrine (NE)*. Several distinguishing features of these neurotransmitters are summarized in Table 9.3. Nerve fibers that release acetylcholine are referred to as *cholinergic* fibers and include all preganglionic fibers of the ANS — sympathetic and parasympathetic systems; all postganglionic fibers of the parasympathetic system; and sympathetic postganglionic

Table 9.3 Distinguishing Features of Neurotransmitters of Autonomic Nervous System

Feature	Acetylcholine	Norepinephrin	Epinephrine[a]
Site of Release	All preganglionic neurons of autonomic nervous system; all postganglionic neurons of parasympathetic system; some sympathetic postganglionic neurons innervating sweat glands; (alpha motor neurons innervating skeletal muscle)[b]	Most sympathetic postganglionic neurons; adrenal medulla (20% of secretion)	Adrenal medulla (80% of secretion)
Receptor	Nicotinic, muscarinic (cholinergic)	α_1, α_2, β_1 (adrenergic)	α_1, α_2, β_1, β_2 (adrenergic)
Termination of Activity	Enzymatic degradation by acetylcholinesterase	Reuptake into nerve terminals; diffusion out of synaptic cleft and uptake at extraneuronal sites; metabolic transformation by monoamine oxidase (within nerve terminal) or catechol-O-methyl-transferase within liver	Metabolic transformation by catechol-O-methyltransferase within liver

[a] Although epinephrine is not a direct neurotransmitter for the autonomic nervous system, its release from the adrenal medulla supplements the effects of a mass sympathetic discharge.

[b] Alpha motor neurons, a component of the somatic nervous system, also release acetylcholine as a neurotransmitter.

fibers innervating sweat glands (see Figure 9.2). Nerve fibers that release norepinephrine are referred to as *adrenergic* fibers. Most sympathetic postganglionic fibers release norepinephrine.

As previously mentioned, the cells of the adrenal medulla are considered modified sympathetic postganglionic neurons. Instead of a neurotransmitter, these cells release *hormones* into the blood. Approximately 20% of the hormonal output of the adrenal medulla is norepinephrine. The remaining 80% is *epinephrine (EPI)*. Unlike true postganglionic neurons in the sympathetic system, the adrenal medulla contains an enzyme that methylates norepinephrine to form epinephrine. The synthesis of epinephrine, also known as *adrenalin*, is enhanced under conditions of stress. These two hormones released by the adrenal medulla are collectively referred to as the *catecholamines*.

9.8   Termination of neurotransmitter activity

For any substance to serve effectively as a neurotransmitter, it must be rapidly removed or inactivated from the synapse or, in this case, the neuroeffector junction. This is necessary in order to allow new signals to get through and influence effector tissue function. Neurotransmitter activity may be terminated by three mechanisms:

- Diffusion out of the synapse
- Enzymatic degradation
- Reuptake into the neuron

The primary mechanism used by cholinergic synapses is *enzymatic degradation*. *Acetylcholinesterase* hydrolyzes acetylcholine to its components choline and acetate; it is one of the fastest acting enzymes in the body and acetylcholine removal occurs in less than 1 msec. The most important mechanism for removal of norepinephrine from the neuroeffector junction is the *reuptake* of this neurotransmitter into the sympathetic neuron that released it. Norepinephrine may then be metabolized intraneuronally by *monoamine oxidase (MAO)*. The circulating catecholamines — epinephrine and norepinephrine — are inactivated by *catechol-O-methyltransferase (COMT)* in the liver.

9.9   Receptors for autonomic neurotransmitters

As discussed in the previous section, all the effects of the ANS in tissues and organs throughout the body, including smooth muscle contraction or relaxation; alteration of myocardial activity; and increased or decreased glandular secretion, are carried out by only three substances: acetylcholine, norepinephrine, and epinephrine. Furthermore, each of these substances may stimulate activity in some tissues and inhibit activity in others. How can this

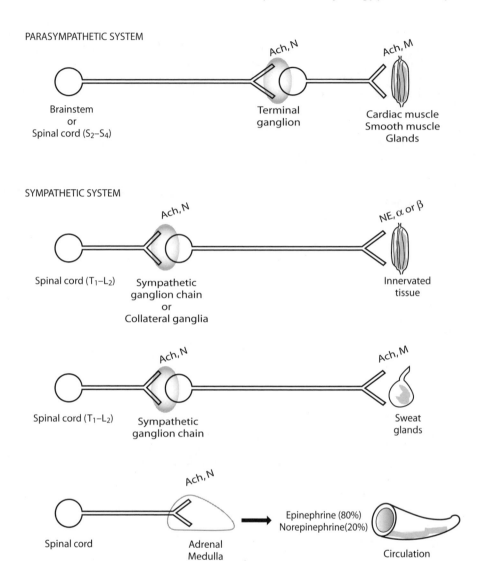

Figure 9.2 Autonomic nerve pathways. All preganglionic neurons release acetylcholine (Ach), which binds to nicotinic receptors (N) on the postganglionic
neurons. All postganglionic neurons in the parasympathetic system and some
sympathetic postganglionic neurons innervating sweat glands release Ach that
binds to muscarinic (M) receptors on the cells of the effector tissue. The remaining postganglionic neurons of the sympathetic system release norepinephrine
(NE), which binds to alpha (α) or beta (β) receptors on cells of the effector tissue.
The cells of the adrenal medulla, which are modified postganglionic neurons in
the sympathetic system, release epinephrine (EPI) and NE into the circulation.

wide variety of effects on many different tissues be carried out by so few neurotransmitters or hormones? The effect caused by any of these substances is determined by receptor distribution in a particular tissue and biochemical properties of the cells in that tissue — specifically, the second messenger and enzyme systems present in the cell.

The neurotransmitters of the ANS and the circulating catecholamines bind to specific receptors on the cell membranes of effector tissue. Each receptor is coupled to a *G protein* also embedded within the plasma membrane. Receptor stimulation causes activation of the G protein and formation of an intracellular chemical, the *second messenger*. (The neurotransmitter molecule, which cannot enter the cell, is the *first messenger*.) The function of intracellular second messenger molecules is to elicit tissue-specific biochemical events within the cell that alter the cell's activity. In this way, a given neurotransmitter may stimulate the same type of receptor on two different types of tissue and cause two different responses due to the presence of different biochemical pathways within each tissue.

Acetylcholine binds to two types of *cholinergic receptors*:

- Nicotinic receptors
- Muscarinic receptors

Nicotinic receptors are found on the cell bodies of all sympathetic and parasympathetic postganglionic neurons in the ganglia of the ANS. Acetylcholine released from the preganglionic neurons binds to these nicotinic receptors and causes a rapid increase in the cellular permeability to Na^+ and Ca^{++} ions. The resulting influx of these two cations causes depolarization and excitation of postganglionic neurons in the ANS pathways. *Muscarinic receptors* are found on cell membranes of effector tissues and are linked to G proteins and second messenger systems that carry out the intracellular effects. Acetylcholine released from all parasympathetic postganglionic neurons, and some sympathetic postganglionic neurons traveling to sweat glands, binds to these receptors. Muscarinic receptors may be inhibitory or excitatory, depending on the tissue upon which they are found. For example, muscarinic receptor stimulation in the myocardium is inhibitory and decreases heart rate, while stimulation of these receptors in the lungs is excitatory and causes contraction of airway smooth muscle and bronchoconstriction.

The two classes of *adrenergic receptors* for norepinephrine and epinephrine are:

- Alpha (α)
- Beta (β)

Furthermore, each class has at least two subtypes of receptors: α_1, α_2, β_1, and β_2. All of these receptors are linked to G proteins and second messenger systems that carry out the intracellular effects.

Alpha receptors are the most abundant of the adrenergic receptors. Of the two subtypes, α_1-receptors are more widely distributed on the effector tissues; these receptors tend to be excitatory. For example, stimulation of α_1-receptors causes contraction of vascular smooth muscle, resulting in vasoconstriction.

Pharmacy application: α_1-adrenergic receptor antagonists

Hypertension, or a chronic elevation in blood pressure, is a major risk factor for coronary artery disease; congestive heart failure; stroke; kidney failure; and retinopathy. An important cause of hypertension is excessive vascular smooth muscle tone or vasoconstriction. Prazosin, an α_1-adrenergic receptor antagonist, is very effective in management of hypertension. Because α_1-receptor stimulation causes vasoconstriction, drugs that block these receptors result in vasodilation and a decrease in blood pressure.

Compared to α_1-receptors, α_2-receptors have only moderate distribution on the effector tissues; however, they have important presynaptic effects. Alpha-one receptors are found on effector tissue cells at the neuroeffector junction; the α_2-receptors are found on the varicosities of the postganglionic neuron. Norepinephrine released from this neuron not only binds to the α_1-receptors on the effector tissue to cause some physiological effect but also binds to the α_2-receptors on the neuron. Alpha-two receptor stimulation results in *"presynaptic inhibition"* or in a decrease in the release of norepinephrine. In this way, norepinephrine inhibits its own release from the sympathetic postganglionic neuron and controls its own activity. Both α_1- and α_2-receptors have equal affinity for norepinephrine released directly from sympathetic neurons as well as circulating epinephrine released from the adrenal medulla.

Beta receptors are also unevenly distributed with β_2-receptors the more common subtype on the effector tissues. Beta-two receptors tend to be inhibitory; for example, β_2-receptor stimulation causes relaxation of vascular smooth muscle and airway smooth muscle, resulting in vasodilation and bronchodilation, respectively. Beta-two receptors have a significantly greater affinity for epinephrine than for norepinephrine. Furthermore, terminations of sympathetic pathways are not found near these receptors, so β_2-receptors are stimulated only indirectly by circulating epinephrine instead of by direct sympathetic nervous activity.

Beta-one receptors are the primary adrenergic receptor on the heart (a small percentage of the adrenergic receptors on the myocardium are β_2). Both subtypes of β-receptors on the heart are excitatory and stimulation leads to an increase in cardiac activity. Beta-one receptors are also found on certain cells in the kidney. Epinephrine and norepinephrine have equal affinity for $β_1$-receptors.

Pharmacy application: sympathomimetic drugs

Sympathomimetic drugs produce effects in a tissue resembling those caused from stimulation by the sympathetic nervous system. An important use for these drugs is in the treatment of bronchial asthma, which is characterized by bronchospasm. As discussed, bronchodilation occurs following $β_2$-adrenergic receptor stimulation. Nonselective β-receptor agonists, such as epinephrine and isoproterenol, are capable of causing bronchodilation. However, a potential problem with these drugs is that they stimulate *all* β-receptors, including β-receptors on the heart. Therefore, an undesirable side effect of treatment with these nonselective agents is an increase in heart rate. Instead, $β_2$-selective drugs such as albuterol are chosen for this therapy because they are equally effective in causing bronchodilation without the adverse effects of nonselective agents.

9.10 Functions of the autonomic nervous system

The two divisions of the ANS are dominant under different conditions: as stated previously, the sympathetic system is activated during emergency "fight-or-flight" reactions and during exercise, and the parasympathetic system is predominant during quiet resting conditions. As such, the physiological effects caused by each system are quite predictable. In other words, all the changes in organ and tissue function induced by the sympathetic system work together to support strenuous physical activity and changes induced by the parasympathetic system are appropriate when the body is resting. Several of the specific effects elicited by sympathetic and parasympathetic stimulation of various organs and tissues are summarized in Table 9.4.

The "fight-or-flight" reaction elicited by the sympathetic system is essentially a whole-body response. Changes in organ and tissue function throughout the body are coordinated so that delivery of well-oxygenated, nutrient-rich blood to the working skeletal muscles increases. Heart rate and myocardial contractility are increased so that the heart pumps more blood per minute. Sympathetic stimulation of vascular smooth muscle causes widespread vasoconstriction, particularly in organs of the gastrointestinal system and in the kidneys. This vasoconstriction serves to "redirect" or redistribute the blood away from these metabolically inactive tissues and toward the contracting muscles. Bronchodilation in the lungs facilitates the movement

Table 9.4 Effects of Autonomic Nerve Activity on Some Effector Tissues

Tissue	Sympathetic receptor	Sympathetic stimulation	Parasympathetic stimulation
Eye			
Radial muscle of iris	α_1	Contraction (mydriasis)	—
Sphincter muscle of iris		—	Contraction (miosis)
Ciliary muscle	β_2	Relaxation for far vision	Contraction for near vision
Heart	β_1, β_2	Increased heart rate	Decreased heart rate
		Increased contractility	—
Arterioles			
Skin	α_1	Strong constriction	—
Abdominal viscera	α_1	Strong constriction	—
Kidney	α_1	Strong constriction	—
Skeletal muscle	α_1, β_2	Weak constriction	—
Lungs			
Airways	β_2	Bronchodilation	Bronchoconstriction
Glands	α_1, β_2	Decreased secretion	Increased secretion
Liver	α_1, β_2	Glycogenolysis	—
		Gluconeogenesis	—
Adipose tissue		Lipolysis	—
Sweat glands	Muscarinic	Generalized sweating	—
	α_1	Localized sweating	—

Adrenal medulla	Nicotinic	Increased secretion of epinephrine and norepineprine	—
Salivary glands	α₁, β	Small volume K⁺ and water secretion	Large volume K⁺ and water secretion / Amylase secretion
Stomach			
Motility	α₁, β₂	Decreased contraction	Increased
Sphincters	α₁		relaxation
Secretion			Stimulation
Intestine			
Motility	α₁, β₂	Decreased contraction	Increased
Sphincters	α₁		relaxation
Secretion			Stimulation
Gall Bladder	β₂	Relaxation	Contraction
Pancreas			
Exocrine	α	Decreased secretion	Increased secretion
Endocrine (Islet β cells)	α	Decreased secretion	Increased secretion
Urinary Bladder			
Detrusor muscle (Bladder wall)	β₂	Relaxation	Contraction
Sphincter	α₁	Contraction	Relaxation
Kidney	β₁	Renin secretion	—

of air in and out of the lungs so that uptake of oxygen from the atmosphere and elimination of carbon dioxide from the body are maximized. An enhanced rate of glycogenolysis (breakdown of glycogen into its component glucose molecules) and gluconeogenesis (formation of new glucose from noncarbohydrate sources) in the liver increases the concentration of glucose molecules in the blood. This is necessary for the brain because glucose is the only nutrient molecule that it can utilize to form metabolic energy. An enhanced rate of lipolysis in adipose tissue increases the concentration of fatty acid molecules in the blood. Skeletal muscles then utilize these fatty acids to form metabolic energy for contraction. Generalized sweating elicited by the sympathetic system enables the individual to thermoregulate during conditions of increased physical activity and heat production. Finally, the eye is adjusted so that the pupil dilates, letting more light in toward the retina (*mydriasis*) and the lens adapts for distance vision.

The parasympathetic system decreases heart rate, which helps to conserve energy under resting conditions. Salivary secretion is enhanced to facilitate swallowing food. Gastric motility and secretion are stimulated to begin processing of ingested food. Intestinal motility and secretion are also stimulated to continue processing and to facilitate absorption of these nutrients. Exocrine and endocrine secretion from the pancreas is promoted. Enzymes released from the exocrine glands of the pancreas contribute to the chemical breakdown of the food in the intestine, and insulin released from the pancreatic islets promotes storage of nutrient molecules within the tissues once they are absorbed into the body. Another bodily maintenance type of function caused by the parasympathetic system is contraction of the urinary bladder, which results in urination. Finally, the eye is adjusted so that the pupil contracts (*miosis*) and the lens adapts for near vision.

Pharmacy application: cholinomimetic drugs

Cholinomimetic drugs produce effects in a tissue resembling those caused from stimulation by the parasympathetic nervous system. These drugs have many important uses including treatment of gastrointestinal and urinary tract disorders that involve depressed smooth muscle activity without obstruction. For example, postoperative ileus is characterized by a loss of tone or paralysis of the stomach or bowel following surgical manipulation. Urinary retention may also occur postoperatively or may be secondary to spinal cord injury or disease (neurogenic bladder). Normally, parasympathetic stimulation of the smooth muscle in each of these organ systems causes contraction to maintain gastrointestinal motility as well as urination. The pharmacotherapy of these disorders has two different approaches. One type of agent is a muscarinic receptor agonist that mimics the effect of the parasympathetic neurotransmitter, acetylcholine, and stimulates smooth muscle contraction. One of the most widely used agents in this category is bethanechol, which can be given subcutaneously. Another approach is to increase the concentration, and therefore activity, of endogenously produced acetylcholine in the neuroeffector synapse. Administration of an acetylcholinesterase inhibitor prevents degradation and removal of neuronally released acetylcholine. In this case, neostigmine is the most widely used agent and may be given subcutaneously or orally.

Pharmacy application: muscarinic receptor antagonists

Inspection of the retina during an ophthalmoscopic examination is greatly facilitated by mydriasis, or the dilation of the pupil. Parasympathetic stimulation of the circular muscle layer in the iris causes contraction and a decrease in the diameter of the pupil. Administration of a muscarinic receptor antagonist such as atropine or scopolamine prevents this smooth muscle contraction. As a result, sympathetic stimulation of the radial muscle layer is unopposed, causing an increase in the diameter of the pupil. These agents are given in the form of eye drops that act locally and limit the possibility of systemic side effects.

9.11 Adrenal medulla

Typically occurring during the "fight-or-flight" response or during exercise, a mass sympathetic discharge involves simultaneous stimulation of organs and tissues throughout the body. Included among these tissues are the adrenal medullae, which release epinephrine and norepinephrine into the blood. In large part, the indirect effects of these catecholamines are similar to, and therefore reinforce, those of direct sympathetic stimulation. However, some important differences in effects of the circulating catecholamines and those of norepinephrine released from sympathetic nerves include:

- Duration of activity
- Breadth of activity
- Affinity for β_2-receptors

Because *duration of activity* of the catecholamines is significantly longer than that of neuronally released norepinephrine, the effects on tissues are more prolonged. This difference has to do with the mechanism of inactivation of these substances. Norepinephrine is immediately removed from the neuroeffector synapse by way of reuptake into the postganglionic neuron. This rapid removal limits duration of the effect of this neurotransmitter. In contrast, no enzymes are in the blood to degrade the catecholamines; instead, they are inactivated by COMT in the liver. As one might expect, hepatic clearance of these hormones from the blood would require several passes through the circulation. Therefore, the catecholamines are available to cause their effects for a comparatively longer period of time (up to 1 to 2 minutes as opposed to milliseconds).

Because catecholamines travel in the blood, organs and tissues throughout the body are exposed to them. Therefore, they are capable of stimulating tissues that are not directly innervated by sympathetic nerve fibers, hepatocytes, and adipose tissue, in particular. As a result, the catecholamines have a much wider *breadth of activity* compared to norepinephrine released from sympathetic nerves.

The third important feature distinguishing catecholamines from neuronally released norepinephrine involves epinephrine's *affinity for β_2-receptors*. Norepinephrine has a very limited affinity for these receptors. Therefore, circulating epinephrine causes effects that differ from those of direct sympathetic innervation, including:

- Greater stimulatory effect on the heart
- Relaxation of smooth muscle
  - Vascular
  - Bronchial
  - Gastrointestinal
  - Genitourinary

Epinephrine and norepinephrine have equal affinity for β_1-receptors, the predominant adrenergic receptors on the heart. However, the human heart also contains a small percentage of β_2-receptors that, like β_1-receptors, are excitatory. Therefore, epinephrine is capable of stimulating a greater number of receptors and causing a *greater stimulatory effect on the myocardium*.

Beta-two adrenergic receptors are also found on smooth muscle in several organ systems. These receptors tend to be inhibitory and cause *relaxation of the smooth muscle*. Vascular smooth muscle in skeletal muscle contains α_1- and β_2-receptors. Norepinephrine, which stimulates only the excitatory α_1-receptors, causes strong vasoconstriction; however, epinephrine, which stimulates both types of receptors, causes only weak vasoconstriction. The vasodilation resulting from β_2-receptor stimulation opposes and therefore weakens vasoconstriction resulting from α_1-receptor stimulation. Given that skeletal muscle may account for 40% of an adult's body weight, the potential difference in vasoconstriction, blood pressure, and distribution of blood flow could be quite significant.

Another noteworthy example of the relaxation of smooth muscle by way of β_2-receptor stimulation involves airways. Bronchodilation, or opening of the airways, facilitates airflow in the lungs. Any direct sympathetic innervation to the lungs is irrelevant in this respect because only circulating epinephrine is capable of stimulating these receptors on airway smooth muscle.

Bibliography

1. Hoffman, B.B., Adrenoceptor-activating and other sympathomimetic drugs, in *Basic and Clinical Pharmacology*, 8th ed., Katzung, B.G., Ed., Lange Medical Books/McGraw–Hill, New York, 2001, chap. 9.
2. Hoffman, B.B., Adrenoceptor antagonist drugs, in *Basic and Clinical Pharmacology*, 8th ed., Katzung, B.G., Ed., Lange Medical Books/McGraw–Hill, New York, 2001, chap. 10.
3. Hoffman, B.B., Lefkowitz, R.J., and Taylor, P., Neurotransmission: the autonomic and somatic motor nervous systems, in *Goodman and Gilman's: The Pharmacological Basis of Therapeutics*, 9th ed., Hardman, J.G. and Limbird, L.E., Eds., McGraw–Hill, New York, 1996, chap. 6.
4. Iversen, S., Iversen, L., and Saper, C., The autonomic nervous system and the hypothalamus, in *Principles of Neuroscience,* 4th ed., Kandel, E.R., Schwartz, J.H., and Jessell, T.M., Eds., McGraw–Hill, New York, 2000, chap. 49.
5. Katzung, B.G., Introduction to autonomic pharmacology, in *Basic and Clinical Pharmacology*, 8th ed., Katzung, B.G., Ed., Lange Medical Books/ McGraw–Hill, New York, 2001, chap. 6.
6. Pappano, A.J., Cholinoceptor-activating and cholinesterase-inhibiting drugs, in *Basic and Clinical Pharmacology*, 8th ed., Katzung, B.G., Ed., Lange Medical Books/McGraw–Hill, New York, 2001, chap. 7.
7. Pappano, A.J., Cholinoceptor-blocking drugs, in *Basic and Clinical Pharmacology*, 8th ed., Katzung, B.G., Ed., Lange Medical Books/McGraw–Hill, New York, 2001, chap. 8.
8. Rhoades, R. and Pflanzer, R., *Human Physiology,* Thomson Learning, Pacific Grove, CA, 2003.
9. Sherwood, L., *Human Physiology from Cells to Systems*, 4th ed., Brooks/Cole, Pacific Grove, CA, 2001.
10. Silverthorn, D., *Human Physiology: An Integrated Approach*, 2nd ed., Prentice Hall, Upper Saddle River, NJ, 2001.
11. *Taber's Cyclopedic Medical Dictionary*, 19th ed., F.A. Davis Co., Philadelphia, PA, 2001.

chapter ten

The endocrine system

Study objectives

Differentiate between the primary functions of the nervous system and the endocrine system

- Describe biochemical and functional distinctions among steroid hormones, protein/peptide hormones, and amine hormones
- Explain beneficial effects of the binding of hormones to plasma proteins
- Distinguish between a trophic and a nontrophic hormone
- Describe the three types of hormone interactions
- Explain the two primary mechanisms by which hormones carry out their effects
- Describe how the effects of hormones are amplified
- Describe how the pituitary gland is formed during embryonic development
- Describe anatomical and functional relationships between the hypothalamus and the pituitary gland
- Explain how negative feedback mechanisms limit release of hormones from the adenohypophysis
- List functions and describe mechanisms regulating release of hormones from the neurohypophysis
- List functions and describe mechanisms regulating release of hormones from the adenohypophysis
- Discuss functions and factors regulating release of the following hormones: thyroid hormones, calcitonin, parathyroid hormone, catecholamines, aldosterone, cortisol, adrenal androgens, insulin, and glucagon

10.1 Introduction

Two major regulatory systems make important contributions to homeostasis: the nervous system and the endocrine system. In order to maintain relatively constant conditions in the internal environment of the body, each of these systems influences the activity of all the other organ systems. The nervous system coordinates fast, precise responses, such as muscle contraction. Electrical impulses generated by this system are very rapid and of short duration (milliseconds). The endocrine system regulates metabolic activity within the cells of organs and tissues. In contrast to the nervous system, this system coordinates activities that require longer duration (hours, days) rather than speed. Examples of such activities include growth; long-term regulation of blood pressure; and coordination of menstrual cycles in females. The endocrine system carries out its effects through the production of *hormones*, chemical messengers that exert a regulatory effect on the cells of the body. Secreted from *endocrine glands*, which are ductless structures, hormones are released directly into the blood. They are then transported by the circulation to the tissues upon which they exert their effects. Because they travel in the blood, the serum concentrations of hormones are very low (10^{-11} to 10^{-9} M); therefore, these molecules must be very potent.

Generally, a single hormone does not affect all of the body's cells. The tissues that respond to a hormone are referred to as the *target tissues*. The cells of these tissues possess specific receptors to which the hormone binds. This receptor binding then elicits a series of events that influences cellular activities.

10.2 Biochemical classification of hormones

Hormones are classified into three biochemical categories (see Table 10.1):

- Steroids
- Proteins/peptides
- Amines

Steroid hormones are produced by the adrenal cortex, testes, ovaries, and placenta. Synthesized from cholesterol, these hormones are lipid soluble; therefore, they cross cell membranes readily and bind to receptors found intracellularly. However, because their lipid solubility renders them insoluble in blood, these hormones are transported in the blood bound to proteins. Furthermore, steroid hormones are not typically preformed and stored for future use within the endocrine gland. Because they are lipid soluble, they could diffuse out of the cells and physiological regulation of their release would not be possible. Finally, steroid hormones are absorbed easily by the gastrointestinal tract and therefore may be administered orally.

Protein/peptide hormones are derived from amino acids. These hormones are preformed and stored for future use in membrane-bound secretory granules. When needed, they are released by exocytosis. Protein/peptide hormones are water soluble, circulate in the blood predominantly in an unbound form, and thus tend to have short half-lives. Because these hormones are unable to cross the cell membranes of their target tissues, they bind to receptors

Table 10.1 Distinguishing Features of Steroid, Protein/Peptide, and Amine Hormones

Feature	Steroid hormones	Protein/peptide hormones	Amine hormones	
			Thyroid hormones	Catecholamines
Synthesis	Synthesized on demand; derived from cholesterol	Synthesized in advance; derived from amino acids	Synthesized in advance; stored as part of thyroglobulin	Synthesized in advance; derived from tyrosine
Transport in blood	Bound to carrier proteins	Soluble in plasma	Bound to carrier proteins	Soluble in plasma
Half-life	Long	Short	Long	Short
Location of receptor	Within cell nucleus	Membrane surface	Within cell nucleus	Membrane surface
Mechanism of action	Gene activation	Second messenger systems	Gene activation	Second messenger systems
Target tissue response	Synthesis of new enzymes	Modification of existing enzymes	Synthesis of new enzymes	Modification of existing enzymes
Sites of production	Adrenal cortex, testes, ovaries, placenta	Hypothalamus, pituitary gland, thyroid gland, parathyroid glands, pancreas	Thyroid gland	Adrenal medulla

on the membrane surface. Protein/peptide hormones cannot be administered orally because they would be digested in the gastrointestinal tract. Instead, they are usually administered by injection (e.g., insulin). Because small peptides are able to cross through mucus membranes, they may be given sublingually or intranasally. For example, Miacalcin®, the synthetic form of the hormone calcitonin, is prepared in the form of a nasal spray.

Amine hormones include the thyroid hormones and the catecholamines. The thyroid hormones tend to be biologically similar to the steroid hormones. They are mainly insoluble in the blood and are transported predominantly (>99%) bound to proteins. As such, these hormones have longer half-lives (triiodothyronine, T_3, = 24 h; thyroxine, T_4, = 7 days). Furthermore, thyroid hormones cross cell membranes to bind with intracellular receptors and may be administered orally (e.g., synthryoid). In contrast to steroid hormones, however, thyroid hormones have the unique property of being stored extracellularly in the thyroid gland as part of the thyroglobulin molecule.

The catecholamines are biologically similar to protein/peptide hormones. These hormones are soluble in the blood and are transported in an unbound form. Therefore, the catecholamines have a relatively short half-life. Because these hormones do not cross cell membranes, they bind to receptors on the membrane surface. Finally, the catecholamines are stored intracellularly in secretory granules for future use.

10.3 Transport of hormones

As discussed in the previous section, steroid and thyroid hormones are transported in the blood bound to plasma proteins. The serum concentrations of free hormone (*H*), plasma protein (*P*), and bound hormone (*HP*) are in equilibrium:

$$[H] \times [P] = [HP]$$

When the concentration of the free form of a hormone decreases, then more of this hormone will be released from the binding proteins. The free hormone is the biologically active form. It binds to the target tissue to cause its actions and is involved with the negative feedback control of its secretion. The binding of hormones to plasma proteins has several beneficial effects, including:

- Facilitation of transport
- Prolonged half-life
- Hormone reservoir

Steroid and thyroid hormones are minimally soluble in the blood. Binding to plasma proteins renders them water soluble and facilitates their transport. Protein binding also prolongs the circulating half-life of these hormones. Because they are lipid soluble, they cross cell membranes easily. As the blood flows through the kidney, these hormones would enter cells or be filtered and lost to the urine if they were not held in the blood by the impermeable plasma proteins. Finally, the protein-bound form of the hormone serves as a "reservoir" of hormone that minimizes the changes in free hormone concentration when hormone secretion from its endocrine gland changes abruptly.

10.4 Functional classification of hormones

Hormones are classified into two functional categories:

- Trophic hormones
- Nontrophic hormones

A *trophic hormone* acts on another endocrine gland to stimulate secretion of its hormone. For example, thyrotropin, or thyroid-stimulating hormone (TSH), stimulates the secretion of thyroid hormones. Adrenocorticotropin, or adrenocorticotropic hormone (ACTH), stimulates the adrenal cortex to secrete the hormone cortisol. Both trophic hormones are produced by the pituitary gland; in fact, many trophic hormones are secreted by the pituitary. The pituitary gland is sometimes referred to as the "master gland" because its hormones regulate the activity of other endocrine glands.

A *nontrophic hormone* acts on nonendocrine target tissues. For example, parathormone released from the parathyroid glands acts on bone tissue to stimulate the release of calcium into the blood. Aldosterone released from the cortical region of the adrenal glands acts on the kidney to stimulate the reabsorption of sodium into the blood.

10.5 Hormone interactions

Multiple hormones may affect a single target tissue simultaneously. Therefore, the response of the target tissue depends not only on the effects of each hormone individually, but also on the nature of the interaction of the hormones at the tissue. The three types of hormone interactions include:

- Synergism
- Permissiveness
- Antagonism

When two hormones interact at the target tissue such that the combination of their effects is more than additive, *synergism* occurs. In other words, their combined effect is greater than the sum of their separate effects. For example, epinephrine, cortisol, and glucagon are three hormones that each increase the level of blood glucose. The magnitude of their individual effects on glucose levels tends to be low to moderate. However, the simultaneous activity of all three hormones results in an increase in blood glucose that is several times greater than the sum of their individual effects.

In *permissiveness*, one hormone enhances the responsiveness of the target tissue to a second hormone; in other words, the first hormone increases the activity of the second. For example, the normal maturation of the reproductive system requires reproductive hormones from the hypothalamus, pituitary, and gonads as well as the presence of thyroid hormone. Although thyroid hormone by itself has no effect on the reproductive system, if it is absent the development of this system is delayed. Therefore, thyroid hormone is considered to have a permissive effect on the reproductive hormones, facilitating their actions causing sexual maturation.

When the actions of one hormone oppose the effects of another, the result is *antagonism*. For example, insulin decreases blood glucose and promotes the formation of fat. Glucagon, on the other hand, increases blood glucose and promotes the degradation of fat. Therefore, the effects of insulin and glucagon are antagonistic.

10.6 Mechanisms of hormone action

The binding of a hormone to its receptor initiates intracellular events that direct the hormone's action. Ultimately, all hormones produce their effects by altering intracellular protein activity. However, the mechanism by which this occurs depends on the location of the hormone receptor. Receptors are typically located on the cell surface or in the cell nucleus. As a result, most hormones carry out their effects by means of two general mechanisms:

- Signal transduction and second messenger systems
- Gene activation

Protein/peptide hormones and the catecholamines are water-soluble substances and, accordingly, are unable to cross the plasma membrane to enter the cell. Therefore, these hormones must bind to their specific receptors on the cell surface. This receptor binding causes a response within the cell by way of *signal transduction* or by the production of intracellular *second messenger molecules*. The original, extracellular hormone is considered the first messenger because it carried the signal to the target tissue.

The most common second messenger activated by protein/peptide hormones and catecholamines is *cyclic adenosine monophosphate (cAMP)*. The pathway by which cAMP is formed and alters cellular function is illustrated in Figure 10.1. The process begins when the hormone binds to its receptor. These receptors are quite large and span the plasma membrane. On the cytoplasmic surface of the membrane, the receptor is associated with a *G protein* that serves as the transducer molecule. In other words, the G protein acts as an intermediary between the receptor and the second messengers that will alter cellular activity. These proteins are referred to as G proteins because they bind with guanosine nucleotides. In an unstimulated cell, the inactive G protein binds guanosine diphosphate (GDP). When the hormone

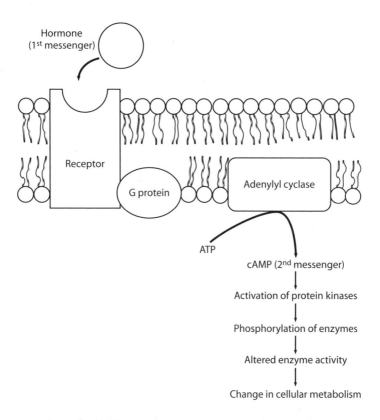

Figure 10.1 The cyclic AMP second messenger system. The most common second messenger system activated by the protein/peptide hormones and the catecholamines involves the formation of cAMP. This multistep process is initiated by binding of the hormone (the first messenger) to its receptor on the cell surface. The subsequent increase in the formation of cAMP (the second messenger) leads to the alteration of enzyme activity within the cell. A change in the activity of these enzymes alters cellular metabolism.

binds to its G protein-associated receptor, the G protein releases GDP and binds with *guanosine triphosphate (GTP)* taken up from the cytoplasm. Upon binding with the GTP, the now activated G protein loses its affinity for the receptor and increases its affinity for the plasma membrane-embedded enzyme, *adenylyl cyclase*. In turn, the adenylyl cyclase becomes activated and splits adenosine triphosphate (ATP) to form cAMP.

The cAMP molecule serves as the second messenger, which carries out the effects of the hormone inside the cell. The primary function of cAMP is to activate *protein kinase A*. This kinase then attaches phosphate groups to specific enzymatic proteins in the cytoplasm. The phosphorylation of these enzymes enhances or inhibits their activity, resulting in the enhancement or inhibition of specific cellular reactions and processes. Either way, cellular metabolism has been altered. Several noteworthy aspects of this mechanism of hormonal action include:

- Onset of hormonal effects
- Multiple systems
- Cellular specificity
- Amplification of effect
- Prolonged action of hormones

The *onset of the response* of cells to the activation of second messenger systems is comparatively rapid (within minutes). This mechanism involves changing the activity of *existing* enzymes rather than production of *new* enzymes, which is a more lengthy process. There are *many signal transduction* and *second messenger pathways*. For example, another signal transduction system involves the opening and closing of ion channels. Furthermore, some tissues use calcium as a second messenger and others use cyclic guanosine monophosphate (cGMP) or inositol triphosphate (IP_3). The *cellular specificity* of a hormone's effect depends on the different kinds of enzyme activity that are ultimately modified in different target tissues. For example, antidiuretic hormone causes reabsorption of water from the kidneys and constriction of smooth muscle in blood vessels: two very different effects in two very different tissues caused by one hormone. Effects elicited by second messenger systems involve a multistep process. This is advantageous because at many of these steps a multiplying or cascading effect takes place that causes *amplification* of the initial signal. For example, one molecule of the hormone epinephrine binding to its receptor on a hepatocyte may result in the production of 10 million molecules of glucose. *Hormone action is prolonged*; once an enzyme is activated, the effects are as long lasting as the enzyme and no longer depend upon the presence of the initiating hormone.

Steroid hormones and thyroid hormone carry out their effects by way of *gene activation*. In contrast to the protein/peptide hormones, which alter existing enzyme activity, these hormones induce the synthesis of new enzymes that then influence cellular metabolism.

Hormones in this category are lipophilic and easily enter the cells of the target tissue by diffusing through the plasma membrane. The hormone continues into the cell nucleus where it binds to its receptor forming a *hormone–receptor complex*. Hormone receptors are also capable of binding to DNA at specific attachment sites referred to as *hormone response elements* (*HRE*). Each of the steroid hormones binds with its receptor and attaches to a different HRE. Binding of the hormone–receptor complex to the DNA activates specific genes within the target cell, resulting in the formation of *mRNA molecules*. The mRNA then diffuses into the cytoplasm and binds to a ribosome where protein synthesis takes place. These new proteins serve as enzymes that regulate cellular reactions and processes.

As with signal transduction and second messenger systems, the mechanism of gene activation allows for amplification of the hormone's effect.

For example, a single hormone-activated gene induces the formation of many mRNA molecules and each mRNA molecule may be used to synthesize many enzyme molecules. Furthermore, the effects of hormones using this mechanism are prolonged. As long as the newly synthesized enzyme is active, the effect of the initiating hormone persists.

10.7 Pituitary gland

The *pituitary gland*, or *hypophysis*, is located at the base of the brain just below the hypothalamus. It is composed of two functionally and anatomically distinct lobes (see Figure 10.2):

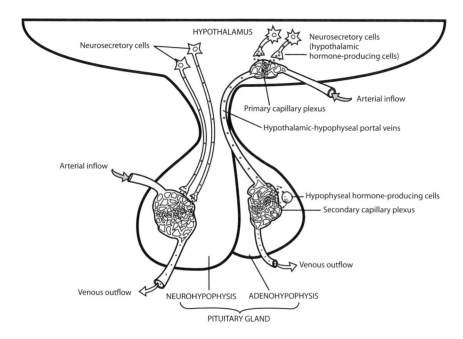

Figure 10.2 Anatomical and functional relationship between the hypothalamus and pituitary gland. The neurohypophysis is derived from the hypothalamus, an anatomical connection that allows the hypothalamus to influence the function of the neurohypophysis directly. Action potentials conducted by neurosecretory cells originating in the hypothalamus cause the release of hormones stored in the neurohypophysis. The adenohypophysis is derived from glandular tissue and therefore has no anatomical connection to the hypothalamus. The release of hormones from the adenohypophysis is regulated by hypothalamic hormones carried to the adenohypophysis through the hypothalamic–hypophyseal portal veins. Hypothalamic hormones enter the tissue of the adenohypophysis and influence production of adenohypophyseal hormones. Hormones released from both regions of the pituitary gland (the neurohypophysis and adenohypophysis) are removed from the pituitary gland by the venous outflow blood and transported to target tissues throughout the body.

- Neurohypophysis (posterior pituitary)
- Adenohypophysis (anterior pituitary)

As its name implies, the *neurohypophysis* is derived embryonically from nervous tissue. It is essentially an outgrowth of the hypothalamus and is composed of bundles of axons, or neural tracts, of neurosecretory cells originating in two hypothalamic nuclei. These neurons are referred to as *neurosecretory cells* because they generate action potentials as well as synthesize hormones. The cell bodies of the neurosecretory cells in the supraoptic nuclei produce primarily antidiuretic hormone (ADH) and the cell bodies of the paraventricular nuclei produce primarily oxytocin. These hormones are then transported down the axons to the neurohypophysis and stored in membrane-bound vesicles in the neuron terminals. Much like neurotransmitters, the hormones are released in response to the arrival of action potentials at the neuron terminal.

The *adenohypophysis* is derived embryonically from glandular tissue, specifically, *Rathke's pouch*. This tissue originates from the oropharynx, or the roof of the mouth. It then migrates toward the embryonic nervous tissue destined to form the neurohypophysis. When these two tissues come into contact, Rathke's pouch loses its connection with the roof of the mouth and the pituitary gland is formed. Unlike the neurohypophysis, which releases hormones originally synthesized in the hypothalamus, the adenohypophysis synthesizes its own hormones in specialized groups of cells. Similar to the neurohypophysis, however, the release of these hormones into the blood is regulated by the hypothalamus.

10.8 Relationship between hypothalamus and pituitary gland

The hypothalamus plays a very important role in the maintenance of homeostasis. It carries out this function, in large part, by regulating the activities of the neurohypophysis and the adenohypophysis. For example, the hypothalamus processes signals from other regions of the nervous system including information regarding pain and emotional states such as depression, anger, and excitement. In addition, because it is not protected by the blood–brain barrier, it monitors the composition of the blood and helps to regulate the concentration of nutrients, electrolytes, water, and hormones. In other words, it is an important processing center for information concerning the internal environment. This information is then used to control the release of hormones from the pituitary. Due to their embryonic origins, the neurohypophysis and the adenohypophysis are regulated by the hypothalamus, using two very different mechanisms:

- Neuronal signals
- Hormonal signals

As discussed previously, the neurohypophysis has a direct anatomical connection to the hypothalamus. Therefore, the hypothalamus regulates the release of hormones from the neurohypophysis by way of *neuronal signals*. Action potentials generated by the neurosecretory cells originating in the hypothalamus are transmitted down the neuronal axons to the nerve terminals in the neurohypophysis and stimulate the release of the hormones into the blood. The tracts formed by these axons are referred to as *hypothalamic-hypophyseal tracts* (see Figure 10.2). The action potentials are initiated by various forms of sensory input to the hypothalamus. Specific forms of sensory input that regulate the release of ADH and oxytocin are described in subsequent sections in this chapter.

The adenohypophysis does not have a direct anatomical connection with the hypothalamus; therefore, regulation of hormone secretion by way of neuronal signals is not possible. Instead, these two structures are associated by a specialized circulatory system and the secretion of hormones from the adenohypophysis is regulated by *hormonal signals* from the hypothalamus (see Figure 10.2). Systemic arterial blood is directed first to the hypothalamus. The exchange of materials between the blood and the interstitial fluid of the hypothalamus takes place at the *primary capillary plexus*. The blood then flows to the adenohypophysis through the *hypothalamic–hypophyseal portal veins*. Portal veins are blood vessels that connect two capillary beds. The second capillary bed in this system is the *secondary capillary plexus* located in the adenohypophysis.

Located in close proximity to the primary capillary plexus in the hypothalamus are specialized neurosecretory cells. In fact, the axons of these cells terminate on the capillaries. The neurosecretory cells synthesize two types of hormones: *releasing hormones* and *inhibiting hormones* (see Table 10.2). Each of these hormones helps to regulate the release of a particular hormone from the adenohypophysis. For example, thyrotropin-releasing hormone produced by the neurosecretory cells of the hypothalamus stimulates secretion of thyrotropin from the thyrotrope cells of the adenohypophysis. The hypothalamic-releasing hormone is picked up by the primary capillary plexus; travels through the hypothalamic–hypophyseal portal veins to the anterior pituitary; leaves the blood by way of the secondary capillary plexus; and exerts its effect on the appropriate cells of the adenohypophysis. The hypophyseal hormone, in this case, thyrotropin, is then picked up by the secondary capillary plexus, removed from the pituitary by the venous blood, and delivered to its target tissue.

A noteworthy feature of this specialized circulation is that the regulatory hypothalamic hormones are delivered directly to the adenohypophysis by the portal system. Therefore, the concentration of these hormones remains very high because they are not diluted in the blood of the entire systemic circulation.

Table 10.2 Summary of Major Hormones

Location	Hormone	Target tissues	Major functions of hormone
Hypothalamus	Releasing and inhibiting hormones (GnRH, TRH, CRH, PRF, PIH, GHRH, GHIH)	Adenohypophysis	Control of release of hormones from the adenohypophysis
	Antidiuretic hormone (ADH)	Kidney	Promotes reabsorption of water
		Arterioles	Vasoconstriction
	Oxytocin	Uterus	Contraction of smooth muscle
		Mammary glands	Ejection of milk
Adenohypophysis	Follicle-stimulating hormone (FSH)	Females: ovaries	Development of follicles; secretion of estrogen
		Males: testes	Spermatogenesis
	Luteinizing hormone (LH)	Females: ovaries	Rupture of follicle and ovulation; secretion of estrogen and progesterone from corpus luteum
		Males: testes	Secretion of testosterone
	Thyroid-stimulating hormone (TSH)	Thyroid gland	Secretion of thyroid hormones (T_3, T_4)
	Adrenocorticotropic hormone (ACTH)	Adrenal cortex	Secretion of cortisol
	Prolactin (PRL)	Mammary glands	Breast development; lactation
	Growth hormone (GH)	Bone, visceral tissues	Growth of skeleton and visceral tissues; increase blood glucose; protein synthesis; increase blood fatty acids
Thyroid gland	Triiodothyronine (T_3) Tetraiodothyronine (T_4)	Most tissues	Growth and maturation, normal neurological development and function; increase in metabolic rate

Gland	Hormone	Target	Effect
Parathyroid glands	Calcitonin	Bone	Decrease blood calcium
	Parathyroid hormone (PTH)	Bone, kidneys, intestine	Increase blood calcium; decrease blood phosphate; activation of vitamin D $_3$
Adrenal medulla	Epinephrine and norepinephrine	Adrenergic receptors throughout the body	"Fight-or-flight" response; reinforces effects of the sympathetic nervous system
Adrenal cortex	Mineralocorticoids (aldosterone)	Kidney	Reabsorption of sodium; excretion of potassium
	Glucocorticoids (cortisol)	Most tissues	Increase blood glucose and fatty acids; adaptation to stress
	Androgens	Various tissues	Secondary sex characteristics in females
Pancreas	Insulin	Most tissues	Cellular uptake, utilization and storage of glucose, fatty acids and amino acids
	Glucagons	Most tissues	Increase blood glucose and fatty acids

10.9 Negative feedback control of hormone release

In many cases, hormones released from the adenohypophysis are part of a three-hormone axis that includes the:

- Hypothalamic hormone
- Adenohypophyseal hormone
- Endocrine gland hormone

The hypothalamic hormone stimulates or inhibits the secretion of the adenohypophyseal hormone. The trophic hormone from the adenohypophysis then stimulates the release of a hormone from another endocrine gland. This final endocrine gland hormone not only carries out its effects on its target tissues, it may also exert a *negative feedback* effect on the release of the hypothalamic and/or adenohypophyseal hormones. In this way, this final hormone regulates its own release (see Figure 10.3). This process is referred to as *long-loop negative feedback*. The adenohypophyseal hormone may also exert a negative feedback effect on the hypothalamic hormone and limit its own release. This process is referred to as *short-loop negative feedback*.

10.10 Hormones of the neurohypophysis

Antidiuretic hormone (ADH), also referred to as *vasopressin*, has two major effects, both of which are reflected by its names: (1) antidiuresis (decrease in urine formation by the kidney); and (2) vasoconstriction of arterioles.

Antidiuretic hormone promotes the reabsorption of water from the tubules of the kidney, or *antidiuresis*. Specifically, it acts on the collecting ducts and increases the number of water channels, which increases the diffusion coefficient for water. This results in the body's conservation of water and the production of a low volume of concentrated urine. The reabsorbed water affects plasma osmolarity and blood volume. This effect of ADH on the kidney occurs at relatively low concentrations. At higher concentrations, ADH causes *constriction of arterioles*, which serves to increase blood pressure. Antidiuretic hormone secretion is regulated by several factors:

- Plasma osmolarity
- Blood volume
- Blood pressure
- Alcohol

The primary factor that influences ADH secretion is a change in *plasma osmolarity. Osmoreceptors* in the hypothalamus are located in close proximity to the ADH-producing neurosecretory cells. Stimulation of these osmoreceptors by an increase in plasma osmolarity results in stimulation of the neurosecretory cells; an increase in the frequency of action potentials in these cells; and the release of ADH from their axon terminals in the neurohypo-

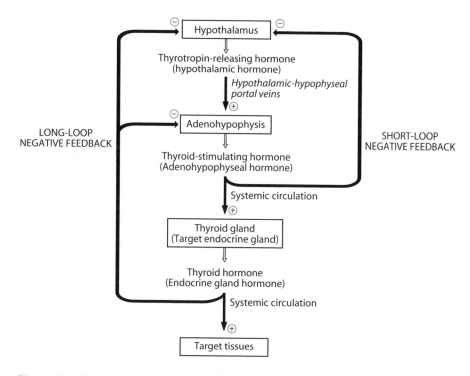

Figure 10.3 Negative-feedback regulation of hormone release. Hormones released from the adenohypophysis are often part of a three-hormone axis that includes the hypothalamic hormone, the adenohypophyseal hormone, and the target endocrine gland hormone. Long-loop negative feedback occurs when the final hormone in the axis inhibits release of hypothalamic and/or adenohypophyseal hormones. Short-loop negative feedback occurs when the adenohypophyseal hormone inhibits release of the hypothalamic hormone. This figure illustrates the thyrotropin-releasing hormone–thyroid-stimulating hormone–thyroid hormone axis.

physis. The water conserved due to the effect of ADH on the kidney helps to reduce plasma osmolarity or dilute the plasma back to normal.

Hypothalamic osmoreceptors have a threshold of 280 mOsM. Below this value, they are not stimulated and little or no ADH is secreted. Maximal ADH levels occur when plasma osmolarity is about 295 mOsM. Within this range, the regulatory system is very sensitive, with measurable increases in ADH secretion occurring in response to a 1% change in plasma osmolarity. Regulation of ADH secretion is an important mechanism by which a normal plasma osmolarity of 290 mOsM is maintained.

Other factors regulating ADH secretion include blood volume and blood pressure. A decrease in *blood volume* of 10% or more causes an increase in ADH secretion sufficient to cause vasoconstriction as well as antidiuresis. A decrease in *mean arterial blood pressure* of 5% or more also causes an increase in ADH secretion. The resulting water conservation and vasoconstriction help increase blood volume and blood pressure back to normal. Furthermore, the effect of blood pressure on ADH secretion may be correlated to the increase in secretion that occurs during sleep, when blood pressure decreases. The result is the production of a low volume of highly concentrated urine that is less likely to elicit the micturition (urination) reflex and interrupt sleep. In contrast, *alcohol* inhibits the secretion of ADH, thus allowing for loss of water from the kidney. Therefore, the consumption of alcoholic beverages may actually lead to excessive water loss and dehydration instead of volume expansion.

Oxytocin also exerts its major effects on two different target tissues. This hormone stimulates:

- Contraction of uterine smooth muscle
- Contraction of myoepithelial cells

Oxytocin stimulates *contraction of the smooth muscle in the wall of the uterus.* During labor, this facilitates the delivery of the fetus and, during intercourse, may facilitate the transport of the sperm through the female reproductive tract. Oxytocin also causes *contraction of the myoepithelial cells* surrounding the alveoli of the mammary glands. This results in *"milk letdown"* or the expulsion of milk from deep within the gland into the larger ducts from which the milk can be obtained more readily by the suckling infant.

The secretion of oxytocin is regulated by *reflexes elicited by cervical stretch and by suckling.* Normally, as labor begins, the fetus is positioned head down. This orientation exerts pressure on the cervix and causes it to stretch. Sensory neurons in the cervix are thus activated to transmit signals to the hypothalamus, which will stimulate the release of oxytocin from the neurohypophysis. This hormone then enhances uterine contraction which causes further pressure and stretch of the cervix, additional oxytocin release, and so on, until pressure has built up adequately so that delivery can take place. In the lactating breast, suckling activates sensory neurons in the nipple to transmit signals to the hypothalamus to stimulate oxytocin release from the neurohypophysis and therefore milk letdown. Interestingly, this reflex may also be triggered through a conditioned response in which the sight or sound of the hungry infant is sufficient to enhance oxytocin secretion. In contrast, the release of oxytocin from the neurohypophysis may be inhibited by pain, fear, or stress.

The function of oxytocin in males is not clearly understood.

10.11 Hormones of the adenohypophysis

The *gonadotropins*, follicle-stimulating hormone and luteinizing hormone, exert their effects on the gonads (ovaries in the female and testes in the male). Taken together, the gonadotropins stimulate the gonads to:

- Produce gametes (ova and sperm)
- Secrete sex hormones (estrogen, progesterone, and testosterone)

Follicle-stimulating hormone (FSH), as its name indicates, stimulates the development of the ovarian follicles in females. It is within the follicles that the ova, or eggs, develop. This hormone also induces the secretion of estrogen from the follicle. In males, FSH acts on the Sertoli cells of the testes, which are involved with production of sperm. *Luteinizing hormone (LH)* is also named for its effects in the female, which are to cause the rupture of the follicle and the release of the ovum and to cause conversion of the ovarian follicle into a *corpus luteum* (Latin, yellow body). This hormone also induces secretion of estrogen and progesterone from the corpus luteum. In males, LH acts on the Leydig cells of the testes to stimulate secretion of testosterone. FSH and LH are produced by the same cell type in the adenohypophysis: the gonadotrope. The release of FSH and LH is regulated by the hypothalamic releasing hormone, *gonadotropin-releasing hormone (GnRH)*.

Thyroid-stimulating hormone (TSH, thyrotropin) regulates the growth and metabolism of the thyroid gland. Furthermore, it stimulates synthesis and release of the thyroid hormones, T_3 and T_4. The release of TSH from the thyrotrope cells of the adenohypophysis is induced by *thyrotropin-releasing hormone (TRH)*. *Adrenocorticotropic hormone (ACTH, adrenocorticotropin)* stimulates growth and steroid production in the adrenal cortex. Specifically, it stimulates secretion of cortisol and other glucocorticoids involved with carbohydrate metabolism. The release of ACTH from the adenohypophysis is influenced by more than one factor. *Corticotropin-releasing hormone (CRH)* from the hypothalamus stimulates the secretion of ACTH. In addition, ACTH secretion follows a *diurnal pattern*, with a peak in the early morning and a valley in the late afternoon.

Prolactin (PRL), produced by the lactotrope cells of the adenohypophysis, is involved with the initiation and maintenance of lactation in females. Its function in males is uncertain. Lactation involves three processes:

- Mammogenesis
- Lactogenesis
- Galactopoeisis

Mammogenesis is the growth and development of the mammary glands that produce the milk. This process requires the actions of many hormones, including estrogens and progestins, in addition to PRL. *Lactogenesis* is the initiation of lactation. During pregnancy, lactation is inhibited by high levels of estrogens and progestins. At delivery, the levels of these two hormones fall, allowing PRL to initiate lactation. *Galactopoeisis* is the maintenance of milk production. This process requires PRL and oxytocin.

The release of prolactin from the adenohypophysis is normally inhibited by *prolactin-inhibiting hormone (PIH, dopamine)* from the hypothalamus. Prolactin secretion is also controlled by *prolactin-releasing factor (PRF)*. The release of PRF from the hypothalamus is mediated by reflexes elicited by suckling and breast stimulation.

Growth hormone (GH, somatotropin) is one of the few hormones that exerts its effects on organs and tissues throughout the body. This hormone is essential for normal growth and development of the skeleton as well as visceral, or soft, tissues from birth until young adulthood. Growth of the skeleton involves an increase in bone thickness and an increase in bone length. The mechanism of this growth involves stimulation of osteoblast (bone-forming cell) activity and proliferation of the epiphyseal cartilage in the ends of the long bones. The growth of visceral tissues occurs by *hyperplasia* (increasing the number of cells) and *hypertrophy* (increasing the size of cells). Growth hormone causes hyperplasia by stimulating cell division and by inhibiting apoptosis (programmed cell death) and cellular hypertrophy by promoting protein synthesis and inhibiting protein degradation.

The growth-promoting effects of GH are carried out by *somatomedins*, which are peptides found in the blood. Two somatomedins have been identified and described. Structurally and functionally similar to insulin, these peptides are referred to as *insulin-like growth factors I and II (IGF-I and IGF-II)*. Growth hormone stimulates the production of IGF-I in the liver, which is the predominant source of that found in the circulation. Local production of IGF-I also occurs in many target tissues. IGF-I is thought to mediate the growth-promoting effects of GH throughout life. Levels of GH and IGF-I increase in parallel during puberty and other periods of growth in children. In contrast, IGF-II production does not depend on GH. Instead, IGF-II is thought to be important during fetal growth and development and is secreted in response to prolactin. The role of IGF-II in the adult is unclear.

Growth hormone also has many metabolic actions in the body:

- Protein metabolism
  - Increase in tissue amino acid uptake
  - Stimulation of protein synthesis
- Lipid metabolism
  - Increase in blood fatty acids
  - Stimulation of lipolysis
  - Inhibition of lipogenesis
- Carbohydrate metabolism
  - Increase in blood glucose
  - Decrease in glucose uptake by muscle
  - Increase in the hepatic output of glucose (glycogenolysis)

The net effects of these actions include enhanced growth due to protein synthesis; enhanced availability of fatty acids for use by skeletal muscle as an energy source; and glucose sparing for the brain, which can use only this nutrient molecule as a source of energy.

The release of GH from the adenohypophysis is regulated by two hypothalamic hormones: *growth hormone-releasing hormone (GHRH)* and *growth hormone-inhibiting hormone (GHIH, somatostatin)*. Any factor or condition that enhances the secretion of GH could do so by stimulating or inhibiting GHRH release or by inhibiting GHIH release. The secretion of GH follows a diurnal rhythm with GH levels low and constant throughout the day and with a marked burst of GH secretion approximately one hour following the onset of sleep (deep or stage III and IV sleep). Other factors that stimulate GH secretion include exercise, stress, hypoglycemia, and increased serum amino acids, particularly arginine and leucine. Factors that inhibit GH secretion include hyperglycemia and aging. In most individuals, production of GH decreases after 30 years of age. This decrease in GH production is likely a critical factor in the loss of lean muscle mass at a rate of 5% per decade and gain of body fat at the same rate after 40 years of age.

10.12 Thyroid gland

The thyroid gland is a butterfly-shaped structure lying over the ventral surface of the trachea just below the larynx. This gland produces two classes of hormones synthesized by two distinct cell types:

- Thyroid hormones (T_3 and T_4) synthesized by follicular cells
- Calcitonin synthesized by parafollicular cells

Thyroid hormones. Internally, the thyroid consists of *follicles*, which are spherical structures with walls formed by a single layer of epithelial cells called *follicular cells*. The center of each follicle contains a homogenous gel referred to as *colloid*. Thyroid hormones are stored here as a component of the larger molecule, *thyroglobulin*. The amount of thyroid hormones stored within the colloid is enough to supply the body for 2 to 3 months.

Derived from the amino acid tyrosine, thyroid hormones are unique because they contain *iodine*. At this time, its incorporation into thyroid hormones is the only known use for iodine in the body. There are two thyroid hormones, named for the number of iodides added to the tyrosine residues of the thyroglobulin: *triiodothyronine* (T_3) and *tetraiodothyronine* (T_4, *thyroxine*). Although significantly more T_4 is synthesized by the thyroid gland, T_3 is the active hormone. At the target tissue, T_4 is deiodoninated to form the more potent T_3.

The thyroid hormones are lipophilic and relatively insoluble in the plasma. Therefore, they are transported throughout the circulation bound to plasma proteins such as *thyroxine-binding globulin* (75%) and albumins (25%). Approximately 99.96% of circulating thyroxine is protein bound. Bound hormone is not available to cause any physiological effects; however, it is in equilibrium with the remaining 0.04% that is unbound. This free form of the hormone is able to bind to receptors on target tissues and cause its effects. Thyroid hormone has many metabolic effects in the body:

- Growth and maturation
  - Perinatal lung maturation
  - Normal skeletal growth

- Neurological
  - Normal fetal and neonatal brain development
  - Regulation of neuronal proliferation and differentiation, myelino-genesis, neuronal outgrowth, and synapse formation
  - Normal CNS function in adults
- Sympathetic nervous system function
  - Increase in the number of β-adrenergic receptors
  - Increase in heart rate
  - Tremor
  - Sweating
- Cardiovascular system
  - Increase in heart rate
  - Increase in myocardial contractility
  - Increase in cardiac output
- Metabolism
  - Increase in basal metabolic rate
  - Stimulation of all metabolic pathways, both anabolic and catabolic
  - Increase in carbohydrate utilization
  - Increase in oxygen consumption
  - Increase in heat production

As mentioned previously, thyroid hormones are secreted at a relatively steady rate. The secretion of hormones from the thyroid gland is regulated by negative feedback in the hypothalamic–pituitary–thyroid axis. The hypothalamus secretes TRH, which stimulates the release of TSH from the adenohypophysis of the pituitary. Thyroid-stimulating hormone then stimulates the release of T_3 and T_4 from the thyroid. In this hormone axis, negative-feedback inhibition is exerted primarily at the level of the pituitary. As the intracellular concentration of T_3 in the thyrotrope cells of the pituitary increases, then the responsiveness of these TSH-producing cells to TRH decreases. The mechanism of this decreased responsiveness involves down-regulation, or decrease in the number, of TRH receptors. This results in a decrease in the secretion of TSH and, consequently, a decrease in the secretion of T_3 and T_4. The excess of intracellular T_3 that elicits the negative feedback control of secretion comes from two sources: 80% from the deiododination of serum T_4 within the thyrotrope cells and 20% from serum T_3.

Calcitonin. This hormone, which is also secreted from the thyroid gland, is synthesized by the *parafollicular cells* (C cells) located between the follicles. The primary effect of *calcitonin* is to decrease the blood levels of calcium and phosphate. The mechanism of action involves the direct inhibition of osteoclast activity, which decreases bone resorption. This results in less demineralization of the bone and therefore a decrease in the release of calcium and phosphate from the bone into the blood. Calcitonin has no direct effect on bone formation by osteoblasts.

The release of calcitonin from the thyroid is regulated by plasma calcium levels through negative feedback. An increase in the level of calcium in the blood stimulates the secretion of calcitonin and a decrease in the level of calcium in the blood inhibits secretion.

Pharmacy application: therapeutic effects of calcitonin

The normal physiological effects of calcitonin are relatively weak; however, when the hormone is used pharmacologically, its effects are very important. Paget's disease is characterized by a significant increase in osteoclast activity and, thus, a high rate of bone turnover and hypercalcemia. Because of minimal species variation, human calcitonin or calcitonin from other species may be used to treat this disorder. Therefore, pharmacological intervention includes administration of synthetic human calcitonin (Cibacalcin®) or salmon calcitonin (Miacalcin), which will depress the bone resorption and ease the symptoms of Paget's. Salmon calcitonin, which is 20 times more potent than human calcitonin, has also been approved for therapeutic use in patients with postmenopausal osteoporosis.

10.13 Parathyroid glands

Four small parathyroid glands are embedded on the posterior surface of the thyroid gland as it wraps around the trachea. *Parathyroid hormone (PTH, parathormone)* is the principal regulator of calcium metabolism. Its overall effects include:

- Increase in blood levels of calcium
- Decrease in blood levels of phosphate

Parathyroid hormone carries out these effects through multiple mechanisms of action:

- Decrease in calcium excretion in the urine
- Increase in phosphate excretion in the urine
- Increase in bone resorption
- Activation of vitamin D_3

Calcium is freely filtered along with other components of the plasma through the nephrons of the kidney. Most of this calcium is reabsorbed into the blood from the proximal tubule of the nephron. However, because the kidneys produce about 180 l of filtrate per day, the amount of calcium filtered is substantial. Therefore, the physiological regulation of even a small percentage of calcium reabsorption may have a significant effect on the amount of calcium in the blood. Parathyroid hormone acts on the Loop of Henle to increase the reabsorption of calcium from this segment of the tubule and decrease the amount excreted in the urine. This activity conserves calcium and increases its concentration in the blood.

Phosphate, which is also freely filtered with plasma through the nephrons of the kidney, is reabsorbed into the blood from the proximal tubule. Parathyroid hormone acts on this segment to decrease phosphate reabsorption and increase the amount excreted in the urine.

Parathyroid hormone stimulates bone resorption by increasing the number and activity of osteoclasts. This demineralization process in the bone releases calcium and phosphate into the blood. Although the action of PTH on the bone appears to increase blood phosphate, its action on the kidney, which increases phosphate excretion in the urine, more than compensates for this increase and the net effect is a decrease in serum phosphate.

The final mechanism of action of PTH involves the activation of vitamin D_3 through the stimulation of 1α-hydroxylase in the kidney. In the gastrointestinal tract, vitamin D_3 is essential for the absorption of calcium. Enhanced absorption of calcium from dietary sources serves to further increase the concentration of calcium in the blood. Many foods, in particular, dairy products, which are rich in calcium, are fortified with vitamin D. The release of PTH from the parathyroid glands is regulated by plasma calcium levels through negative feedback. A decrease in the level of calcium in the blood stimulates the secretion of PTH and an increase in the calcium level in the blood inhibits it.

10.14 Adrenal glands

There are two adrenal glands, one located on top of each kidney. These glands are composed of two distinct functional regions:

- Adrenal medulla
- Adrenal cortex

Adrenal medulla. Derived from neural crest tissue, the adrenal medulla forms the inner portion of the adrenal gland. It is the site of production of the *catecholamines*, epinephrine and norepinephrine, which serve as a circulating counterpart to the sympathetic neurotransmitter, norepinephrine, released directly from sympathetic neurons to the tissues. As such, the adrenal medulla and its hormonal products play an important role in the activity of the sympathetic nervous system. This is fully discussed in Chapter 9, which deals with the autonomic nervous system.

Adrenal cortex. The adrenal cortex forms the outer portion of the adrenal gland and accounts for 80 to 90% of the weight of the gland. It is the site of synthesis of many types of steroid hormones such as:

- Mineralocorticoids
- Glucocorticoids
- Adrenal androgens

Mineralocorticoids. The primary mineralocorticoid is *aldosterone*. The actions of this hormone include:

- Stimulation of renal retention of sodium
- Promotion of renal excretion of potassium

Aldosterone acts on the distal tubule of the nephron to increase sodium reabsorption. The mechanism of action involves an increase in the number of sodium-permeable channels on the luminal surface of the distal tubule and an increase in the activity of the Na^+–K^+ ATPase pump on the basilar surface of the tubule. Sodium diffuses down its concentration gradient out of the lumen and into the tubular cells. The pump then actively removes the sodium from cells of the distal tubule and into the extracellular fluid so that it may diffuse into the surrounding capillaries and return to the circulation. Due to its osmotic effects, the retention of sodium is accompanied by the retention of water. In other words, wherever sodium goes, water follows. As a result, aldosterone is very important in regulation of blood volume and blood pressure. The retention of sodium and water expands the blood volume and, consequently, increases mean arterial pressure.

The retention of sodium is coupled to the excretion of potassium. For every three Na^+ ions reabsorbed, two K^+ ions and one H^+ ion are excreted.

The release of aldosterone from the adrenal cortex is regulated by two important factors:

- Serum potassium levels
- The renin–angiotensin system

The mechanism by which potassium regulates aldosterone secretion is unclear; however, this ion appears to have a direct effect on the adrenal cortex. An increase in the level of potassium in the blood stimulates the release of aldosterone. The effect of aldosterone on the kidney then decreases the level of potassium back to normal.

Angiotensin II (Ag II) is a potent stimulus for the secretion of aldosterone. The formation of Ag II occurs by the following process:

Angiotensinogen

↓ renin

Angiotensin I

↓ ACE

Angiotensin II

This multistep process is initiated by the enzyme renin. Angiotensinogen is a precursor peptide molecule released into the circulation from the liver.

In the presence of renin, an enzyme produced by specialized cells in the kidney, angiotensinogen is split to form angiotensin I. This prohormone is then acted upon by angiotensin-converting enzyme (ACE) as the blood passes through the lungs to form Ag II. Angiotensin II acts directly on the adrenal cortex to promote aldosterone secretion.

Because this process requires renin in order to occur, it is important to understand the factors involved in its release from the kidney. These factors include:

- Decrease in blood volume
- Decrease in blood pressure
- Sympathetic stimulation

A decrease in blood volume or blood pressure may result in a decrease in the blood flow to the kidney. The kidney monitors renal blood flow by way of stretch receptors in the vessel walls. A decrease in renal blood flow stimulates the release of renin. The subsequent secretion of aldosterone causes retention of sodium and water and, therefore, an increase in blood volume and blood pressure back to normal. An increase in renal blood flow tends to cause the opposite effect.

Sympathetic nerve activity causes an increase in blood pressure through many mechanisms, including an increase in cardiac activity and vasoconstriction. Activation of the sympathetic system also causes the stimulation of β_1-adrenergic receptors on the renin-producing cells, which promotes renin release.

Glucocorticoids. The primary glucocorticoid is *cortisol*. Receptors for the glucocorticoids are found in all tissues. The overall effects of these hormones include:

- Increase in blood glucose
- Increase in blood free fatty acids

Cortisol increases blood glucose by several mechanisms of action including:

- Decrease in glucose utilization by many peripheral tissues (especially muscle and adipose tissue)
- Increase in availability of gluconeogenic substrates
  - Increase in protein catabolism (especially muscle)
  - Increase in lipolysis
- Increase in hepatic gluconeogenesis

Cortisol-induced lipolysis not only provides substrates for gluconeogenesis (formation of glucose from noncarbohydrate sources) but it also increases the amount of free fatty acids in the blood. As a result, the fatty acids are used by muscle as a source of energy and glucose is spared for the brain to use to form energy.

The release of cortisol from the adrenal cortex is regulated by several factors including:

- Circadian rhythm
- Stress
- Negative-feedback inhibition by cortisol

Corticotropin-releasing hormone (CRH) secreted from the hypothalamus stimulates the release of ACTH from the adenohypophysis. This pituitary hormone then stimulates the release of cortisol from the adrenal cortex. The hormones of this hypothalamic–pituitary–adrenocortical axis exhibit marked diurnal variation. This variation is due to the diurnal secretion of CRH. The resulting secretion of ACTH increases at night and peaks in the early morning just before rising (4 A.M. to 8 A.M.). The levels of ACTH then gradually fall during the day to a low point late in the evening, between 12 P.M. and 4 P.M. This rhythm is influenced by many factors, including light–dark patterns, sleep–wake patterns, and eating. After an individual changes time zones, it takes about 2 weeks for this rhythm to adjust to the new time schedule; this may account for some aspects of jet lag.

Cortisol is an important component of the body's response to physical and psychological stress. Nervous signals regarding stress are transmitted to the hypothalamus and the release of CRH is stimulated. The resulting increase in cortisol increases levels of glucose, free fatty acids, and amino acids in the blood, providing the metabolic fuels that enable the individual to cope with the stress. A potent inhibitor of this system is cortisol itself. This hormone exerts a negative-feedback effect on the hypothalamus and the adenohypophysis and inhibits the secretion of CRH and ACTH, respectively.

Pharmacy application: therapeutic effects of corticosteroids

When administered in pharmacological concentrations (greater than physiological), cortisol and its synthetic analogs (hydrocortisone, prednisone) have potent anti-inflammatory and immunosuppressive effects. In fact, these steroids inhibit almost every step of the inflammatory response resulting in the decreased release of vasoactive and chemoattractive factors, decreased secretion of lipolytic and proteolytic enzymes, decreased extravasation of leukocytes to areas of injury, and, ultimately, decreased fibrosis. Typically, the inflammatory response is quite beneficial in that it limits the spread of infection. However, in many clinical conditions, such as rheumatoid arthritis and asthma, the response becomes a destructive process. Therefore, although glucocorticoids have no effect on the underlying cause of disease, the suppression of inflammation by these agents is very important clinically.

Corticosteroids also exert inhibitory effects on the overall immune process. These drugs impair the function of the leukocytes responsible for antibody production and destruction of foreign cells. As a result, corticosteroids are also used therapeutically in the prevention of organ transplant rejection.

Adrenal androgens. The predominant androgens produced by the adrenal cortex are *dehydroepiandrosterone* (*DHEA*) and *androstenedione*. These steroid hormones are weak androgens; however, in peripheral tissues they can be converted to more powerful androgens, such as testosterone, or even to estrogens. The quantities of these hormones released from the adrenal cortex are very small. Therefore, the contribution of this source of these hormones to androgenic effects in the male is negligible compared to that of the testicular androgens. However, the adrenal gland is the major source of androgens in females. These hormones stimulate pubic and axillary (underarm) hair development in pubertal females. In pathological conditions in which adrenal androgens are overproduced, masculinization of females may occur.

10.15 Pancreas

The pancreas is an exocrine gland and an endocrine gland. The exocrine tissue produces a bicarbonate solution and digestive enzymes. These substances are transported to the small intestine where they play a role in the chemical digestion of food. These functions are fully discussed in Chapter 18 on the digestive system.

Scattered throughout the pancreas and surrounded by exocrine cells are small clusters of endocrine cells referred to as the *islets of Langerhans*. These islets make up only 2 to 3% of the mass of the pancreas; however, their blood supply has been modified so that they receive 5 to 10 times more blood than the exocrine pancreas. Furthermore, this blood carrying the pancreatic hormones is then transported through the hepatic portal vein and delivered directly to the liver where the hormones, in a relatively high concentration, carry out many of their metabolic effects. The most important hormones produced by the pancreas that regulate glucose metabolism are insulin and glucagon.

Insulin. *Insulin* is a peptide hormone produced by β-cells of the islets of Langerhans. It is an important anabolic hormone secreted at times when the concentration of nutrient molecules in the blood is high, such as periods following a meal. Its overall effects include allowing the body to use carbohydrates as an energy source and to store nutrient molecules. Specifically, insulin exerts its important actions on the following tissues:

- Liver
  - Increase in glucose uptake

- Increase in glycogenesis (formation of glycogen, the storage form of glucose)
- Increase in lipogenesis (formation of triglycerides, the storage form of lipids)
- Adipose tissue
  - Increase in glucose uptake
  - Increase in free fatty acid uptake
  - Increase in lipogenesis
- Muscle
  - Increase in glucose uptake
  - Increase in glycogenesis
  - Increase in amino acid uptake
  - Increase in protein synthesis

Insulin is the only hormone that lowers blood glucose (epinephrine, growth hormone, cortisol, and glucagon increase blood glucose). It does so by stimulating the uptake of glucose from the blood into the liver, adipose tissue, and muscle. This glucose is first used as an energy source and then stored in the form of glycogen in the liver and in muscle. Excess glucose is stored as fat in adipose tissue.

Insulin also plays a role in fat metabolism. In humans, most fatty acid synthesis takes place in the liver. The mechanism of action of insulin involves directing excess nutrient molecules toward metabolic pathways leading to fat synthesis. These fatty acids are then transported to storage sites, predominantly adipose tissue. Finally, insulin stimulates the uptake of amino acids into cells where they are incorporated into proteins.

The secretion of insulin from the pancreas is regulated primarily by the circulating concentration of glucose. When serum glucose increases, secretion of insulin is stimulated; when it decreases, insulin secretion is inhibited. Secretion typically begins to increase within 10 minutes following the ingestion of food and reaches a peak in 30 to 45 minutes. This increased insulin stimulates the uptake of glucose into the body's cells and lowers serum glucose levels back to normal. Other factors affecting insulin secretion include: circulating amino acids and free fatty acids; several gastrointestinal hormones, including gastrin, secretin, and cholecystokinin; and the parasympathetic nervous system. Each of these factors stimulates the secretion of insulin. Sympathetic nervous stimulation inhibits insulin secretion.

Glucagon. Also a peptide hormone, *glucagon* is produced by α-cells of the islets of Langerhans. The overall effects of glucagon include:

- Increase in hepatic glucose production
  - Glycogenolysis
  - Gluconeogenesis
- Stimulation of lipolysis in the liver and in adipose tissue

The effects of glucagon on glucose metabolism are generally opposite to those of insulin. Acting primarily on the liver, glucagon stimulates glycogenolysis (breakdown of glycogen, the storage form of glucose) and gluconeogenesis, which increase blood glucose levels. This hormone also stimulates lipolysis, which increases the circulating concentration of free fatty acids. These molecules may then be used as an alternative energy source by muscle or serve as gluconeogenic substrates in the liver. Finally, glucagon stimulates the hepatic uptake of amino acids, which also serve as substrates for gluconeogenesis.

Factors that stimulate glucagon secretion include: a decrease in blood glucose; an increase in blood amino acids; sympathetic nervous stimulation; stress; and exercise. Factors that inhibit glucagon secretion include insulin and an increase in blood glucose. Table 10.2 summarizes the major functions of the hormones discussed in this chapter.

Bibliography

1. Iversen, S., Iversen, L., and Saper, C.B., The autonomic nervous system and the hypothalamus, in *Principles of Neural Science*, 4th ed., Kandel, E.R., Schwartz, J.H., and Jessell, T.M., Eds., McGraw–Hill, New York, 2000, chap. 49.
2. Kettyle, W.M. and Arky, R.A., *Endocrine Pathophysiology*, Lippincott-Raven Publishers, Philadelphia, 1998.
3. Marcus, R., Agents affecting calcification and bone turnover: calcium, phosphate, parathyroid hormone, vitamin D, calcitonin, and other compounds, in *Goodman and Gilman's: The Pharmacological Basis of Therapeutics*, 9th ed., Hardman, J.G. and Limbird, L.E., Eds., McGraw–Hill, New York, 1996, chap. 61.
4. Porterfield, S.P., *Endocrine Physiology*, 2nd ed., C.V. Mosby, St. Louis, 2001.
5. Schimmer, B.P. and Parker, K.L., Adrenocorticotropic hormone; adrenocortical steroids and their synthetic analogs; inhibitors of the synthesis and actions of adrenocortical hormones, in *Goodman and Gilman's: The Pharmacological Basis of Therapeutics*, 9th ed., Hardman, J.G. and Limbird, L.E., Eds., McGraw–Hill, New York, 1996, chap. 59.
6. Sherwood, L., *Human Physiology from Cells to Systems*, 4th ed., Brooks/Cole, Pacific Grove, CA, 2001.
7. Silverthorn, D.U., *Human Physiology: An Integrated Approach*, 2nd ed., Prentice- Hall, Upper Saddle River, NJ, 2001.

chapter eleven

Skeletal muscle

Study objectives

- Discuss the functions of skeletal muscle
- Distinguish between isometric and isotonic contractions
- Describe the components of the thick filaments and thin filaments
- Explain the functions of the following: myosin crossbridges, troponin, tropomyosin, sarcomeres, Z lines, neuromuscular junction, transverse tubules, and sarcoplasmic reticulum
- Describe the sliding filament theory of skeletal muscle contraction
- Explain how creatine phosphate, oxidative phosphorylation, and glycolysis provide energy for skeletal muscle contraction
- List the factors that influence the onset of muscle fatigue
- Describe the factors that lead to development of muscle fatigue
- Describe the metabolic processes that lead to oxygen debt
- Distinguish among the three types of muscle fibers: slow-twitch oxidative, fast-twitch oxidative, and fast-twitch glycolytic
- Describe the factors that influence the strength of skeletal muscle contraction including: multiple motor unit summation, asynchronous motor unit summation, frequency of nerve stimulation, length–tension relationship, and diameter of the muscle fiber

11.1 Introduction

Skeletal muscle comprises the largest group of tissues in the human body and accounts for up to 40% of total body weight. This type of muscle, which is innervated by the somatic nervous system, is under voluntary control. Skeletal muscle performs many important functions in the body, including:

- Movement of body parts
- Heat production
- Breathing
- Speaking

Most skeletal muscles are attached to bones, which enables them to *control body movements*, such as walking. These muscles are also responsible for the manipulation of objects, such as writing with a pencil or eating with a fork. Furthermore, eye movement is carried out by several pairs of skeletal muscles. Finally, the contractions of certain groups of muscles referred to as "antigravity" muscles are needed to maintain posture and provide body support. Only about 20 to 30% of the nutrient energy consumed during skeletal muscle activity is actually converted into purposeful work. The remaining 70 to 80% is given off as *heat*. Therefore, because of its large mass, skeletal muscle is the tissue most responsible for maintaining and increasing body temperature. Although it typically occurs subconsciously, *breathing* is a voluntary activity. The diaphragm and other muscles of inspiration and expiration are skeletal muscles. As such, breathing can be voluntarily controlled to some extent (see Chapter 17). *Speaking*, and other forms of vocalization, depend upon the coordinated contraction of skeletal muscles.

11.2 Isometric vs. isotonic contraction

The two primary types of muscle contraction are:

- Isometric
- Isotonic

Isometric contraction occurs when the muscle develops tension and exerts force on an object, but does not shorten. In other words, it refers to muscle contraction during which the length of the muscle remains constant. For example, supporting an object in a fixed position, such as carrying a book or a backpack, requires isometric contraction. This type of contraction also occurs when attempting to move an object that is too heavy to shift or reposition. In this case, the muscle may exert maximal force against the object; however, because the object does not move, the length of the contracting muscle does not change. Finally, the antigravity muscles of the back and legs perform submaximal isometric contractions while maintaining posture and for body support.

Isotonic contraction occurs when the muscle shortens under a constant load. For example, when an object is lifted, the muscle contracts and becomes shorter although the weight of the object remains constant. In addition to moving external objects, isotonic contractions are performed for movements of the body, such as moving the legs when walking.

Many activities require both types of muscle contraction. An example is running: when one of the legs hits the ground, isometric contraction of the muscles within this limb keep it stiff and help to maintain body support. At the same time, isotonic contractions in the opposite leg move it forward to take the next stride.

11.3 Structure of skeletal muscle

A whole muscle is composed of muscle cells, or *muscle fibers*. Muscle fibers are elongated, cylindrical cells. Due to fusion of many smaller fibers during embryonic development, muscle fibers are the largest cells in the body, with several nuclei near their surface. Muscle fibers lie parallel to each other and extend along the entire length of the muscle. These fibers may be a few millimeters in length (muscles of the eyes) or up to 2 or more feet in length (muscles of the legs).

Muscle fibers are incapable of mitosis. In fact, the number of muscle fibers per muscle is likely determined by the second trimester of fetal development. Therefore, enlargement of a whole muscle is not due to an increase in the number of fibers in the muscle, but rather to the hypertrophy of existing fibers. Because muscle fibers have no gap junctions between them, electrical activity cannot spread from one cell to the next. Therefore, each muscle fiber is innervated by a branch of an alpha motor neuron. A *motor unit* is defined as an alpha motor neuron and all of the muscle fibers that it innervates.

Internally, muscle fibers are highly organized. Each fiber contains numerous *myofibrils* — cylindrical structures that also lie parallel to the long axis of the muscle. The myofibrils are composed of *thick filaments* and *thin filaments*. It is the arrangement of these filaments that creates alternating light and dark bands observed microscopically along the muscle fiber. Thus, skeletal muscle is also referred to as *striated muscle*.

Sarcomeres. The thick and thin filaments are organized into repeating segments referred to as *sarcomeres*, which are the functional units of skeletal muscle. (In other words, the sarcomere is the smallest contractile unit within skeletal muscle.) A myofibril is composed of hundreds or thousands of sarcomeres in series along its length. When a muscle is stimulated, each of these sarcomeres contracts and becomes shorter. As a result, the entire muscle contracts and becomes shorter. Therefore, the function of the sarcomere determines whole muscle function. A sarcomere is the area between two *Z lines* (see Figure 11.1, panel c). The function of the Z line is to anchor the thin filaments in place at either end of the sarcomere. The thick filaments are found in the central region of the sarcomere. Ultimately, interaction between the thick and thin filaments causes shortening of the sarcomere.

Thick filaments. Each thick filament contains 200 to 300 *myosin* molecules. Each myosin molecule is made up of two identical subunits shaped like golf clubs: two long shafts wound together with a *myosin head*, or *crossbridge*, on the end of each. These molecules are arranged so that the shafts are bundled together and oriented toward the center of the thick filament. The myosin heads project outward from either end of the thick filament (see Figure 11.1, panel a).

Thin filaments. The thin filaments are composed of three proteins:

- Actin
- Tropomyosin
- Troponin

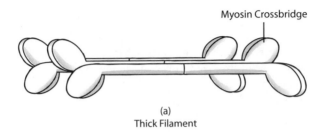

(a)
Thick Filament

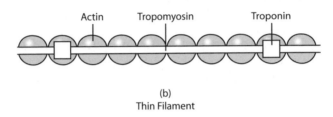

(b)
Thin Filament

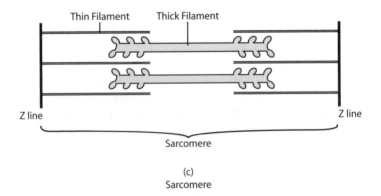

(c)
Sarcomere

Figure 11.1 Components of the sarcomere. (a) The thick filament is composed of myosin molecules shaped like golf clubs and consisting of a long shaft with a globular portion at one end. The myosin is arranged so that the shafts are in the center of the thick filament and the globular portions, or myosin crossbridges, protrude from each end of the thick filament. The myosin crossbridges bind to the actin of the thin filament. (b) The thin filament consists of three proteins. Globular actin molecules join together to form two strands of fibrous actin that twist around each other. Tropomyosin is a filamentous protein found on the surface of the actin, physically covering the binding sites for the myosin cross-bridges. Troponin molecules stabilize the tropomyosin filaments in position on the actin. (c) Sarcomere — the thick and thin filaments are highly organized. They are arranged to form the sarcomere that is the functional unit of skeletal muscle. The sarcomere is the region between two Z lines.

The predominant protein, *actin*, consists of spherical subunits (globular actin) arranged into two chains twisted around each other (fibrous actin). *Tropomyosin* is a long, thread-like protein found on the outer surface of the actin chain. Each tropomyosin molecule is associated with six to seven actin subunits. The function of tropomyosin is to cover binding sites for myosin on the actin subunits when the muscle is in the resting state. This prevents the interaction between actin and myosin that causes muscle contraction. *Troponin* is a smaller protein consisting of three subunits. One subunit binds to actin, another binds to tropomyosin, and the third binds with calcium. When the muscle is relaxed, troponin holds the tropomyosin in its blocking position on the surface of the actin (see Figure 11.1, panel b).

11.4 Neuromuscular junction

Each muscle fiber is innervated by a branch of an alpha motor neuron. The synapse between the somatic motor neuron and the muscle fiber is referred to as the *neuromuscular junction*. Action potentials in the motor neuron cause release of the neurotransmitter *acetylcholine*. Binding of acetylcholine to its receptors on the muscle fiber causes an increase in the permeability to Na$^+$ and K$^+$ ions. The ensuing depolarization generates an action potential that travels along the surface of the muscle fiber in either direction that is referred to as a *propagated action potential*. This action potential elicits the intracellular events that lead to muscle contraction.

11.5 Mechanism of contraction

As mentioned previously, skeletal muscle fibers are very large cells with a wide diameter; the action potential is readily propagated, or transmitted, along the surface of the muscle fiber. However, a mechanism is needed to transmit the electrical impulse into the central region of the muscle fiber as well. The *transverse tubules* (*T tubules*) are invaginations of the cell membrane penetrating deep into the muscle fiber and surrounding each myofibril. (Imagine poking fingers into an inflated balloon.) As the action potential travels along the surface of the fiber, it is also transmitted into the T tubules. As a result, all regions of the muscle fiber are stimulated by the action potential.

All types of muscle require *calcium* for contraction. In skeletal muscle, Ca^{++} ions are stored within an extensive membranous network referred to as the *sarcoplasmic reticulum*. This network is found throughout the muscle fiber and surrounds each myofibril. Furthermore, segments of the sarcoplasmic reticulum lie adjacent to each T tubule that, with a segment of sarcoplasmic reticulum on either side of it, is referred to as a *triad*. As the action potential is transmitted along the T tubule, it stimulates the release of Ca^{++} ions from the sarcoplasmic reticulum. The only source of calcium for skeletal muscle contraction is the sarcoplasmic reticulum.

The mechanism of skeletal muscle contraction is described by the *Sliding Filament Theory* (see Figure 11.2). This mechanism begins with the *"priming"*

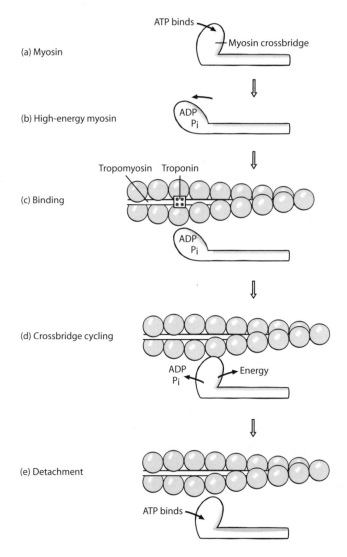

Figure 11.2 Mechanism of skeletal muscle contraction. (a) Myosin — the myosin crossbridge has a binding site for ATP. (b) High-energy myosin — within the crossbridge, myosin ATPase splits ATP into ADP and inorganic phosphate (P_i). As a result, the crossbridge swivels outward and energy is stored. (c) Binding — in the presence of calcium, which binds to troponin, tropomyosin is repositioned into the groove between the two strands of actin. As a result, binding sites for myosin on the actin are uncovered and the crossbridges attach to actin. (d) Crossbridge cycling — energy stored within the myosin crossbridge is released and the crossbridge swivels inward, pulling the actin inward. The ADP and P_i are released. (e) Detachment — binding of a new molecule of ATP to the myosin crossbridge allows myosin to detach from actin and the process begins again.

of the myosin crossbridge, a process that requires energy, which is supplied by adenosine triphosphate (ATP). Each myosin crossbridge contains *myosin ATPase*. When ATP attaches to its binding site on the myosin crossbridge, it is split by the myosin ATPase to yield adenosine diphosphate (ADP) and inorganic phosphate (P_i). The ADP and P_i remain tightly bound to the myosin crossbridge. Energy released by this process causes the myosin crossbridge to swivel outward toward the end of the thick filament. When the crossbridge is in this conformation, it is "primed" and referred to as the *high-energy form of myosin*; this form of myosin is capable of binding to actin. However, this interaction is prevented by tropomyosin, which physically covers the binding sites for myosin on the actin subunits. In order to uncover these binding sites, calcium is needed.

In a stimulated muscle fiber, Ca^{++} ions are released from the sarcoplasmic reticulum and bind to troponin. As a result, the troponin–actin linkage is weakened, allowing the tropomyosin to be repositioned such that the myosin-binding sites are uncovered. The myosin crossbridge now binds to the actin, causing the energy previously stored within the myosin to be discharged and the crossbridge to swivel inward toward the center of the thick filament. This process is referred to as *crossbridge cycling*. As the myosin crossbridge swivels inward, it pulls the actin inward as well. It is important to note that the interaction between actin and myosin causes the thin filaments to slide inward over the thick filaments toward the center of the sarcomere. Consequently, the sarcomeres shorten and the whole muscle shortens or contracts. It is for this reason that this process is referred to as the Sliding Filament Theory of muscle contraction.

When the myosin crossbridge binds with the actin, ADP and P_i are released from the myosin. This opens the binding site to another molecule of ATP. In fact, the myosin remains attached to the actin until another ATP molecule binds to the myosin. Binding of a new ATP causes the myosin to release the actin. This ATP is split by the ATPase and the myosin crossbridge swivels outward once again, returning the myosin to its high-energy state. As long as Ca^{++} ions are present and the binding sites on the actin are uncovered, crossbridge cycling continues. The crossbridges of the thick filament pull the thin filaments inward incrementally so that the sarcomeres become even shorter and the muscle contracts further.

Interestingly, the myosin crossbridges do not all cycle at the same time. At any given moment, some crossbridges remain attached to the actin and others are in the process of releasing the actin in order to cycle once again. In other words, myosin crossbridge cycling is staggered. This process maintains the shortening of the sarcomere and prevents thin filaments from slipping back to their original positions in between cycles.

In the absence of ATP, myosin crossbridges are unable to release the actin. As a result, the sarcomeres, and therefore the muscle, remain contracted. This phenomenon is referred to as *rigor mortis*. Following death, the concentration of intracellular calcium increases. This calcium allows the contractile process between the previously formed high-energy myosin and the actin to take place. However, the muscle stores of ATP are rapidly depleted, the myosin remains attached to the actin, and stiffness ensues.

When the action potentials in the alpha motor neuron cease, stimulation of muscle fiber is ended. Ca^{++} ions are pumped back into the sarcoplasmic reticulum and troponin and tropomyosin return to their original positions. As a result, the myosin-binding sites on the actin are covered once again. The thin filaments return passively to their original positions, resulting in muscle relaxation.

11.6 Sources of ATP for muscle contraction

Skeletal muscle uses only ATP as a source of energy for contraction. However, intracellular stores of ATP are quite limited. In fact, the amount of ATP normally found in skeletal muscle is enough to sustain only a few seconds of contraction. Therefore, metabolic pathways to form additional ATP are needed. These pathways include:

- Creatine phosphate
- Oxidative phosphorylation
- Glycolysis

Energy may be transferred from *creatine phosphate* to ADP by way of the following reaction:

$$\text{Creatine phosphate} + \text{ADP} \xleftarrow{\text{CK}} \text{Creatine} + \text{ATP}$$

The enzyme creatine kinase (CK) facilitates the transfer of phosphate and energy to a molecule of ADP to form ATP. Stores of creatine phosphate are sufficient to sustain approximately 15 more seconds of muscle contraction. Because this is a single-step process, it provides ATP very rapidly and is the first pathway for formation of ATP to be accessed.

The second pathway to be utilized in the formation of ATP is *oxidative phosphorylation*. This process involves the metabolic breakdown of glucose and fatty acids. Because it requires oxygen, oxidative phosphorylation provides energy at rest and under conditions of mild (walking) to moderate (jogging) exercise. This pathway is advantageous because it produces a large amount of energy (36 molecules of ATP) from each molecule of glucose; however, oxidative phosphorylation is comparatively slow due to the number of steps involved. Furthermore, this process requires enhanced blood flow to the active muscles for continuous delivery of oxygen as well as nutrient molecules. Although glucose may be obtained by way of glycogenolysis within the skeletal muscle fibers, these glycogen stores are limited. Glycogenolysis in the liver and lipolysis in the adipose tissues yield additional molecules of glucose and fatty acids for energy formation. As exercise is sustained, skeletal muscle relies more upon fatty acids as a source of fuel for the oxidative phosphorylation pathway. In this way, glucose is spared for the brain.

During intense exercise, when the oxygen supply cannot keep pace with the oxygen demand, skeletal muscle produces ATP anaerobically by way of *glycolysis*. Although this pathway provides ATP more rapidly, it produces much less energy (2 molecules of ATP) from each molecule of glucose. Furthermore, glycolysis results in production of lactic acid in the muscle tissue. The accumulation of lactic acid may lead to pain as well as to muscle fatigue.

11.7 Muscle fatigue

Muscle fatigue is defined as the inability of a muscle to maintain a particular degree of contraction over time. The onset of fatigue is quite variable and influenced by several factors, including:

- Intensity and duration of contractile activity
- Utilization of aerobic vs. anaerobic metabolism for energy
- Composition of the muscle
- Fitness level of the individual

Although the exact mechanisms leading to muscle fatigue remain somewhat unclear, several factors have been implicated:

- Depletion of energy reserves
- Accumulation of lactic acid
- Increase in inorganic phosphate

Depletion of glycogen stores within contracting skeletal muscles fibers is associated with the onset of fatigue. Interestingly, this occurs even though the muscle may be utilizing fatty acids as its primary energy source. The *accumulation of lactic acid* lowers the pH within the muscle and the change in pH may ultimately alter the activity of enzymes involved with energy production as well as crossbridge cycling. The breakdown of creatine phosphate causes an *increase in concentration of inorganic phosphate*. Fatigue associated with elevated inorganic phosphate may be due to slowed release of P_i from myosin and therefore a decreased rate of crossbridge cycling. It may also involve decreased sensitivity of the contractile proteins to calcium, which would also impair crossbridge cycling.

11.8 Oxygen debt

Hyperventilation persists for a period of time following cessation of exercise and is due to the *oxygen debt* incurred during exercise. Specifically, oxygen is needed for the following metabolic processes:

- Restoration of creatine phosphate reserves
- Metabolism of lactic acid
- Replacement of glycogen stores

During the recovery period from exercise, ATP (newly produced by way of oxidative phosphorylation) is needed to replace the *creatine phosphate reserves* — a process that may be completed within a few minutes. Next, the *lactic acid* produced during glycolysis must be metabolized. In the muscle, lactic acid is converted into pyruvic acid, some of which is then used as a substrate in the oxidative phosphorylation pathway to produce ATP. The remainder of the pyruvic acid is converted into glucose in the liver that is then stored in the form of *glycogen* in the liver and skeletal muscles. These later metabolic processes require several hours for completion.

11.9 Types of muscle fibers

Two major differences between the types of muscle fibers are:

- Speed of contraction
- Metabolic pathway used to form ATP

As such, three types of muscle fibers (see Table 11.1) exist:

- Slow-twitch oxidative
- Fast-twitch oxidative
- Fast-twitch glycolytic

Table 11.1 Features of Skeletal Muscle Fiber Types

Feature	Slow-twitch oxidative	Fast-twitch oxidative	Fast-twitch glycolytic
Myosin ATPase activity	Slow	Fast	Fast
Speed of contraction	Slow	Fast	Fast
Removal of calcium	Slow	Fast	Fast
Duration of contraction	Long	Short	Short
Mitochondria	Many	Many	Few
Capillaries	Many	Many	Few
Myoglobin content	High	High	Low
Color of fiber	Dark red	Red	Pale
Diameter of fiber	Small	Intermediate	Large
Source of ATP	Oxidative phosphorylation	Oxidative phosphorylation; glycolysis	Glycolysis
Glycogen content	Low	Intermediate	High
Onset of fatigue	Delayed	Intermediate	Rapid

Fast-twitch muscle fibers develop tension two to three times faster than slow-twitch muscle fibers because of more rapid splitting of ATP by *myosin ATPase*. This enables the myosin crossbridges to cycle more rapidly. Another factor influencing the speed of contraction involves the rate of *removal of calcium* from the cytoplasm. Muscle fibers remove Ca^{++} ions by pumping them back into the sarcoplasmic reticulum. Fast-twitch muscle fibers remove Ca^{++} ions more rapidly than slow-twitch muscle fibers, resulting in quicker twitches that are useful in fast precise movements. The contractions generated in slow-twitch muscle fibers may last up to 10 times longer than those of fast-twitch muscle fibers; therefore, these twitches are useful in sustained, more powerful movements.

Muscle fibers also differ in their ability to resist fatigue. Slow-twitch muscle fibers rely primarily on oxidative phosphorylation for the production of ATP. Accordingly, these muscle fibers have a greater number of *mitochondria*, the organelles in which these metabolic processes are carried out. These fibers also have an *extensive capillary network* for delivery of oxygen. Furthermore, the *high myoglobin content* within slow-twitch muscle fibers facilitates diffusion of oxygen into the cells from the extracellular fluid. Myoglobin imparts the characteristic red color to these muscle fibers; thus, they are referred to as *"red muscle."*

Finally, slow-twitch muscle fibers have a *small diameter*. This facilitates the diffusion of oxygen through the fiber to the mitochondria where it is utilized. Taken together, each of these characteristics enhances the ability of these fibers to utilize oxygen. Therefore, in slow-twitch oxidative muscle fibers *oxidative phosphorylation predominates* and *fatigue is delayed*.

Fast-twitch muscle fibers fall into two categories. Fast-twitch glycolytic muscle fibers have fewer mitochondria, fewer capillaries, less myoglobin, and large diameters. As a result, these fibers rely primarily on glycolysis for the production of ATP. The resulting accumulation of lactic acid and decrease in pH hastens the onset of fatigue. Because this type of muscle fiber has less myoglobin, it has a much paler appearance than the slow-twitch oxidative muscle fibers. Therefore, it is referred to as *"white muscle."* Fast-twitch oxidative muscle fibers have many mitochondria and capillaries, a significant amount of myoglobin, and intermediate-sized diameters. These muscle fibers utilize a combination of oxidative and glycolytic metabolism to produce ATP. As a result, fast-twitch oxidative muscle fibers are more resistant to fatigue than fast-twitch glycolytic muscle fibers.

11.10 Muscle mechanics

A *muscle twitch* is a brief, weak contraction produced in a muscle fiber in response to a single action potential. While the action potential lasts 1 to 2 msec, the resulting muscle twitch lasts approximately 100 msec. However, a muscle twitch in a single muscle fiber is too brief and too weak to be useful or to perform any meaningful work. In fact, hundreds or thousands of muscle fibers are organized into whole muscles. In this way, the fibers may work together to produce muscle contractions strong enough and of sufficient duration to be productive. Furthermore, muscles must be able to generate contractions of variable strengths. Different tasks require different degrees of contraction or tension development within the whole muscle. The *strength of skeletal muscle contraction* depends on two major factors:

- Number of muscle fibers contracting
- Amount of tension developed by each contracting muscle fiber

Number of muscle fibers contracting. As the *number of contracting muscle fibers* increases, the strength of skeletal muscle contraction increases. Two major factors determine the number of muscle fibers activated at any given moment:

- Multiple motor unit summation
- Asynchronous motor unit summation

A *motor unit* is defined as an alpha motor neuron and all of the skeletal muscle fibers it innervates. The number of muscle fibers innervated by an alpha motor neuron varies considerably, depending upon the function of the muscle. For example, the muscles of the eyes and hands have very small motor units. In other words, each alpha motor neuron associated with these muscles synapses with only a few muscle fibers. As a result, each of these muscles is innervated by a comparatively large number of alpha motor neurons. Densely innervated muscles are capable of carrying out more precise, complex motor activities. On the other hand, antigravity muscles have very large motor units. For example, the gastrocnemius muscle of the calf has about 2000 muscle fibers in each motor unit. Muscles with large motor units tend to be more powerful and more coarsely controlled.

Multiple motor unit summation involves recruitment of motor units. As the number of motor units stimulated at any given moment increases, the strength of contraction increases. *Asynchronous motor unit summation* refers to the condition in which motor unit activation within a muscle is alternated. In other words, at one moment, some of the motor units within the muscle are activated, while other motor units are relaxed. This is followed by the relaxation of previously activated motor units and activation of previously relaxed motor units. Consequently, only a fraction of the motor units within the muscle generate tension at any given moment. Therefore, this type of summation may generate submaximal contractions only.

An advantage of asynchronous motor unit summation is that the onset of muscle fatigue is significantly delayed because each motor unit has alternating periods of relaxation in which there is time for the restoration of energy supplies. The antigravity muscles of the back and legs employ asynchronous motor unit summation. These muscles are required to generate sustained submaximal contractions in order to maintain posture and body support over the course of the day.

Amount of tension developed by each contracting muscle fiber. As the amount of tension developed by each individual muscle fiber increases, the overall strength of skeletal muscle contraction increases. Three major factors determine the amount of tension developed by a contracting muscle fiber:

- Frequency of nerve stimulation
- Length of muscle fiber at the onset of contraction
- Diameter of muscle fiber

As mentioned previously, a single action potential lasting only 2 msec causes a muscle twitch that lasts approximately 100 msec. If the muscle fiber has adequate time to completely relax before it is stimulated by another action potential, the subsequent muscle twitch will be of the same magnitude as the first. However, if the muscle fiber is restimulated before it has completely relaxed, then the tension generated during the second muscle twitch is added to that of the first (see Figure 11.3). In fact, the *frequency of nerve impulses* to a muscle fiber may be so rapid that there is no time for relaxation in between stimuli. In this case, the muscle fiber attains a state of smooth, sustained maximal contraction referred to as *tetanus*.

The amount of tension developed by a muscle fiber during tetanic contraction can be as much as three to four times greater than that of a single muscle twitch. The mechanism involved with this increased strength of contraction involves the concentration of cytosolic calcium. Each time muscle fiber is stimulated by an action potential, Ca^{++} ions are released from the sarcoplasmic reticulum. However, as soon as the these ions are released, a

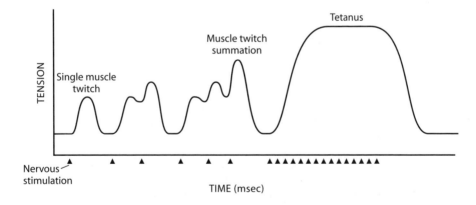

Figure 11.3 Muscle twitch summation and tetanus. A single action potential (represented by ▲) generates a muscle twitch. Because duration of the action potential is so short, subsequent action potentials may restimulate the muscle fiber before it has completely relaxed, leading to muscle twitch summation and greater tension development. When the frequency of stimulation becomes so rapid that no relaxation occurs between stimuli, tetanus occurs. Tetanus is a smooth, sustained, maximal contraction.

continuously active calcium pump begins returning Ca⁺⁺ ions to the sarcoplasmic reticulum. Consequently, fewer Ca⁺⁺ ions are available to bind with
troponin and only a portion of binding sites on the actin become available
to the myosin crossbridges. Each subsequent stimulation of muscle fiber
results in release of more Ca⁺⁺ ions from the sarcoplasmic reticulum. In other
words, as the frequency of nerve stimulation increases, the rate of Ca⁺⁺ ion
release exceeds the rate of Ca⁺⁺ ion removal. Therefore, the cytosolic concentration of calcium remains elevated. A greater number of Ca⁺⁺ ions bind with
troponin, resulting in a greater number of binding sites on the actin available
to myosin crossbridges. As the number of cycling crossbridges increases, the
amount of tension developed increases.

The amount of tension developed by a stimulated muscle fiber is highly
dependent upon *length of the muscle fiber at onset of contraction.* This association between the resting length of the muscle fiber and tension development
is referred to as the *length–tension relationship.* The sarcomere length at which
maximal tension can be developed is termed the *optimal length* (L_o). In skeletal
muscle, optimal length is between 2.0 and 2.2 µm. At this point, the actin
filaments have overlapped all of the myosin crossbridges on the thick filaments (see Figure 11.4, point a). In other words, the potential for crossbridge
cycling and tension development upon stimulation has been maximized.

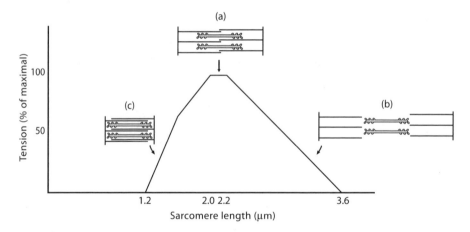

Figure 11.4 The length–tension relationship. The length of the sarcomere prior to
stimulation influences the amount of tension that may be developed in the muscle
fiber. (a) The optimal length of the sarcomere is between 2.0 and 2.2 µm. At this
length, actin overlaps all of the myosin crossbridges. The potential for crossbridge
cycling and the tension that may be developed upon stimulation of the muscle
fiber are maximized. (b) When the sarcomere is overstretched so that actin does
not overlap the myosin crossbridges, then crossbridge cycling cannot take place
and tension cannot be developed in the muscle fiber. (c) When the sarcomere is
shortened prior to stimulation, thin filaments overlap each other and thick filaments abut the Z lines. Further shortening and tension development upon stimulation are markedly impaired.

If the muscle fiber is stretched prior to stimulation such that the actin filaments have been pulled out to the end of the thick filaments, no overlap is present between actin and the myosin crossbridges (see Figure 11.4, point b). In this case, no crossbridge cycling occurs and tension development is zero. Tension development is also impaired when the muscle fiber is allowed to shorten prior to stimulation (see Figure 11.4, point c). If the actin filaments overlap each other, fewer binding sites are available for the myosin crossbridges. Also, if the thick filaments are forced up against the Z lines, further shortening cannot take place.

Interestingly, the range of resting sarcomere lengths is limited by the attachment of skeletal muscles to the bones. Because of this fixed orientation, skeletal muscles cannot overstretch or overshorten prior to stimulation. Typically, these muscles are within 70 to 130% of their optimal length. In other words, attachment to the bones ensures that the overlap of actin and myosin is such that crossbridge cycling approaches the maximum. As the number of cycling crossbridges increases, the strength of muscle contraction increases.

The *diameter of the muscle fiber* is influenced by two major factors:

- Resistance training
- Testosterone

Repeated bouts of anaerobic, high-intensity *resistance training* such as weight lifting cause muscle hypertrophy and increase the diameter of the muscle fiber. This form of training promotes synthesis of actin and myosin filaments and, as a result, the number of crossbridges available to cycle and develop tension is increased. Thus, larger muscles are capable of developing more powerful contractions.

Because muscle fibers in males are thicker than those found in females, these muscles are larger and stronger, even without the benefit of resistance training. This enlargement is due to effects of *testosterone*, a sex hormone found primarily in males. Testosterone promotes the synthesis of actin and myosin filaments in muscle fibers.

Bibliography

1. Guyton, A.C. and Hall, J.E., *Textbook of Medical Physiology*, 10th ed., W.B. Saunders, Philadelphia, 2000.
2. McArdle, W.D., Katch, F.I., and Katch, V.L., *Exercise Physiology, Energy, Nutrition and Human Performance*, 4th ed., Williams & Wilkins, Baltimore, 1996.
3. Robergs, R.A. and Roberts, S.O., *Exercise Physiology, Exercise, Performance, and Clinical Applications*, C.V. Mosby, St. Louis, 1997.
4. Sherwood, L., *Human Physiology from Cells to Systems*, 4th ed., Brooks/Cole, Pacific Grove, CA, 2001.
5. Silverthorn, D.U., *Human Physiology: An Integrated Approach*, 2nd ed., Prentice-Hall, Upper Saddle River, NJ, 2001.

chapter twelve

Smooth muscle

Study objectives

- Describe the morphological differences between skeletal muscle and smooth muscle
- Explain how contraction of smooth muscle occurs
- Explain how relaxation of smooth muscle occurs
- Explain why smooth muscle contraction is slow and prolonged
- Distinguish between multiunit smooth muscle and single-unit smooth muscle
- Compare and contrast pacemaker and slow-wave potentials
- List the factors that may alter smooth muscle contractile activity
- Explain how intracellular calcium concentration may be increased
- Describe the length–tension relationship in smooth muscle

12.1 Introduction

Although skeletal muscle comprises the bulk of muscle tissue in the body, *smooth muscle* is far more important in terms of homeostasis. Most smooth muscle is found in the walls of tubes and hollow organs. Contraction and relaxation of the smooth muscle in these tissues regulates the movement of substances within them. For example, contraction of the smooth muscle in the wall of a blood vessel narrows the diameter of the vessel and leads to a decrease in the flow of blood through it. Contraction of the smooth muscle in the wall of the stomach exerts pressure on its contents and pushes these substances forward into the small intestine. Smooth muscle functions at a subconscious level and is *involuntary*. It is innervated by the *autonomic nervous system*, which regulates its activity.

12.2 Structure of smooth muscle

Smooth muscle cells are small and spindle shaped (thin and elongated; see Table 12.1). Similar to skeletal muscle, the contractile apparatus in smooth

Table 12.1 Comparison of Skeletal and Smooth Muscle

Feature	Skeletal muscle	Multiunit smooth muscle	Single unit smooth muscle
Location	Attached to bones; openings of some hollow organs (sphincters)	Large blood vessels; eyes; hair follicles	Walls of hollow organs of digestive, reproductive, and urinary tracts; small blood vessels
Thick filaments	Myosin	Myosin	Myosin
Thin filaments	Actin, tropomyosin, troponin	Actin, tropomyosin	Actin, tropomyosin
Filament arrangement	Sarcomeres	Diamond-shaped lattice	Diamond-shaped lattice
Microscopic appearance	Striated	Smooth	Smooth
Control	Voluntary	Involuntary	Involuntary
Innervation	Somatic nervous system	Autonomic nervous system	Autonomic nervous system
Contraction	Neurogenic	Neurogenic	Myogenic
Role of nervous system	Initiate contraction	Initiate contraction	Modify contraction
Morphology	Large, cylindrical	Small, spindle-shaped	Small, spindle-shaped
Transverse tubules	Yes	No	No
Sarcoplasmic reticulum	Well developed	Very little	Very little
Source of calcium	Sarcoplasmic reticulum	Extracellular fluid (most); sarcoplasmic reticulum (some)	Extracellular fluid (most); sarcoplasmic reticulum (some)
Site of calcium binding	Troponin	Calmodulin	Calmodulin
Function of calcium	Reposition troponin/tropomyosin to uncover myosin binding sites on actin	Phosphorylate and activate myosin to bind with actin	Phosphorylate and activate myosin to bind with actin
Regulation of tension development	Alter number of contacting motor units; frequency of nerve stimulation	Alter number of contracting muscle cells; alter intracellular Ca^{++} concentration	Alter intracellular Ca^{++} concentration
Length-tension relationship	Narrow	Broad	Broad

muscle consists of thick filaments composed of *myosin* and thin filaments composed of *actin*. However, in contrast to skeletal muscle, these filaments are not organized into sarcomeres. As such, this muscle has no striations, resulting in a "smooth" appearance.

Because there are no sarcomeres in smooth muscle, there are no Z lines. Instead, the actin filaments are attached to *dense bodies*. These structures, which contain the same protein as Z lines, are positioned throughout the cytoplasm of the smooth muscle cell as well as attached to the internal surface of the plasma membrane. Myosin filaments are associated with the actin filaments, forming contractile bundles oriented in a diagonal manner. This arrangement forms a *diamond-shaped lattice* of contractile elements throughout the cytoplasm. Consequently, the interaction of actin and myosin during contraction causes the cell to become shorter and wider.

The action potential easily penetrates all regions of these small cells. Therefore, smooth muscle does not have *transverse tubules*. Furthermore, smooth muscle cells have very little *sarcoplasmic reticulum*, so intracellular storage of calcium is limited. Instead, the calcium needed for contraction is obtained primarily from the extracellular fluid. The influx of Ca^{++} ions through their channels in the cell membrane stimulates the release of a small amount of Ca^{++} ions from the sarcoplasmic reticulum.

12.3 Calcium and the mechanism of contraction

In skeletal muscle, calcium binds to troponin and causes the repositioning of tropomyosin. As a result, the myosin-binding sites on the actin become uncovered and crossbridge cycling takes place. Although an increase in cytosolic calcium is also needed in smooth muscle, its role in the mechanism of contraction is very different. Three major steps are involved in *smooth muscle contraction*:

- Calcium binding with calmodulin
- Activation of myosin kinase
- Phosphorylation of myosin

Upon entering the smooth muscle cell, Ca^{++} ions bind with *calmodulin*, an intracellular protein with a chemical structure similar to that of troponin. The resulting Ca^{++}–calmodulin complex binds to and activates *myosin kinase*. This activated enzyme then *phosphorylates myosin*. Crossbridge cycling in smooth muscle may take place only when myosin has been phosphorylated.

Relaxation of smooth muscle involves two steps:

- Removal of calcium ions
- Dephosphorylation of myosin

Calcium ions are actively pumped back into the extracellular fluid as well as the sarcoplasmic reticulum. When the concentration of calcium falls below a certain level, steps one and two of the contractile process reverse. Calcium no longer binds with calmodulin and myosin kinase is no longer activated.

The dephosphorylation of myosin requires the activity of *myosin phosphatase*. Located in cytoplasm of the smooth muscle cell, this enzyme splits the phosphate group from the myosin. Dephosphorylated myosin is inactive; crossbridge cycling no longer takes place and the muscle relaxes.

12.4 Smooth muscle contraction is slow and prolonged

Contraction of smooth muscle is significantly slower than that of skeletal muscle. Furthermore, smooth muscle contraction is quite prolonged (3000 msec) compared to that in skeletal muscle (100 msec). The slow onset of contraction as well as its sustained nature is due to the slowness of attachment and detachment of the myosin crossbridges with the actin. Two factors are involved:

- Myosin ATPase activity
- Rate of calcium removal

In smooth muscle, myosin crossbridges have less *myosin ATPase activity* than those of skeletal muscle. As a result, the splitting of ATP that provides energy to "prime" the crossbridges, preparing them to interact with actin, is markedly reduced. Consequently, the rates of crossbridge cycling and tension development are slower. Furthermore, a slower *rate of calcium removal* causes the muscle to relax more slowly.

Interestingly, the reduction in myosin ATPase activity causes smooth muscle to be more *economical*. In other words, it can maintain contraction with significantly less ATP consumption. This benefits tissues, such as the blood vessels, that maintain tonic contraction with little energy consumption and without developing fatigue. Furthermore, prolonged attachment of myosin crossbridges to the actin results in an equal, if not greater, *force of contraction*. Smooth muscle is capable of developing a force of 4 to 6 kg/cm^2 in cross-sectional area compared to 3 to 4 kg/cm^2 in skeletal muscle.

12.5 Types of smooth muscle

The two major types of smooth muscle (although many smooth muscles exhibit properties of each type) are:

- Multiunit smooth muscle
- Single-unit smooth muscle

Multiunit smooth muscle is located in the large blood vessels, eyes (iris and ciliary muscle of the lens), and piloerector muscles at the base of hair follicles. This type of muscle consists of discrete smooth muscle cells or units that function independently. Each of these units is innervated by the autonomic nervous system. In fact, like skeletal muscle, this type of smooth muscle must be stimulated by these nerves in order to initiate contraction. Therefore, this muscle is referred to as *neurogenic*. Interestingly, nerve stimulation elicits graded potentials only. Action potentials do not occur in this muscle. The amount of ion flux that occurs in a single muscle cell is inadequate to depolarize the muscle to threshold; however, the graded potentials are sufficient to cause smooth muscle contraction. The contractile response of the whole muscle results from the sum of the responses of multiple individual units.

Most smooth muscle is *single-unit smooth muscle*. Also referred to as *visceral smooth muscle*, it is found in the walls of tubes and hollow organs in the digestive, reproductive, and urinary systems, as well as in the walls of small blood vessels. The cells of this type of smooth muscle are connected electrically by *gap junctions* so that electrical activity can spread from one cell to the next, forming a *functional syncytium*. Any change in electrical activity in one region of the muscle quickly spreads throughout the muscle layer such that the cells of the muscle function as one, or as a "single unit."

Action potentials are generated in single-unit smooth muscle. Simultaneous depolarization of 30 to 40 smooth muscle cells is required to generate a propagated action potential; the presence of gap junctions allows this to occur readily. Because single-unit smooth muscle is *self-excitable* and capable of generating action potentials without input from the autonomic nervous system, it is referred to as *myogenic*. In this muscle, the function of the autonomic nervous system is to modify contractile activity only. Input is not needed to elicit contraction.

The ability to depolarize spontaneously is related to the unstable resting membrane potentials in single-unit smooth muscle. Two types of spontaneous depolarizations may occur:

- Pacemaker potentials
- Slow-wave potentials

A *pacemaker potential* involves gradual depolarization of the cell membrane to threshold. The subsequent generation of an action potential causes smooth muscle contraction. This type of spontaneous depolarization is referred to as a "pacemaker potential" because it creates a regular rhythm of contraction.

Slow-wave potentials also involve gradual depolarization of the cell membrane, but these depolarizations do not necessarily reach threshold. Therefore, the depolarization may simply be followed by repolarization back to the initial membrane potential. These slow "wave-like" potentials occur rhythmically and do not lead to smooth muscle contraction. The peak-to-peak amplitude of the slow-wave potential is in the range of 15 to 30 mV. Therefore, under the appropriate conditions, the depolarization phase of the slow-wave potential may, in fact, reach threshold. When this occurs, a burst of action potentials is generated, resulting in muscle contraction.

The mechanism of the slow-wave potential is unclear. One hypothesis is that the rate at which sodium ions are actively transported out of the cell rhythmically increases and decreases. A decrease in the outward movement of Na^+ ions allows positive charges to accumulate along the internal surface of the cell membrane and depolarization takes place. This is followed by an increase in the outward movement of Na^+ ions, which causes the internal surface of the cell membrane to become more negative, and repolarization takes place.

12.6 Factors influencing contractile activity of smooth muscle

Many factors influence the contractile activity of smooth muscle. The strength of contraction of multiunit smooth muscle may be enhanced by *stimulation of a greater number of cells*, or contractile units. This mechanism is directly comparable to motor-unit recruitment employed by skeletal muscle. As the number of contracting muscle cells increases, so does the strength of contraction. However, this mechanism is of no value in single-unit smooth muscle. Due to the presence of gap junctions, all of the muscle cells in the tissue are activated at once.

Other factors that influence contractile activity include:

- Autonomic nervous system
- Hormones and blood-borne substances
- Locally produced substances
- Intracellular calcium concentration

The autonomic nervous system (ANS) modifies contractile activity of both types of smooth muscle. As discussed in Chapter 9, the ANS innervates the smooth muscle layer in a very diffuse manner, so neurotransmitter is released over a wide area of muscle. Typically, the effects of sympathetic and parasympathetic stimulation in a given tissue oppose each other; one system enhances contractile activity while the other inhibits it. The specific effects (excitatory or inhibitory) that the two divisions of the ANS have on a given smooth muscle depend upon its location.

Many *hormones and other blood-borne substances* (including drugs) also alter contractile activity of smooth muscle. Some of the more important substances include: epinephrine; norepinephrine; angiotensin II; vasopressin; oxytocin; and histamine. *Locally produced substances* that may alter contraction in the tissue in which they are synthesized include: nitric oxide; prostaglandins; leukotrienes; carbon dioxide; and hydrogen ion.

All of these factors (ANS stimulation, blood-borne and locally produced substances) alter smooth muscle contractile activity by altering the *intracellular concentration of calcium*. An increase in cytosolic calcium leads to an increase in crossbridge cycling and therefore an increase in tension development. The concentration of calcium within the cytoplasm of the smooth muscle cell may be increased by several mechanisms, including:

- Voltage-gated Ca^{++} channels
- Ligand-gated Ca^{++} channels
- IP_3-gated Ca^{++} channels
- Stretch-activated Ca^{++} channels

Voltage-gated Ca^{++} channels open when the smooth muscle cell is depolarized. Calcium then enters the cell down its electrochemical gradient. *Ligand-gated Ca^{++} channels* are associated with various hormone or neurotransmitter receptors. Binding of a given substance to its receptor causes the ligand-gated Ca^{++} channel to open and, once again, Ca^{++} ions enter the cell. This process, which occurs without a significant change in membrane potential (due to a simultaneous increase in Na^+ ion removal from the cell), is referred to as *pharmacomechanical coupling*.

Inositol triphosphate (IP_3)-gated channels are also associated with membrane-bound receptors for hormones and neurotransmitters. In this case, binding of a given substance to its receptor causes activation of another membrane-bound protein, phospholipase C. This enzyme promotes hydrolysis of phosphatidylinositol 4,5-diphosphate (PIP_2) to IP_3. The IP_3 then diffuses to the sarcoplasmic reticulum and opens its calcium channels to release Ca^{++} ions from this intracellular storage site.

Finally, an increase in volume or pressure within a tube or hollow organ causes stretch or distortion of the smooth muscle in the organ wall. This may cause activation of *stretch-activated Ca^{++} channels*. The subsequent influx of calcium initiates contraction of the smooth muscle. This process is referred to as *myogenic contraction* and is common in blood vessels.

12.7 Length–tension relationship

The length of smooth muscle prior to stimulation has little influence on subsequent tension development. This is in marked contrast to skeletal muscle which exhibits a strong length–tension relationship. As discussed in Chapter 11, the influence of resting muscle length on the tension developed in skeletal muscle is based upon the arrangement of thick and thin filaments into sarcomeres. Any change in muscle length alters the degree of overlap of these filaments and therefore the number of crossbridges cycling and the amount of tension developed.

The contractile elements in smooth muscle are not organized into sarcomeres. Furthermore, the resting length of smooth muscle is much shorter than its optimal length. In other words, this muscle can be significantly stretched and the amount of tension developed may actually increase because the muscle is closer to its optimal length. Finally, thick filaments are longer in smooth muscle than they are in skeletal muscle. As a result, overlap of thick and thin filaments still occurs, even when the muscle has been stretched out.

This very broad length–tension relationship in smooth muscle is physiologically advantageous. Tubes and hollow organs may be stretched considerably as substances pass through them. Regardless, the smooth muscle must retain its ability to contract forcefully and regulate the movement of these substances through the organs.

Bibliography

1. Costanzo, L. *Physiology*, W.B. Saunders, Philadelphia, 1998.
2. Guyton, A.C. and Hall, J.E., *Textbook of Medical Physiology*, 10th ed., W.B. Saunders, Philadelphia, 2000.
3. Lombard, J.H. and Rusch, N.J., Cells, nerves and muscles, in *Physiology Secrets*, Raff, H., Ed., Hanley and Belfus, Inc., Philadelphia, 1999, chap. 1.
4. Rhoades, R. and Pflanzer, R., *Human Physiology*, 4th ed., Brooks/Cole, Pacific Grove, CA, 2003.
5. Sherwood, L., *Human Physiology from Cells to Systems*, 4th ed., Brooks/Cole, Pacific Grove, CA, 2001.
6. Silverthorn, D.U., *Human Physiology: An Integrated Approach*, 2nd ed., Prentice-Hall, Upper Saddle River, NJ, 2001.
7. Sperelakis, N., *Essentials of Physiology*, 2nd ed., Sperelakis, N. and Banks, R.O., Eds., Little, Brown, Boston, 1996.

chapter thirteen

Cardiac physiology

Study objectives

- Compare functions of the right side and the left side of the heart
- Compare the functions of the arterial system and venous system
- Describe the functions of the three major mechanical components of the heart: atria, ventricles, and valves
- Describe the route of blood flow through the heart
- Discuss the functions of the chordae tendinae and the papillary muscles
- Explain why the thickness of the myocardium varies between the different heart chambers
- Compare and contrast the functional and structural features of cardiac muscle and skeletal muscle
- Understand the physiological importance of the myocardial syncytium
- Describe the components of the specialized electrical conduction system of the heart
- Explain how the pacemaker of the heart initiates the heart beat
- Understand the physiological importance of the AV nodal delay
- Describe the mechanism and physiological significance of rapid electrical conduction through the Purkinje fibers
- Compare and contrast the action potentials generated by the SA node and ventricular muscle cells
- Discuss the mechanism and physiological significance of the effective refractory period
- List the types of information obtained from an electrocardiogram
- Describe each of the components of the electrocardiogram
- Define tachycardia and bradycardia
- Understand how arrhythmias may be treated pharmacologically
- Define systole and diastole
- Describe the mechanical events, status of the valves, and pressure changes that take place during each phase of the cardiac cycle

13.1 Introduction

The cardiovascular system includes the *heart*, which serves as a pump for the blood, and the *blood vessels*, which transport blood throughout the body. Under normal conditions, this system is a continuous, closed circuit, meaning that the blood is found only in the heart and blood vessels.

The heart actually consists of two separate pumps. The right side of the heart pumps blood to the lungs through the pulmonary circulation so that gas exchange, uptake of oxygen and elimination of carbon dioxide can take place. The left side of the heart pumps blood to the rest of the tissues of the body through the systemic circulation. In this way, oxygen and nutrients are delivered to the tissues to sustain their activities and carbon dioxide and other metabolic waste products are removed from the tissues. In both circulations, blood vessels of the *arterial system*, arteries and arterioles, carry blood away from the heart and toward the tissues. The arterioles deliver blood to the *capillaries* where the exchange of substances between the blood and the tissues takes place. From the capillaries, blood flows into the vessels of the *venous system*, veins and venules, which carry blood back to the heart.

The human heart begins pumping approximately 3 weeks after conception and must continue this activity without interruption all day, every day, for an entire lifetime. In a typical individual, this means the heart pumps over 100,000 times per day and propels about 2000 gallons of blood through almost 65,000 miles of blood vessels. This function of the heart will be discussed here as well as in the following chapter on cardiac output. The function of the blood vessels will be considered in the chapter on the circulatory system.

13.2 Functional anatomy of the heart

The heart is located in the center of the thoracic cavity. It sits directly above the muscles of the diaphragm, which separates the thorax from the abdomen, and lies beneath the sternum between the two lungs. The heart is enclosed and anchored in place by a double-walled fibrous sac referred to as the *pericardium*. The membranes of the pericardium produce a small amount of *pericardial fluid* that minimizes friction produced by the movement of the heart when it beats. To function mechanically as a pump, the heart must have:

- Receiving chambers
- Delivery chambers
- Valves

The *atria* (sing. *atrium*) are chambers that receive blood returning to the heart through the veins. The blood then moves to the *ventricles*, or delivery chambers, of the heart. The powerful contractions of the ventricles generate a force sufficient to propel blood through the systemic or the pulmonary circulations. *Valves* ensure the one-way, or forward, flow of the blood.

The route of blood flow through the heart begins with the venae cavae, which return blood from the peripheral tissues to the right side of the heart (see Figure 13.1; Table 13.1). The *superior vena cava* returns blood from the head and arms to the heart and the *inferior vena cava* returns blood from the trunk of the body and the legs to the heart. As this blood has already passed through the tissues of the body, it is low in oxygen. Blood from the venae cavae first enters the *right atrium* and then the *right ventricle*. Contraction of the right ventricle propels this blood to the lungs through the pulmonary circulation by way of the *pulmonary artery*. As it flows through the lungs, blood becomes enriched with oxygen and eliminates carbon dioxide to the

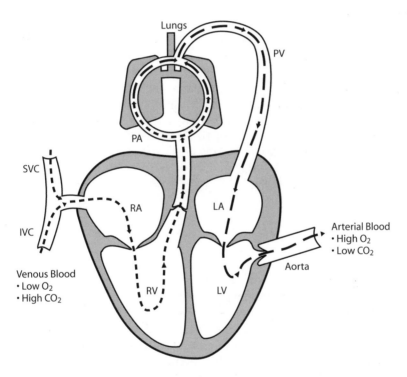

Figure 13.1 Route of blood flow through the heart. Systemic blood returns to the heart by way of the superior (SVC) and inferior (IVC) venae cavae. This blood, which is low in oxygen and high in carbon dioxide, enters the right atrium (RA) and then the right ventricle (RV). The right ventricle pumps the blood through the pulmonary artery (PA) to the pulmonary circulation. It is within the lungs that gas exchange takes place. Next, this blood, which is high in oxygen and low in carbon dioxide, returns to the heart by way of the pulmonary veins (PV). It enters the left atrium (LA) and then the left ventricle (LV). The left ventricle pumps the blood through the aorta to the systemic circulation and the peripheral tissues.

Table 13.1 Route of Blood Flow through the Heart

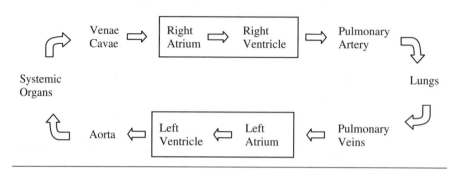

atmosphere. Blood then returns to the heart through the *pulmonary veins*. The blood first enters the *left atrium* and then the *left ventricle*. Contraction of the left ventricle propels the blood back to the peripheral tissues through systemic circulation by way of the *aorta*, the largest arterial vessel.

In summary, the heart is a single organ consisting of two pumps; the right heart delivers blood to the lungs and the left heart delivers blood to the rest of the body. Both pumps work simultaneously. The atria fill with blood and then contract at the same time and the ventricles fill with blood and then contract at the same time. Contraction of the atria occurs prior to contraction of the ventricles in order to ensure proper filling of the ventricles with blood.

Two sets of valves in the heart maintain the one-way flow of blood as it passes through the heart chambers:

- Atrioventricular (AV) valves
- Semilunar valves

Each of these valves consists of thin flaps of flexible but tough fibrous tissue whose movements are passive. The *atrioventricular (AV) valves* are found between the atria and the ventricles. The right AV valve is a tricuspid valve and has three cusps or leaflets. The left AV valve (also referred to as the *mitral valve*) is a bicuspid valve because it has two cusps. When the ventricles contract, the pressure within them increases substantially, creating a pressure gradient for blood flow from the ventricles back into the atria where the pressure is very low. Closure of the AV valves prevents this potential backward flow of blood. However, what prevents this increased ventricular pressure from causing eversion of the valves or opening of the valves in the opposite direction, which would also allow blood to flow backward into the atria? Strong fibrous ligaments, the *chordae tendinae*, are attached to the flaps of the valves. The chordae tendinae arise from cone-shaped *papillary muscles* that protrude into the ventricles. These muscles are continuous with the ventricular muscle so, when the ventricles are stimulated to contract, the papillary muscles also contract, pulling downward on the chordae tendinae. In this way, the flaps of the valves are not pushed open into the atria, but instead are held in place in the closed position. Blood is now forced to continue its forward progression and move from the ventricles into their respective arteries.

The *semilunar valves* separate the ventricles from their associated arteries. The *pulmonary valve* is found between the right ventricle and the pulmonary artery and the *aortic valve* is found between the left ventricle and the aorta. These valves prevent backward flow of blood from the pulmonary artery or the aorta into their preceding ventricles when the ventricles relax. The semilunar valves also have three cusps. There are no valves between the venae cavae or the pulmonary veins and the atria into which they deliver blood. The closure of the valves causes the "lub-dub" associated with the heart beat. The *first heart sound*, or the "lub," occurs when the ventricles contract and the AV valves close. The *second heart sound*, or the "dub," occurs when the ventricles relax and the semilunar valves close.

The wall of the heart has three layers:

- Epicardium
- Endocardium
- Myocardium

The outermost layer, the *epicardium*, is the thin membrane on the external surface of the heart. The innermost layer, the *endocardium*, consists of a thin delicate layer of cells lining the chambers of the heart and the valve leaflets. The endocardium is continuous with the *endothelium*, which lines the blood vessels.

The middle layer is the *myocardium*, which is the muscular layer of the heart. This is the thickest layer, although the thickness varies from one chamber to the next. Thickness of the myocardium is related to the amount of work that a given chamber must perform when pumping blood. The atria, which serve primarily as receiving chambers, perform little pumping action. Under normal resting conditions, most of the blood (75%) moves passively along a pressure gradient (higher pressure to lower pressure) from the veins, into the atria and ventricles where the pressure is close to zero. Therefore, it follows that the atria have relatively thin layers of myocardium because powerful contractions are not necessary. On the other hand, when the ventricles contract, they must develop enough pressure to force open the semilunar valves and propel the blood through the entire pulmonary or systemic circulations. Under normal resting conditions, between heart beats, the pressure in the pulmonary artery is approximately 8 mmHg and pressure in the aorta is approximately 80 mmHg. Therefore, in order to eject blood into the pulmonary artery, the right ventricle must generate a pressure greater than 8 mmHg and, in order to eject blood into the aorta, the left ventricle must generate a pressure greater than 80 mmHg. Because the left ventricle performs significantly more work, its wall is much thicker than that of the right ventricle.

Table 13.2 Distinguishing Features of Cardiac Muscle and Skeletal Muscle

Cardiac muscle	Skeletal muscle
Organized into sarcomeres	Organized into sarcomeres
Sliding-filament mechanism of contraction	Sliding-filament mechanism of contraction
Source of calcium: Sarcoplasmic reticulum Tranverse tubules	Source of calcium: Sarcoplasmic reticulum
Resting length of sarcomere *less than* optimal length	Resting length of sarcomere *equal* to optimal length
Gap junctions provide electrical communication between cells, forming a functional syncytium	No gap junctions
Myogenic	Neurogenic
Contraction *modified* by autonomic nervous system	Contraction *elicited* by somatic nervous system

Cardiac muscle has many structural and functional similarities with skeletal muscle (Chapter 11; also see Table 13.2). The contractile elements, composed of thin actin filaments and thick myosin filaments, are organized into *sarcomeres*. Therefore, as with skeletal muscle, tension development within the myocardium occurs by way of the *sliding filament mechanism*. As the action potential travels along the surface of the muscle cell membrane, the impulse also spreads into the interior of the cell along the *transverse (T) tubules*. This stimulates the release of calcium from the *sarcoplasmic reticulum*. Calcium promotes the interaction of actin and myosin resulting in cross-bridge cycling and muscle shortening. Unlike skeletal muscle whose only source of calcium is the sarcoplasmic reticulum, cardiac muscle also obtains calcium from the T tubules, which are filled with extracellular fluid. This added calcium results in a much stronger contraction.

The arrangement of the myofilaments into sarcomeres renders the cardiac muscle subject to the *length–tension relationship*. When the resting sarcomere length is altered, the amount of tension developed by the myocardium upon stimulation is altered as well. In the heart, the resting sarcomere length is determined by the volume of blood within the ventricle immediately prior to contraction. This length–tension relationship is described by the *Frank–Starling mechanism* and is discussed in more detail in the next chapter on cardiac output.

Skeletal and cardiac muscles also have important differences. Skeletal muscle cells are elongated and run the length of the entire muscle; furthermore, these cells have no electrical communication between them. Cardiac muscle cells, on the other hand, branch and interconnect with each other. Intercellular junctions found where adjoining cells meet end-to-end are referred to as *intercalated discs*. Two types of cell-to-cell junctions exist within these discs. *Desmosomes* hold the muscle cells together and provide the structural support needed when the heart beats and exerts a mechanical stress that would tend to pull the cells apart. *Gap junctions* are areas of very low electrical resistance (1/400 of the resistance of the outside membrane) that allow free diffusion of ions. It is through the gap junctions that the electrical impulse, or heart beat, spreads rapidly from one cell to another. As a result, the myocardium is a *syncytium* in which the initiation of a heart beat in one region of the heart results in stimulation and contraction of all cardiac muscle cells at essentially the same time. The heart is actually composed of two syncytiums: atrial and ventricular. In each case, but particularly in the ventricles, simultaneous stimulation of all the muscle cells results in a more powerful contraction, facilitating the pumping of blood.

Skeletal muscle is neurogenic and requires stimulation from the somatic nervous system to initiate contraction. Because no electrical communication takes place between these cells, each muscle fiber is innervated by a branch of an alpha motor neuron. Cardiac muscle, however, is *myogenic*, or self-excitatory; this muscle spontaneously depolarizes to threshold and generates action potentials without external stimulation. The region of the heart with the fastest rate of inherent depolarization initiates the heart beat and determines the heart rhythm. In normal hearts, this *"pacemaker"* region is the sinoatrial node.

13.3 Electrical activity of the heart

The specialized excitation and electrical conduction system in the heart consists of:

- Sinoatrial node
- Interatrial pathway
- Internodal pathway
- Atrioventricular node
- Bundle of His
- Bundle branches
- Purkinje fibers

The *sinoatrial (SA) node* is located in the wall of the right atrium near the entrance of the superior vena cava. The specialized cells of the SA node spontaneously depolarize to threshold and generate 70 to 75 heart beats/min. The "resting" membrane potential, or *pacemaker potential*, is different from that of neurons, which were discussed in Chapter 3 (Membrane Potential). First of all, this potential is approximately –55 mV, which is less negative than that found in neurons (–70 mV; see Figure 13.2, panel A). Second, pacemaker potential is unstable and slowly depolarizes toward threshold (*phase 4*). Two important ion currents contribute to this slow depolarization. These cells are inherently leaky to sodium. The resulting influx of Na^+ ions occurs through channels that differ from the fast Na^+ channels that cause rapid depolarization in other types of excitable cells. Toward the end of phase

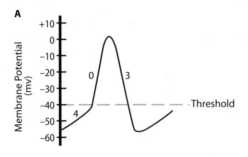

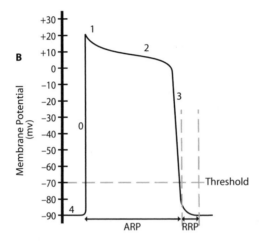

Figure 13.2 Cardiac action potentials. Panel A: sinoatrial (SA) node; during phase 4 (the pacemaker potential), the cells of the SA node depolarize toward threshold due to the influx of Na$^+$ and Ca^{++} ions. The upward swing of the action potential, phase 0, results from the influx of calcium through slow Ca^{++} channels. Repolarization (phase 3) is due to the efflux of K$^+$ ions. Panel B: ventricular muscle; the resting membrane potential (phase 4) is very negative due to the high permeability of the K$^+$ channels. The upward swing of the action potential (phase 0) results from the rapid influx of sodium through fast Na$^+$ channels. The brief repolarization that occurs during phase 1 is due to the abrupt closure of the channels. The plateau of the action potential, phase 2, results from the influx of calcium through slow Ca^{++} channels. Finally, repolarization (phase 3) is due to the efflux of K$^+$ ions. The absolute, or effective, refractory period (ARP) persists until the fast Na$^+$ channels return to their resting state (–70 mV). No new action potentials may be generated during this period. This is followed by the relative refractory period (RRP).

4, Ca^{++} channels start to become activated allowing Ca^{++} ion influx, which continues to depolarize the membrane toward threshold.

Phase 0 begins when the membrane potential reaches threshold (–40 mV). Recall that the upstroke of the action potential in neurons is due to increased permeability of fast Na$^+$ channels, resulting in a steep, rapid depolarization.

However, in the SA node, the action potential develops more slowly because the fast Na⁺ channels do not play a role. Whenever the membrane potential is less negative than –60 mV for more than a few milliseconds, these channels become inactivated. With a resting membrane potential of –55 mV, this is clearly the case in the SA node. Instead, when the membrane potential reaches threshold in this tissue, many slow Ca⁺⁺ channels open, resulting in the depolarization phase of the action potential. The slope of this depolarization is less steep than that of neurons.

Phase 3 begins at the peak of the action potential. At this point, the Ca⁺⁺ channels close and K⁺ channels open. The resulting efflux of K⁺ ions causes the repolarization phase of the action potential.

Because cardiac muscle is myogenic, nervous stimulation is not necessary to elicit the heart beat. However, the heart rate is modulated by input from the autonomic nervous system. The sympathetic and parasympathetic systems innervate the SA node. Sympathetic stimulation causes an increase in heart rate or an increased number of beats/min. Norepinephrine, which stimulates β_1-adrenergic receptors, increases the rate of pacemaker depolarization by increasing the permeability to Na⁺ and Ca⁺⁺ ions. If the heart beat is generated more rapidly, then the result is more beats per minute.

Parasympathetic stimulation causes a decrease in heart rate. Acetylcholine, which stimulates muscarinic receptors, increases the permeability to potassium. Enhanced K⁺ ion efflux has a twofold effect. First, the cells become hyperpolarized and therefore the membrane potential is farther away from threshold. Second, the rate of pacemaker depolarization is decreased because the outward movement of K⁺ ions opposes the effect of the inward movement of Na⁺ and Ca⁺⁺ ions. The result of these two effects of potassium efflux is that it takes longer for the SA node to reach threshold and generate an action potential. If the heart beat is generated more slowly, then fewer beats per minute are elicited.

From the SA node, the heart beat spreads rapidly throughout both atria by way of the gap junctions. As mentioned previously, the atria are stimulated to contract simultaneously. An *interatrial conduction pathway* extends from the SA node to the left atrium. Its function is to facilitate conduction of the impulse through the left atrium, creating the atrial syncytium (see Figure 13.3).

An *internodal conduction pathway* also extends from the SA node and transmits the impulse directly to the *atrioventricular (AV) node*. This node is located at the base of the right atrium near the interventricular septum, which is the wall of myocardium separating the two ventricles. Because the atria and ventricles are separated from each other by fibrous connective tissue, the electrical impulse cannot spread directly to the ventricles. Instead, the AV node serves as the only pathway through which the impulse can be transmitted to the ventricles. The speed of conduction through the AV node is slowed, resulting in a slight delay (0.1 sec). The cause of this *AV nodal delay* is partly due to the smaller fibers of the AV node. More importantly, however, fewer gap junctions exist between the cells of the node, which

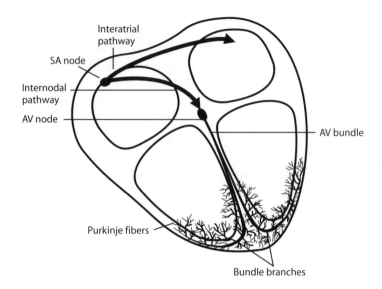

Figure 13.3 Route of excitation and conduction in the heart. The heart beat is initiated in the sinoatrial (SA) node, or the pacemaker, in the right atrium of the heart. The electrical impulse is transmitted to the left atrium through the interatrial conduction pathway and to the atrioventricular (AV) node through the internodal pathway. From the AV node, the electrical impulse enters the ventricles and is conducted through the AV bundle, the left and right bundle branches, and, finally, the Purkinje fibers, which terminate on the true cardiac muscle cells of the ventricles.

increases the resistance to current the flow. The physiological advantage of the AV nodal delay is that it allows atria to complete their contraction before ventricular contraction begins. This timing ensures proper filling of the ventricles prior to contraction.

From the AV node, the electrical impulse spreads through the *AV bundle* or the *bundle of His*. This portion of the conduction system penetrates the fibrous tissue separating the atria from the ventricles and enters the interventricular septum where it divides into the *left and right bundle branches*. The bundle branches travel down the septum toward the apex of the heart and then reverse direction, traveling back toward the atria along the outer ventricle walls. This route of conduction of the impulse facilitates ejection of blood from the ventricles. If the impulse were to be conducted directly from the atria to the ventricles, the ventricular contraction would begin at the top of the chambers and proceed downward toward the apex. This would trap the blood at the bottom of the chambers. Instead, the wave of ventricular electrical stimulation and, therefore, contraction moves from the apex of the heart toward the top of the chambers where the semilunar valves are located and ejection takes place.

The final portion of the specialized conduction system consists of the *Purkinje fibers* that extend from the bundle branches. These fibers, which spread throughout the myocardium, terminate on the true cardiac muscle cells of the ventricles. The rate of conduction of the impulse through the Purkinje fibers is very rapid and results in the functional syncytium of the ventricles discussed earlier. The entire ventricular myocardium is stimulated almost simultaneously, which strengthens its pumping action. The increased rate of conduction (six times the rate of other ventricular muscle cells) is due in part to the large diameter of the Purkinje fibers. Furthermore, the gap junctions have a very high level of permeability, which decreases the resistance to current flow. It is estimated that Purkinje fibers conduct impulses at a velocity of 1.5 to 4.0 m/sec.

The action potential generated in the ventricular muscle is very different from that originating in the SA node. The resting membrane potential is not only stable; it is much more negative than that of the SA node. Second, the slope of the depolarization phase of the action potential is much steeper. Finally, there is a lengthy plateau phase of the action potential in which the muscle cells remain depolarized for approximately 300 msec. The physiological significance of this sustained depolarization is that it leads to sustained contraction (also about 300 msec), which facilitates ejection of blood. These disparities in the action potentials are explained by differences in ion channel activity in ventricular muscle compared to the SA node.

At rest, the permeability to K^+ ions in ventricular muscle cells is significantly greater than that of Na^+ ions. This condition results in a stable resting membrane potential that approaches the equilibrium potential for K^+ of –90 mV (*phase 4*) (see Figure 13.2, panel B). Upon stimulation by an electrical impulse, the voltage-gated fast Na^+ channels open, causing a marked increase in the permeability to Na^+ ions and a rapid and profound depolarization of the membrane potential toward +30 mV (*phase 0*). These voltage-gated Na^+ channels remain open very briefly and within 1 msec are inactivated. The resulting decrease in sodium permeability causes a small repolarization (*phase 1*). The ventricular muscle cells do not completely repolarize immediately as do neurons and skeletal muscle cells. Instead, a plateau phase of the action potential (*phase 2*) occurs. During this phase, permeability to K^+ ions decreases and permeability to Ca^{++} ions increases. Like the voltage-gated Na^+ channels, the voltage-gated Ca^{++} channels are also activated by depolarization; however, they open much more slowly. The combination of decreased K^+ ion efflux and increased Ca^{++} ion influx causes prolonged depolarization. Repolarization (*phase 3*) occurs when the Ca^{++} channels close and K^+ channels open, allowing for rapid efflux of K^+ ions and a return to the resting membrane potential.

As in neurons, cardiac muscle cells undergo an absolute or *effective refractory period* in which, at the peak of the action potential, the voltage-gated fast Na^+ channels become inactivated and incapable of opening regardless of further stimulation. Therefore, the fast Na^+ channels cannot reopen, Na^+ ions cannot enter the cell, and another action potential cannot be generated. These channels do not return to their resting position and become capable of opening in sufficient numbers to generate a new action potential until the cardiac muscle cell has repolarized to approximately –70 mV. As a result, the absolute refractory period lasts almost as long as the duration of the associated contraction — about 250 msec. The physiological significance of this phenomenon is that it prevents the development of tetanus or spasm of the ventricular myocardium. By the time the cardiac muscle cell can be stimulated to generate another action potential, the contraction from the previous action potential is over. Therefore, tension from sequential action potentials cannot accumulate and become sustained. This is in contrast to skeletal muscle where tetanic contractions readily occur in order to produce maximal strength (Chapter 11). The pumping action of the heart, however, requires alternating contraction and relaxation so that the chambers can fill with blood. Sustained contraction or tetanus would preclude ventricular filling.

The effective refractory period is followed by a *relative refractory period* that lasts for the remaining 50 msec of the ventricular action potential. During this period, action potentials may be generated; however, the myocardium is more difficult than normal to excite.

13.4 Electrocardiogram

A portion of the electrical current generated by the heart beat flows away from the heart through the surrounding tissues and reaches the body surface. Using electrodes placed on the skin, this current can be measured and used to produce a recording referred to as an *electrocardiogram (ECG)*. An important point to remember regarding the ECG is that it represents the sum of all electrical activity throughout the heart at any given moment, not individual action potentials. Therefore, an upward deflection of the recording does not necessarily represent depolarization, nor does a downward deflection represent repolarization. Furthermore, a recording is made only when current is flowing through the heart during the actual process of depolarization or repolarization. No recording is made when the heart is completely depolarized (during the plateau phase of the ventricular action potential) or completely repolarized (between heart beats). The ECG provides information concerning:

- Relative size of heart chambers
- Various disturbances of rhythm and electrical conduction
- Extent and location of ischemic damage to the myocardium
- Effects of altered electrolyte concentrations
- Influence of certain drugs (e.g., digitalis and antiarrhythmic drugs)

The ECG provides no information concerning contractility or, in other words, the mechanical performance of the heart as a pump.

The normal ECG is composed of (Figure 13.4):

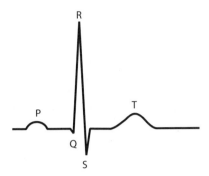

Figure 13.4 Electrocardiogram. The electrocardiogram (ECG) is a measure of the overall electrical activity of the heart. The P wave is caused by atrial depolarization, the QRS complex is caused by ventricular depolarization, and the T wave is caused by ventricular repolarization.

- *P wave*, caused by atrial depolarization
- *QRS complex*, caused by ventricular depolarization
- *T wave*, caused by ventricular repolarization

The ECG has several noteworthy characteristics. First, the firing of the SA node, which initiates the heart beat, precedes atrial depolarization and therefore should be apparent immediately prior to the P wave. However, due to its small size, it does not generate enough electrical activity to spread to the surface of the body and be detected by the electrodes. Therefore, there is no recording of the depolarization of the SA node.

Second, the area under the curve of the P wave is small compared to that of the QRS complex. This is related to the muscle mass of the chambers. The ventricles have significantly more muscle than the atria and therefore generate more electrical activity. Furthermore, although it may not appear to be the case given the spike-like nature of the QRS complex, areas under the QRS complex and the T wave are approximately the same. This is because these recordings represent electrical activity of the ventricles even though one is caused by depolarization and the other by repolarization. Either way, the muscle mass involved is the same.

Third, no recording takes place during the PR segment when the electrical impulse is being conducted through the AV node. As with the SA node, not enough tissue is involved to generate sufficient electrical activity to be detected by the electrodes. The length of the PR segment is determined by the duration of the AV nodal delay.

Finally, no recording occurs during the ST segment — the period between ventricular depolarization and ventricular repolarization. In other words, the ventricles are completely depolarized and the muscle cells are in the plateau phase of the action potential. As mentioned earlier, unless current is actually flowing through the myocardium, there is no recording.

Using the ECG, the heart rate may be determined by calculating the time from the beginning of one P wave to the beginning of the next P wave, or from peak to peak of the QRS complexes. A normal resting heart rate in adults is approximately 70 beats/min. A heart rate of less than 60 beats/min is referred to as *bradycardia* and a heart rate of more than 100 beats/min is referred to as *tachycardia*.

Pharmacy application: antiarrhythmic drugs

Normal cardiac contraction depends on the conduction of electrical impulses through the myocardium in a highly coordinated fashion. Any abnormality of the initiation or propagation of the impulse is referred to as an *arrhythmia*. These disorders are the most common clinical problem encountered by a cardiologist. There is a wide range of types of arrhythmias with multiple etiologies and a variety of symptoms. In this section, two types of cardiac tachyarrhythmias are discussed. The most common treatment for these conditions is drug therapy.

Verapamil (Class IV antiarrhythmic drug) is an effective agent for atrial or supraventricular tachycardia. A Ca^{++} channel blocker, it is most potent in tissues where the action potentials depend on calcium currents, including slow-response tissues such as the SA node and the AV node. The effects of verapamil include a decrease in heart rate and in conduction velocity of the electrical impulse through the AV node. The resulting increase in duration of the AV nodal delay, which is illustrated by a lengthening of the PR segment in the ECG, reduces the number of impulses permitted to penetrate to the ventricles to cause contraction.

Procainamide (Class IA antiarrhythmic drug) is an effective agent for ventricular tachycardia. Its mechanism of action involves blockade of the fast Na^+ channels responsible for phase 0 in the fast response tissue of the ventricles. Therefore, its effect is most pronounced in the Purkinje fibers. The effects of this drug's activity include a decrease in excitability of myocardial cells and in conduction velocity. Therefore, a decrease in the rate of the phase 0 upstroke and a prolonged repolarization are observed. As a result, duration of the action potential and the associated refractory period is prolonged and the heart rate is reduced. These effects are illustrated by an increase in the duration of the QRS complex.

13.5 Cardiac cycle

The *cardiac cycle* is the period of time from beginning of one heart beat to beginning of the next. As such, it consists of two alternating phases:

- *Systole*, in which the chambers contract and eject the blood
- *Diastole*, in which the chambers relax allowing blood to fill them

Atria and ventricles undergo phases of systole and diastole; however, the duration of each phase in the chambers differs. In the atria, whose primary function is to receive blood returning to the heart from the veins, diastole is the predominant phase, lasting for almost 90% of each cardiac cycle at rest. In the ventricles, whose primary function is to develop enough force to eject blood into the pulmonary or systemic circulations, systole is much longer lasting and accounts for almost 40% of each cycle at rest.

A discussion of the cardiac cycle requires the correlation of pressure changes; ventricular volume changes; valve activity; and heart sounds. In this section, the focus will be on the left side of the heart (see Table 13.3). Identical events occur simultaneously on the right side of the heart; however, the pressures are lower.

Ventricular filling. This process occurs during ventricular diastole. When the ventricle has completely relaxed and pressure in the ventricle is lower than pressure in the atrium, the AV valve opens. The pressure in the atrium at this time is greater than that of the ventricle due to the continuous return of blood from the veins. The initial phase of filling is rapid because blood had accumulated in the atrium prior to the opening of the AV valve; once this valve opens, the accumulated blood rushes in. The second phase of filling is slower as blood continues to flow from the veins into the atrium and then into the ventricle. This phase of filling is referred to as *diastasis*. Up to this point, ventricular filling has occurred *passively*, and at rest approximately 75% of the blood entering the ventricle does so in this manner. The third phase of ventricular filling results from atrial contraction. At this time, the remaining 25% of the blood is forced into the ventricle by this *active* process. The volume of blood in the ventricles at the end of the filling period is referred to as the *end-diastolic volume (EDV)* and is approximately 120 to 130 ml at rest. Note that during the entire diastolic filling period, the aortic (semilunar) valve is closed. The ventricular pressure during the filling phase is very low (0 to 10 mmHg) and pressure in the aorta during diastole is approximately 80 mmHg. Therefore, the aortic valve remains closed to prevent the backward flow of blood from the aorta into the ventricle during ventricular diastole.

Ventricular contraction. This process occurs during ventricular systole. When the ventricular myocardium begins to contract and squeeze down on the blood within the chamber, the pressure increases rapidly. In fact, ven-

Table 13.3 Summary of Events Occurring during Cardiac Cycle

	Filling	Isovolumetric contraction	Ejection	Isovolumetric relaxation
Period	Diastole	Systole	Systole	Diastole
Pressures	$P_A > P_V < P_{aorta}$ $P_A, P_V \approx$ 0–10 mmHg $P_{aorta} \approx$ 80 mmHg	$P_A < P_V < P_{aorta}$ P_v increases toward 80 mmHg	$P_A < P_V > P_{aorta}$ $P_V P_{aorta} \approx$ 120 mmHg	$P_A < P_V < P_{aorta}$ P_V decreases toward 0 mmHg
AV valve	Open	Closed	Closed	Closed
Aortic valve	Closed	Closed	Open	Closed
Ventricular volume	Increases from 60 ml (ESV) to 130 ml (EDV)	No change	Decreases from 130 ml (EDV) to 60 ml (ESV)	No change
ECG	TP segment P wave PR segment	QRS complex	ST segment	T wave
Heart sounds	None	First heart sound	None	Second heart sound

tricular pressure is almost instantly greater than atrial pressure. As a result, the AV valve closes to prevent the backward flow of blood from the ventricle into the atrium during ventricular systole. The closure of this valve results in the first heart sound ("lub"). The ventricle continues its contraction and its build-up of pressure; however, during a period of several milliseconds ventricular pressure is climbing toward that of the aorta (from less than 10 mmHg up toward 80 mmHg). Until ventricular pressure exceeds aortic pressure, the aortic valve remains closed. As a result, both valves leading into and out of the chamber are closed and this period is referred to as *isovolumetric contraction*. During this phase neither filling of the ventricle nor ejection of blood from the ventricle occurs, so blood volume does not change. Eventually, the build-up of ventricular pressure overtakes the aortic pressure and the aortic valve is pushed open. At this point, *ejection*, or ventricular emptying, takes place. It is important to note that the chamber does not eject all of the blood within it. Some blood remains in the ventricle following contraction and this volume, referred to as *end-systolic volume (ESV)*, is approximately 50 to 60 ml at rest. Therefore, the volume of blood pumped out of each ventricle per beat, or the *stroke volume (SV)*, is about 70 ml in a healthy adult heart at rest.

After systole, the ventricles abruptly relax and ventricular pressure decreases rapidly. Pressure in the aorta, which has peaked at 120 mmHg during systole, remains above 100 mmHg at this point. Therefore, the blood in the distended artery is immediately pushed back toward the ventricle down the pressure gradient. The backward movement of blood snaps the aortic valve shut, resulting in the second heart sound ("dub"). During this portion of ventricular diastole, there is a period of several milliseconds where ventricular pressure is dissipating and falling back toward zero. Because atrial pressure is close to zero, the AV valve remains closed. Therefore, during this phase of *isovolumetric relaxation*, both valves leading into and out of the chamber are closed. As with isovolumetric contraction, no change takes place in the blood volume of the ventricle during this phase of isovolumetric relaxation. When the ventricular pressure falls to a point at which it is once again exceeded by atrial pressure, the AV valve opens, ventricular filling occurs, and the cardiac cycle begins again.

Due to the alternating phases of systole and diastole, the heart pumps blood intermittently. It contracts to pump the blood into the arteries and then it relaxes so it can once again fill with blood. However, capillary blood flow is not interrupted by this cycle because blood flow to the tissues is continuous. This steady blood flow is due to the elastic properties of the arterial walls. When the stroke volume is ejected into the arterial system, some of the blood is pushed forward toward the tissues. The remainder of the stroke volume is retained in the arteries. These large blood vessels are characterized by an abundance of collagen fibers and elastin fibers. These connective tissue fibers allow the arteries to be quite strong, capable of withstanding high pressures but also reasonably distensible. The rapid addition of the stroke volume causes arterial distension, or stretch, resulting in "storage" of a portion of this blood in these vessels. During diastole, when the heart relaxes, the arteries recoil and regain their original shape. This recoil squeezes down on the stored blood and pushes it forward toward the tissues. Therefore, blood flow is continuous during ventricular systole and diastole.

Bibliography

1. Berne, R.M. and Levy, M.N., *Cardiovascular Physiology*, 8th ed., C.V. Mosby, St. Louis, 2001.
2. Du Pont Pharma, *Introduction to Nuclear Cardiology*, 3rd ed., Du Pont Pharma Radiopharmaceuticals, 1993.
3. Guyton, A.C. and Hall, J.E., *Textbook of Medical Physiology*, 10th ed., W.B. Saunders, Philadelphia, 2000.
4. Lilly, L.S., *Pathophysiology of Heart Disease*, Lea & Febiger, Malvern, PA, 1993, chaps. 11 and 17.
5. Rhoades, R. and Pflanzer, R., *Human Physiology*, Thomson Learning, Pacific Grove, CA, 2003.
6. Rodin, D.M., Antiarrhythmic drugs, in *Goodman and Gilman's: The Pharmacological Basis of Therapeutics*, 9th ed., Hardman, J.G. and Limbird, L.E., Eds., McGraw–Hill, New York, 1996, chap. 35.
7. Sherwood, L., *Human Physiology from Cells to Systems*, 3rd ed., Brooks/Cole, Pacific Grove, CA, 2001.
8. Silverthorn, D.U., *Human Physiology: An Integrated Approach*, 2nd ed., Prentice-Hall, Upper Saddle River, NJ, 2001.
9. Smith, E.R., Pathophysiology of cardiac electrical disturbances, in *Physiopathology of the Cardiovascular System*, Alpert, J.S., Ed., Little, Brown, Boston, 1984, chap. 14.

chapter fourteen

Cardiac output

Study objectives

- Describe the factors that determine cardiac output
- Distinguish among cardiac output, cardiac reserve, and cardiac index
- Discuss the factors that control heart rate
- Distinguish between the terms chronotropic and inotropic
- Discuss the factors that control stroke volume
- Distinguish between preload and afterload
- Describe the Frank–Starling law of the heart
- Understand how the cardiac function curve is generated
- Explain the mechanism of action of diuretics in congestive heart failure and hypertension
- Define ejection fraction
- Describe how cardiac output varies in a sedentary individual vs. an endurance-trained athlete

14.1 Introduction

The primary function of the heart is to deliver a sufficient volume of blood (oxygen and nutrients, etc.) to the tissues so that they may carry out their functions effectively. As the metabolic activity of a tissue varies, so will its need for blood. An important factor involved in meeting this demand is *cardiac output (CO)* or the volume of blood pumped into the aorta per minute. Cardiac output is determined by heart rate multiplied by stroke volume:

Cardiac output (CO) = heart rate (HR) × stroke volume (SV)

An average adult at rest may have a heart rate of 70 beats per minute and a stroke volume of 70 ml per beat. In this case, the cardiac output would be:

CO = 70 beats/min × 70 ml/beat = 4900 ml/min ≈ 5 l/min

Table 14.1 Factors Affecting Cardiac Output

Heart rate
Autonomic nervous system
Catecholamines (epinephrine and norepinephrine)
Body temperature

Stroke volume
Length of diastole
Venous return (preload)
Contractility of the myocardium
Afterload
Heart rate

Miscellaneous
Activity level
Body size
Age

This is approximately equal to the total blood volume in the body. Therefore, the entire blood volume is pumped by the heart each minute.

Many factors are involved in determining cardiac output in a given individual (see Table 14.1):

- Activity level
- Body size
- Age

A primary determinant is the *level of activity* of the body. During intense exercise in an average sedentary person, cardiac output may increase to 18 to 20 l/min. In a trained athlete, the increase in cardiac output is even greater and may be as much as 30 to 35 l/min. *Cardiac reserve* is the difference between the cardiac output at rest and the maximum volume of blood that the heart is capable of pumping per minute. The effect of endurance training is to increase cardiac reserve significantly so that a greater volume of blood can be pumped to the working muscles. In this way, exercise performance is maximized and muscle fatigue is delayed. On the other hand, patients with heart conditions such as congestive heart failure or mitral valve stenosis are not able to increase their cardiac output as much, if at all, during exercise. Therefore, these patients are forced to limit their level of exertion as the disease process progresses.

The *size of the body* is another factor that determines cardiac output. Healthy young men have a cardiac output of about 5.5 to 6.0 l/min; the cardiac output in women averages 4.5 to 5.0 l/min. This difference does not involve gender per se, but rather the mass of body tissue that must be perfused with blood. *Cardiac index* normalizes cardiac output for body size and is calculated by the cardiac output per square meter of body surface

area. An average person weighing 70 kg has a body surface area of approximately 1.7 square meters. Therefore:

$$\text{Cardiac index} = 5 \text{ l/min} \div 1.7 \text{ m}^2 = 3 \text{ l/min/m}^2$$

Cardiac output also varies with *age*. Expressed as cardiac index, it rapidly
rises to a peak of more than 4 l/min/m² at age 10 and then steadily declines
to about 2.4 l/min/m² at the age of 80. This decrease in cardiac output is a
function of overall metabolic activity and therefore indicative of declining
activity with age.

14.2 Control of heart rate

Heart rate varies considerably, depending upon a number of variables. In
normal adults at rest, the typical average heart rate is about 70 beats per
minute; however, in children the resting heart rate is much greater. Heart
rate will increase substantially (greater than 100 beats per minute) during
emotional excitement and exercise and will decrease by 10 to 20 beats per
minute during sleep. In endurance-trained athletes, the resting heart rate
may be 50 beats per minute or lower. This condition, referred to as *training-induced bradycardia*, is beneficial because it reduces the workload of the
heart. Chronotropism refers to changes in the heart rate. A factor resulting
in a *positive chronotropic effect* is one that increases heart rate and a factor
resulting in a *negative chronotropic effect* decreases heart rate. In this section,
three factors that control heart rate will be discussed:

- Autonomic nervous system influence
- Catecholamines
- Body temperature

The *autonomic nervous system* exerts the primary control on heart rate.
Because the sympathetic and parasympathetic systems have antagonistic
effects on the heart, heart rate at any given moment results from the balance
or sum of their inputs. The SA node, which is the pacemaker of the heart
that determines the rate of spontaneous depolarization, and the AV node are
innervated by the sympathetic and parasympathetic systems. The specialized ventricular conduction pathway and ventricular muscle are innervated
by the sympathetic system only.

Sympathetic stimulation increases heart rate. Norepinephrine, the neurotransmitter released from sympathetic nerves, binds to the β-adrenergic
receptors in the heart and causes the following effects:

- Increased rate of discharge of the SA node
- Increased rate of conduction through the AV node
- Increased rate of conduction through the bundle of His and the
  Purkinje fibers

The mechanism of these effects involves enhanced depolarization of these cells due to decreased potassium permeability and increased sodium and calcium permeability. With fewer K$^+$ ions leaving the cell and with more Na$^+$ and Ca^{++} ions entering the cell, the inside of the cell becomes less negative and approaches threshold more rapidly. In this way, action potentials are generated faster and travel through the conduction pathway more quickly so that the heart can generate more heartbeats per minute (see Figure 14.1).

Parasympathetic stimulation decreases heart rate. Acetylcholine, the neurotransmitter released from the vagus nerve (the parasympathetic nerve to the heart), binds to muscarinic receptors and causes the following effects:

- Decreased rate of discharge of the SA node
- Decreased rate of conduction through the AV node

The mechanism of these effects involves the increased permeability to potassium. The enhanced efflux of K$^+$ ions has two effects on the action potential of the SA node. First, the cells become hyperpolarized so that the membrane potential is further away from threshold (from a normal resting potential of –55 mV down toward –65 mV). As a result, greater depolarization is now needed to reach threshold and generate an action potential. Second, the rate of depolarization during the pacemaker potential is reduced. The outward movement of positively charged K$^+$ ions opposes the depolarizing effect of Na$^+$- and Ca^{++}-ion influx. In this way, action potentials are generated more slowly and fewer heartbeats are generated per minute (see Figure 14.1).

At rest, the parasympathetic system exerts the predominant effect on the SA node and therefore on heart rate. In a denervated heart, such as a trans-

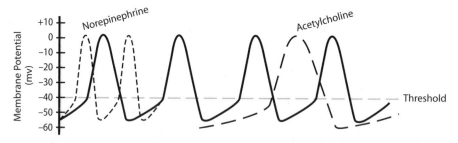

Figure 14.1 Effect of autonomic nervous system stimulation on action potentials of the sinoatrial (SA) node. A normal action potential generated by the SA node under resting conditions is represented by the solid line; the positive chronotropic effect (increased heart rate) of norepinephrine released from sympathetic nerve fibers is illustrated by the short dashed line; and the negative chronotropic effect (decreased heart rate) of acetylcholine released from parasympathetic nerve fibers is illustrated by the long dashed line.

planted heart, the resting heart rate is 100 beats per minute. This indicates that the SA node, without any input from the autonomic nervous system, has an inherent rate of depolarization of 100 beats per minute. However, the intact or fully innervated heart generates only 70 beats per minute. Therefore, it is evident that the rate of spontaneous discharge by the SA node is suppressed by the influence of the parasympathetic system. In contrast, the sympathetic system dominates during exercise. Maximal heart rate during intense exercise is approximately 195 beats per minute in all individuals, regardless of exercise training.

The second factor that exerts control on heart rate is the release of the *catecholamines*, epinephrine and norepinephrine, from the adrenal medulla. Circulating catecholamines have the same effect on heart rate as direct sympathetic stimulation, which is to increase heart rate. In fact, in the intact heart, the effect of the catecholamines serves to supplement this direct effect. In a denervated heart, circulating catecholamines serve to replace the effect of direct sympathetic stimulation. In this way, patients who have had a heart transplant may still increase their heart rate during exercise.

Body temperature also affects heart rate by altering the rate of discharge of the SA node. An increase of 1°F in body temperature results in an increase in heart rate of about 10 beats per minute. Therefore, the increase in body temperature during a fever or that which accompanies exercise serves to increase heart rate and, as a result, cardiac output. This enhanced pumping action of the heart delivers more blood to the tissues and supports the increased metabolic activity associated with these conditions.

14.3 Control of stroke volume

Many factors contribute to the regulation of stroke volume. Factors discussed in this section include:

- Length of diastole
- Venous return (preload)
- Contractility of the myocardium
- Afterload
- Heart rate

Two important concepts to keep in mind throughout this discussion are that (1) the heart can only pump what it gets; and (2) a healthy heart pumps all of the blood returned to it. The SA node may generate a heartbeat and cause the ventricles to contract; however, these chambers must be properly filled with blood in order for this activity to be effective. On the other hand, the volume of blood that returns to the heart per minute may vary considerably. The heart has an intrinsic ability to alter its strength of contraction in order to accommodate these changes in volume.

Diastole is the period in the cardiac cycle in which relaxation of the myocardium and ventricular filling take place. In an individual with a resting heart rate of 75 beats per minute, the length of the cardiac cycle is 0.8 sec and the length of ventricular diastole is 0.5 sec. As mentioned in the previous chapter, the end-diastolic volume is approximately 130 ml and the resulting stroke volume is about 70 ml. Consider a case in which the heart rate is increased. Given that cardiac output is determined by heart rate multiplied by stroke volume, an increase in either of these variables should result in an increase in cardiac output.

In general, this is quite true; however, the effect of increased heart rate on cardiac output is limited by its effect on the length of diastole. As heart rate increases, the length of the cardiac cycle and therefore the length of diastole or the time for filling will decrease. At very high heart rates, this may result in a decrease in ventricular filling or end-diastolic volume; a decrease in stroke volume; and a decrease in cardiac output. Once again, "the heart can only pump what it gets." If time for filling is inadequate, then despite an increase in heart rate, cardiac output will actually decrease. This explains why the maximal heart rate during exercise is about 195 beats per minute in all individuals. Beyond this rate, the ventricles are unable to fill with blood properly and the positive effect of increased heart rate on cardiac output is lost.

Venous return is defined as the volume of blood returned to the right atrium per minute. Assuming a constant heart rate and therefore a constant length of diastole, an increase in venous return, or the rate of blood flow into the heart, will increase ventricular filling, end-diastolic volume, stroke volume, and cardiac output. Ventricular blood volume prior to contraction is also referred to as *preload*. Once again, "a healthy heart pumps all of the blood returned to it." In fact, cardiac output is equal to venous return. The heart has an inherent, self-regulating mechanism by which it can alter its force of contraction based upon the volume of blood that flows into it. This *intrinsic mechanism*, the *Frank–Starling law of the heart*, states that when ventricular filling is increased, this increased volume of blood stretches the walls of these chambers and, as a result, the ventricles contract more forcefully. The stronger contraction results in a larger stroke volume.

This concept is illustrated by the *cardiac function curve* (see Figure 14.2). As end-diastolic volume increases, stroke volume and therefore cardiac output increase. This phenomenon is based on the length–tension relationship of cardiac muscle. Recall in the discussion of skeletal muscle in Chapter 11 that the resting length of the sarcomere determines the amount of tension generated by the muscle upon stimulation. Due to their attachments to the bones, the resting lengths of skeletal muscles do not vary greatly. Therefore, the sarcomeres are normally at their optimal length of 2.2 μm, resulting in maximal tension development. At this point, the overlap of the actin and myosin filaments in the sarcomere is such that the greatest amount of cross-bridge cycling to generate tension takes place. The myocardium of the heart, however, is not limited by attachment to any bones. Therefore, the resting length of the sarcomeres of these muscle cells may vary substantially due to changes in ventricular filling.

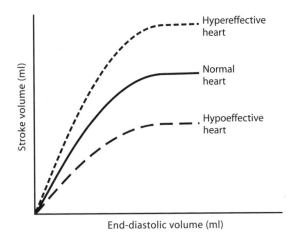

Figure 14.2 Cardiac function curve. This curve illustrates the stroke volume pumped by the heart for a given end-diastolic volume within the ventricle. As ventricular filling (end-diastolic volume) increases, stroke volume increases. Factors causing a positive inotropic effect (increased contractility) result in greater stroke volume for a given amount of filling compared to the normal heart. This "hypereffective" heart is illustrated by the short dashed line shifted to the left of that of the normal heart. Factors causing a negative inotropic effect (decreased contractility) result in reduced stroke volume for a given amount of filling. This "hypoeffective" heart is illustrated by the long dashed line shifted to the right of that of the normal heart.

Interestingly, at a normal resting end-diastolic volume of 130 ml, the amount of ventricular filling and resting cardiac muscle fiber length is *less than the optimal length*. Therefore, as filling increases, muscle fibers and their component sarcomeres are stretched and move closer to the optimal length for crossbridge cycling and tension development. This results in a stronger ventricular contraction and an increase in stroke volume. In other words, a healthy heart operates on the ascending portion of the cardiac function curve, so an increase in preload results in an increase in stroke volume.

Pharmacy application: diuretics and cardiac output

Diuretics are a group of therapeutic agents designed to reduce the volume of body fluids. Their mechanism of action is at the level of the kidney and involves an increase in the excretion of Na^+ and Cl^- ions and, consequently, an increase in urine production. As discussed in Chapter 2, sodium is the predominant extracellular cation and, due to its osmotic effects, a primary determinant of extracellular fluid volume. Therefore, if more sodium is excreted in the urine, then more water is also lost, thus reducing the volume of extracellular fluids including the plasma.

As plasma volume decreases, less blood is available for ventricular filling.

It is this reduction in preload that, in some cases, is beneficial to patients experiencing heart failure or hypertension. Unlike a healthy heart, a failing heart is unable to pump all of the blood returned to it. Instead, the blood dams up and overfills the chambers of the heart. This results in congestion and increased pressures in the heart and venous system and the formation of peripheral edema. Because the failing heart is operating on the flat portion of a depressed cardiac function curve (see Figure 14.2), treatment with diuretics will relieve the congestion and edema, but have little effect on stroke volume and cardiac output.

Hypertension (blood pressure >140/90 mmHg) may be caused by an elevation in cardiac output or excessive vasoconstriction. Diuretics are used in these patients to reduce cardiac output. Assume that the hearts of these individuals are operating on the ascending portion of the cardiac function curve. As the plasma volume is reduced in response to treatment with diuretic drugs, venous return and preload are reduced, as are ventricular filling and stroke volume, and cardiac output, thus bringing blood pressure back within the normal range.

Stimulation of the ventricular myocardium by the sympathetic system will also increase stroke volume by increasing *contractility* of the muscle. At any given end-diastolic volume, norepinephrine released from the sympathetic nerves to the heart will cause a more forceful contraction resulting in the ejection of more blood from the ventricles or an increase in stroke volume and in cardiac output (see Figure 14.2). In other words, the cardiac function curve shifts to the left. Epinephrine released from the adrenal medulla has the same effect on contractility as direct sympathetic stimulation. The mechanism involves the stimulation of β-adrenergic receptors and the subsequent increase in permeability to calcium. An increase in intracellular calcium results in increased crossbridge cycling and greater tension development. Sympathetic stimulation, circulating catecholamines, or any other factor that increases contractility has a *positive inotropic effect* on the heart. Therapeutic agents, such as β-adrenergic receptor blockers and calcium channel blockers that inhibit calcium influx and therefore contractility, have a *negative inotropic effect*.

The contractility of the myocardium determines the *ejection fraction* of the heart, which is the ratio of the volume of blood ejected from the left ventricle per beat (stroke volume) to the volume of blood in the left ventricle at the end of diastole (end-diastolic volume):

$$\text{Ejection fraction} = SV \div EDV$$

Under normal resting conditions in which the end-diastolic volume is 120 to 130 ml and the stroke volume is 70 ml/beat, the ejection fraction is 55 to 60%:

Ejection fraction = 70 ml/beat ÷ 120ml = 58%

During exercise when sympathetic stimulation to the heart is increased, the ejection fraction may increase to more than 80% resulting in greater stroke volume and cardiac output.

Another factor determining cardiac performance is *afterload*, or the pressure in the artery leading from the ventricle. When the ventricle contracts, it must develop a pressure greater than that in the associated artery in order to push open the semilunar valve and eject the blood (see Chapter 13). Typically, diastolic blood pressure in the aorta is 80 mmHg; therefore, the left ventricle must develop a pressure slightly greater than 80 mmHg to open the aortic valve and eject the stroke volume. A dynamic exercise such as running may cause only a small increase in diastolic pressure (up to 90 mmHg), although a resistance exercise such as weight lifting, which has a much greater impact on blood pressure and diastolic pressure, may be as high as 150 to 160 mmHg.

A healthy heart can easily contract vigorously enough to overcome any increases in afterload associated with exercise or other types of physical exertion. In contrast, however, a diseased heart or one weakened by advanced age may not be able to generate enough force to overcome a significantly elevated afterload effectively. In this case, stroke volume and cardiac output would be reduced. In addition, a sustained or chronic increase in afterload, as observed in patients with hypertension, will also have a detrimental effect on cardiac workload. Initially, the left ventricle will hypertrophy and chamber walls will become thicker and stronger to compensate for this excess workload. However, eventually the balance between the oxygen supply and oxygen demand of the heart is disrupted, leading to decreased stroke volume, decreased cardiac output, and heart failure.

Changes in *heart rate* also affect the contractility of the heart. As heart rate increases, so does ventricular contractility. The mechanism of this effect involves the gradual increase of intracellular calcium. When the electrical impulse stimulates the myocardial cell, permeability to calcium is increased and calcium enters the cell, allowing it to contract. Between beats, the calcium is removed from the intracellular fluid and the muscle relaxes. When heart rate is increased, periods of calcium influx occur more frequently and time for calcium removal is reduced. The net effect is an increase in intracellular calcium, an increased number of crossbridges' cycling, and an increase in tension development.

Pharmacy application: cardiac glycosides and cardiac output

A patient is considered to be in heart failure when cardiac output is insufficient to meet the metabolic demands of his body. The most effective method to improve cardiac output is to enhance myocardial contractility, which will increase stroke volume. Because of their positive inotropic effect, the cardiac glycosides, including digoxin, have been used for many years to treat heart failure. Digoxin binds to and inhibits the Na^+–K^+ ATPase in the myocardial cell membrane, ultimately leading to an increase in the intracellular concentration of calcium. As described previously, any increase in calcium will increase myocardial contractility, stroke volume, and cardiac output.

14.4 Effect of exercise on cardiac output

Endurance training such as running alters the baseline or tonic activity of the sympathetic and parasympathetic systems. In a trained athlete, dominance of the parasympathetic system is even greater than it is in a sedentary individual, resulting in training-induced bradycardia. Although the resting heart rate is 70 to 75 beats/min in a sedentary person, in a trained athlete it may be 50 beats/min or lower. Due to the decrease in heart rate in these individuals, the length of diastole is increased. Assuming a constant rate of venous return, this longer filling period results in a greater end-diastolic volume and an increased stroke volume (40 to 50% greater in the elite athlete compared to the untrained individual). Therefore, at rest when their bodies' metabolic demands are similar, cardiac output in a sedentary person and an athlete is also similar (see Table 14.2).

During exercise, cardiac output increases substantially to meet increased metabolic demand of the working muscles. However, endurance training results in significantly greater increases in cardiac output, which improves oxygen and nutrient delivery to the working muscles (18 to 20 l/min in sedentary individuals; 30 to 35 l/min in trained athletes). As a result, exercise performance is enhanced and fatigue is delayed.

In order to increase cardiac output, heart rate and stroke volume are increased. The maximum heart rate in all individuals is about 195 beats/min; therefore, the difference in cardiac output in trained vs. untrained people during exercise involves stroke volume. This volume increases approximately 50 to 60% during exercise. Because the athlete has a much larger stroke volume at rest, the increase in stroke volume during exercise is that much greater (see Table 14.2). In this way, even with a similar maximal heart rate, the endurance-trained athlete pumps a significantly greater volume of blood per minute. In order to accommodate these larger stroke volumes, the ventricles of these athletes hypertrophy such that the chambers become larger and increase their diameters.

Table 14.2 Effect of Exercise on Cardiac Output

	Sedentary individual	Endurance-trained athlete
Rest		
Heart rate	71 beats/min	50 beats/min
Stroke volume	70 ml/beat	100 ml/beat
Cardiac output	5000 ml/min	5000 ml/min
Exercise		
Heart rate	195 beats/min	195 beats/min
Stroke volume	1000 ml/beat	160 ml/beat
Cardiac output	19,500 ml/min	31,200 ml/min

Bibliography

1. Berne, R.M. and Levy, M.N., *Cardiovascular Physiology*, 8th ed., C.V. Mosby, St. Louis, 2001.
2. Guyton, A.C. and Hall, J.E., *Textbook of Medical Physiology*, 10th ed., W.B. Saunders, Philadelphia, 2000.
3. Jackson, E.K., Diuretics, in *Goodman and Gilman's: The Pharmacological Basis of Therapeutics*, 9th ed., Hardman, J.G. and Limbird, L.E., Eds., McGraw–Hill, New York, 1996, chap. 29.
4. Kelly, R.A. and Smith, T.W., Pharmacological treatment of heart failure, in *Goodman and Gilman's: The Pharmacological Basis of Therapeutics*, 9th ed., Hardman, J.G. and Limbird, L.E., Eds., McGraw–Hill, New York, 1996, chap. 34.
5. McArdle, W.D., Katch, F.I., and Katch, V.L., *Exercise Physiology: Energy, Nutrition, and Human Performance*, 4th ed., Williams & Wilkins, Baltimore, 1996.
6. Oates, J.A., Antihypertensive agents and the drug therapy of hypertension, in *Goodman and Gilman's: The Pharmacological Basis of Therapeutics*, 9th ed., Hardman, J.G. and Limbird, L.E., Eds., McGraw–Hill, New York, 1996, chap. 33.
7. Rhoades, R. and Pflanzer, R., *Human Physiology*, Thomson Learning, Pacific Grove, CA, 2003.
8. Rowell, L.B., *Human Cardiovascular Control*, Oxford University Press, New York, 1993.
9. Sherwood, L., *Human Physiology from Cells to Systems*, 4th ed., Brooks/Cole, Pacific Grove, CA, 2001.
10. Silverthorn, D.U., *Human Physiology: An Integrated Approach*, 2nd ed., Prentice-Hall, Upper Saddle River, NJ, 2001.
11. *Taber's Cyclopedic Medical Dictionary*, 19th ed., F.A. Davis Co., Philadelphia, 2001.
12. Urban, N. and Porth, C.M., Heart failure and circulatory shock, in *Pathophysiology: Concepts of Altered Health States*, 5th ed., Porth, C.M., Ed., Lippincott–Raven Publishers, Philadelphia, 1998, chap. 20.

chapter fifteen

The circulatory system

Study objectives

- List the functions of the circulatory system
- Describe how the volume of blood flow to individual tissues differs according to specific tissue function
- Explain the function of each component of the blood vessel wall
- Distinguish among arteries, arterioles, capillaries, and veins in terms of their anatomical characteristics and their functions
- Distinguish among diastolic pressure, systolic pressure, and pulse pressure
- Understand the method by which mean arterial pressure is calculated
- Describe how blood pressure changes as blood flows through the circulatory system
- Understand Ohm's law and describe the relationship among blood flow, blood pressure, and vascular resistance
- List the factors that affect vascular resistance and explain their physiological significance
- Explain why mean arterial pressure must be closely regulated
- Explain how the autonomic nervous system alters cardiac output, total peripheral resistance, and therefore mean arterial pressure
- List sources of input to the vasomotor center
- Describe the mechanism of action and physiological significance of the baroreceptor reflex, chemoreceptor reflex, and low-pressure reflex
- Indicate the source, factors regulating the release, and physiological significance of the following vasoconstrictors: catecholamines, angiotensin II, vasopressin, endothelin, and thromboxane A_2
- Indicate the source, factors regulating the release, and physiological significance of the following vasodilators: prostacyclin, nitric oxide, and atrial natriuretic peptide
- Compare and contrast the compliance of systemic arteries and systemic veins
- List specific blood reservoirs and their common characteristics

- Explain how blood volume, sympathetic stimulation of the veins, skeletal muscle activity, and respiratory activity influence venous return
- Describe the effects of gravity on the circulatory system
- Describe the mechanism of active hyperemia
- Define autoregulation of blood flow
- Explain how the myogenic mechanism causes autoregulation of blood flow
- Describe effects of acute exercise on the circulatory system
- Explain how blood flow through capillaries is regulated by vasomotion
- Describe the physiological significance of the Starling principle
- Explain how hydrostatic forces and osmotic forces regulate the bulk flow of fluid across the capillary wall
- Describe the four general conditions that can lead to edema formation

15.1 Introduction

The *circulatory system* carries out many important functions that contribute to homeostasis. It obtains oxygen from the lungs; nutrients from the gastrointestinal tract; and hormones from the endocrine glands; and it delivers these substances to the tissues that need them. Furthermore, it removes metabolic waste products, such as carbon dioxide, lactic acid, and urea, from the tissues. Finally, it contributes to the actions of the immune system by transporting antibodies and leukocytes to areas of infection. Overall, the circulatory system plays a vital role in maintenance of optimal conditions for cell and tissue function.

All tissues are *perfused*, that is, all tissues receive blood flow. The amount of blood that flows through each tissue, however, depends upon that tissue's function. For example, many tissues, such as the heart, brain, and skeletal muscles, receive blood flow sufficient to supply their metabolic needs. When metabolic activity increases, as it does during exercise, blood flow to these tissues increases accordingly. Other tissues, however, receive blood flow in significant excess of their metabolic needs. These tissues, including the kidneys, organs of the digestive system, and skin, have important homeostatic functions. Among other vital activities, kidneys filter the blood and remove waste products; the organs of the digestive system absorb nutrients into the blood; and thermoregulation involves control of blood flow to the body surface where heat can be eliminated.

These functions are carried out most effectively and efficiently when the involved tissues receive an abundant blood flow. Under normal resting conditions, the kidneys, which account for only 1% of the body's weight, receive 20% of the cardiac output (CO); the gastrointestinal tract receives approximately 27% of the CO; and the skin receives 6 to 15% of the blood pumped by the heart per minute. Because these tissues receive more blood than they need to support metabolic activity, they can easily tolerate a sustained decrease in blood flow. During exercise, when the metabolic demand of the working skeletal muscles and the heart increases substantially, blood flow is directed away from the kidneys and organs of the digestive system and toward the skeletal and cardiac muscles.

15.2 Blood vessels

The walls of blood vessels may contain varying amounts of fibrous tissue, elastic tissue, and smooth muscle. All blood vessels are lined with a single layer of endothelial cells forming the endothelium. The *fibrous connective tissue* provides structural support and stiffens the vessel. The *elastic connective tissue* allows vessels to expand and hold more blood. It also allows the vessels to recoil and exert pressure on blood within the vessels, which pushes this blood forward. Most blood vessels contain *smooth muscle* arranged in circular or spiral layers. Therefore, contraction of vascular smooth muscle, or *vasoconstriction*, narrows the diameter of the vessel and decreases the flow of blood through it. Relaxation of vascular smooth muscle, or *vasodilation*, widens the diameter of the vessel and increases the flow of blood through it. The smooth muscle of the vessel is innervated by the autonomic nervous system and is, therefore, physiologically regulated. Furthermore, this is where endogenous vasoactive substances and pharmacological agents exert their effects. The *endothelium* has several important physiological functions, including contributing to the regulation of blood pressure, blood vessel growth, and the exchange of materials between blood and the interstitial fluid of the tissues.

The circulatory system is composed of several anatomically and functionally distinct blood vessels including: (1) arteries, (2) arterioles, (3) capillaries, and (4) veins.

Arteries carry blood away from the heart (see Figure 15.1). These vessels contain fibrous connective tissue that strengthens them and enables them to withstand the high blood pressures generated by the heart. In general, the arteries function as a system of *conduits*, or pipes, transporting the blood under high pressure toward the tissues. There is little smooth muscle and therefore little physiological regulation of vessel diameter in these vessels.

Another noteworthy anatomical feature of the arteries is the presence of elastic connective tissue. When the heart contracts and ejects the blood, a portion of the stroke volume flows toward the capillaries. However, much of the stroke volume ejected during systole is retained in the distensible arteries. When the heart relaxes, the arteries recoil and exert pressure on the blood within them, forcing this "stored" blood to flow forward. In this way, a steady flow of blood toward the capillaries is maintained throughout the entire cardiac cycle.

As the arteries travel toward the peripheral organs and tissues, they branch and become smaller. Furthermore, the walls of the vessels become less elastic and more muscular. The smallest arterial vessels, *arterioles*, are composed almost entirely of smooth muscle with a lining of endothelium.

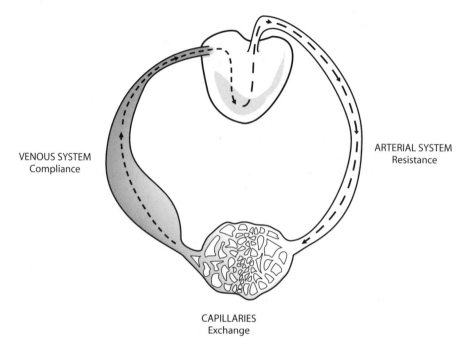

VENOUS SYSTEM
Compliance

ARTERIAL SYSTEM
Resistance

CAPILLARIES
Exchange

Figure 15.1 The circulatory system. Arteries carry blood away from the heart. The smallest arterial vessels, the arterioles, are composed mainly of smooth muscle and are the major resistance vessels in the circuit. The capillaries are the site of exchange between blood and tissues. Veins carry blood back toward the heart. The small veins are the major compliance vessels in the circuit and, under resting conditions, contain 64% of the blood volume.

Therefore, depending upon the degree of constriction of the vascular smooth muscle, these vessels may alter their diameter, and consequently their blood flow, across a very wide range. For this reason, the arterioles are the major *resistance vessels* in the circulatory system. In fact, the primary function of arterioles is to regulate the distribution of the cardiac output and to determine which tissues receive more blood and which receive less, depending upon the tissue's and the body's needs.

From the arterioles, blood flows through *capillaries*, the smallest vessels in the circulatory system. The capillaries are the *site of exchange* between blood and the interstitial fluid surrounding the cells of the tissues. The primary mechanism of exchange is simple diffusion as substances move across the capillary walls "down" their concentration gradients, or from an area of high concentration to an area of low concentration. Two important factors influencing the process of diffusion include surface area and thickness of the barrier. As the surface area increases, so does diffusion. Approximately 10 billion capillaries are in the adult human body with a total exchange surface area of more than 6300 square meters — the equivalent of almost two football fields. Furthermore, most tissue cells are not more than 20 µm away from the nearest capillary. The capillaries also have the thinnest walls of all the blood vessels; they are composed of only a flat layer of endothelium, one cell thick, supported by a thin acellular matrix referred to as the *basement membrane*, with a total thickness of only 0.5 µm. As such, the anatomical characteristics of the capillaries, which maximize the exchange surface area and minimize the thickness of the barrier, render these vessels ideally suited for the exchange of materials by simple diffusion.

Following the exchange of substances with the tissues, blood begins its route back to the heart through the venous system. Blood flows from the capillaries into the *venules*, small vessels consisting mainly of a layer of endothelium and fibrous connective tissue. From the venules, the blood flows into *veins* that become larger as they travel toward the heart. As with the arteries, the walls of these vessels consist of a layer of endothelium, elastic connective tissue, smooth muscle, and fibrous connective tissue. However, veins have much thinner walls and wider diameters than the arteries they accompany. These vessels are very distensible and are capable of holding large volumes of blood at a very low pressure. For this reason, the veins are the major *compliance vessels* of the circulatory system (see Figure 15.1). In fact, approximately 64% of the blood volume is contained within the veins under resting conditions. During exercise, the pumping action of the contracting skeletal muscles and the smooth muscle in the walls of the veins forces this blood toward the heart and increases venous return. Therefore, the veins are referred to as *blood reservoirs* and play an important role in regulation of venous return and, consequently, cardiac output.

Another important anatomical characteristic of veins is the presence of *valves*, which ensure the one-way flow of blood back toward the heart. They are most abundant in the lower limbs, where the effects of gravity on the circulatory system are most prevalent and would tend to cause pooling of blood in the feet and ankles. Finally, the large veins and the *venae cavae* return blood to the right atrium of the heart. As with the large arteries and aorta, these vessels function primarily as conduits. There is little smooth muscle and therefore little physiological regulation of their diameter.

15.3 Blood pressure throughout systemic circulation

The pressure generated by left ventricular contraction is the driving force for the flow of blood through the entire systemic circulation, from the aorta all of the way back to the right atrium. The mean pressure in the aorta and large arteries is typically very high (90 to 100 mmHg) due to the continual addition of blood to the system by the pumping action of the heart. However, this pressure is *pulsatile*; in other words, it fluctuates because of the alternating contraction and relaxation phases of the cardiac cycle. In a healthy resting adult, *systolic pressure* is approximately 120 mmHg and *diastolic pressure* is approximately 80 mmHg (see Figure 15.2). The *pulse pressure* is the difference between the systolic and diastolic pressures:

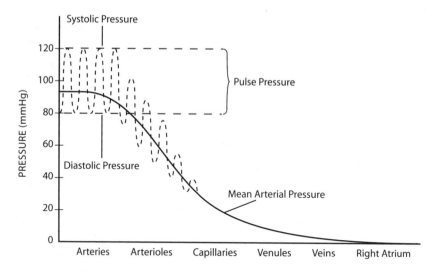

Figure 15.2 Pressures throughout the systemic circulation. At rest, blood pressure in the aorta and the other large arteries fluctuates between a low pressure of 80 mmHg during diastole and a high pressure of 120 mmHg during systole. The difference between diastolic and systolic pressure is the pulse pressure. Mean arterial pressure in these arteries is approximately 93 mmHg. As the blood continues forward and flows through the arterioles, the pulse pressure is dampened. Because of the high resistance to blood flow in these vessels, the overall pressure drops dramatically. Furthermore, fluctuations between diastolic and systolic pressure are eliminated so that the blood pressure becomes nonpulsatile. Blood pressure continues to decline, although at a slower rate, as blood flows through the capillaries and veins back toward the heart.

Systolic pressure – diastolic pressure = pulse pressure

Therefore, using the average values of 120 mmHg (systolic) and 80 mmHg (diastolic), the pulse pressure is 40 mmHg:

120 mmHg – 80 mmHg = 40 mmHg

The *mean arterial pressure (MAP)* is calculated as follows:

MAP = diastolic pressure + 1/3 (pulse pressure)

Therefore, using these same values, the MAP is 93 mmHg:

MAP = 80 mmHg + 1/3 (40 mmHg)

At rest, the MAP is closer to the diastolic pressure because the diastolic phase of the cardiac cycle lasts almost twice as long as the systolic phase. During exercise when heart rate increases and the length of diastole decreases, systolic pressure contributes more to the MAP.

As blood flows through the rest of the system, pressure continually falls (see Figure 15.2). Furthermore, the pulsatile nature of blood pressure is lost as blood flows through the arterioles. The pulse pressure is damped out by the considerable resistance offered to blood flow by the arterioles. At the arteriolar end of the capillaries, the blood pressure is 30 to 35 mmHg; at the venular end, the capillary pressure is approximately 10 mmHg. It is important that capillary pressure remain low so as to avoid leakage of fluid out of the capillaries into the tissues. Venous pressure is approximately 6 to 8 mmHg and pressure in the right atrium is close to zero.

15.4 Blood flow through a vessel

The *flow of blood through a vessel* is determined by two factors:

- Pressure gradient
- Vascular resistance

The relationship among blood flow (Q, ml/min), the pressure gradient (ΔP, mmHg), and vascular resistance (R, mmHg/ml/min) is described by *Ohm's law*:

$$Q = \frac{\Delta P}{R}$$

The *pressure gradient* is the difference between the pressure at the beginning of a blood vessel and the pressure at the end. The inflow pressure is always greater than the outflow pressure because substances, including blood and air, must flow "down" their pressure gradients; in other words, from an area of higher pressure to an area of lower pressure. The inflow pressure is initially generated by the contraction of the heart. As discussed previously, blood pressure falls continuously as the blood flows through the circulatory system. This loss of driving pressure is due to the friction generated as the components of the flowing blood come into contact with the vessel wall as well as each other. Blood flow through a vessel is directly proportional to the pressure gradient; in other words, the greater the difference between inflow pressure and outflow pressure is, the greater the flow of blood through the vessel.

The second factor that determines the flow of blood through a vessel is *resistance*. In contrast to the pressure gradient, blood flow through a vessel is indirectly proportional to the resistance. In other words, resistance impedes or opposes blood flow. Three factors affect vascular resistance:

- Blood viscosity
- Vessel length
- Vessel radius

Viscosity describes the friction developed between the molecules of a fluid as they interact with each other during flow. More simply put, the "thicker" the fluid, then the greater its viscosity. Viscosity and resistance are directly proportional so that, as the viscosity of the fluid increases, the resistance to flow increases. In the case of blood flow through the circulatory system, erythrocytes, or red blood cells, suspended in the blood are the primary factor determining viscosity. *Hematocrit*, the percentage of the blood that consists of red blood cells, is 40 to 54% (average = 47%) for an adult male and 37 to 47% (average = 43%) for an adult female. Under normal physiological conditions, hematocrit and blood viscosity do not vary considerably within an individual. Only pathological conditions, such as chronic hypoxia, sickle cell anemia, and excess blood fibrinogen, may result in hyperviscosity and, consequently, impaired blood flow.

Friction also develops as blood contacts the vessel wall while flowing through it. Therefore, the greater the vessel surface area in contact with the blood, the greater the amount of friction developed and the greater is the resistance to blood flow. Two factors determine the vessel surface area: length of the vessel and vessel radius.

The longer the vessel, the more the blood comes into contact with the vessel wall and the greater the resistance is. However, *vessel length* in the body remains constant. Therefore, as with blood viscosity, it is not a variable factor causing changes in resistance.

The most important physiological variable determining the resistance to blood flow is *vessel radius*. A given volume of blood comes into less contact with the wall of a vessel with a large radius compared to a vessel with a small radius. Therefore, as the radius of a vessel increases, the resistance to blood flow decreases. In other words, blood flows more readily through a larger vessel than it does through a smaller vessel.

Small changes in vessel radius result in significant changes in vascular resistance and in blood flow because the resistance is inversely proportional to the fourth power of the radius:

$$R \propto 1/r^4$$

If this equation is substituted into Ohm's law, then blood flow may be calculated as follows:

$$Q = \frac{\Delta P}{1/r^4}$$

Assume two blood vessels of equal length, each has a pressure gradient of 1 mmHg. However, blood vessel *A* has a radius of 1 mm and blood vessel *B* has a radius of 2 mm. The flow of blood through vessel *A* is 1 ml/min and the flow of blood through vessel *B* is 16 ml/min. Simply doubling vessel radius causes a 16-fold increase in blood flow.

As mentioned previously, the arterioles are the major resistance vessels in the circulatory system. Because the walls of these vessels contain primarily smooth muscle, they are capable of significant changes in their radius. Therefore, regulation of blood flow to the tissues is carried out by the arterioles.

Ohm's law may be rewritten to include the three factors that affect vascular resistance: blood viscosity (η), vessel length (L), and vessel radius (r). The following equation is known as *Poiseuille's law*:

$$Q = \frac{\pi \Delta P r^4}{8\eta L}$$

15.5 Regulation of arterial pressure

Mean arterial pressure (MAP) is the driving force for blood flow through the body's organs and tissues. The MAP must be closely monitored and regulated for several reasons. It must be high enough to provide a force sufficient to propel blood through the entire systemic circuit: from the heart to the top of the head, to the tips of the toes, and back to the heart again. *Hypotension*, or a fall in blood pressure, may cause insufficient blood flow to the brain causing dizziness and, perhaps, fainting. However, *hypertension*, or blood pressure that is too high, may be detrimental to the cardiovascular system. An increase in diastolic pressure increases the afterload on the heart and increases cardiac workload. Furthermore, chronic elevation in blood pressure increases the risk of various types of vascular damage, such as atherosclerosis and the rupture of small blood vessels. Atherosclerosis will often occur in arteries that supply the heart and brain and it impairs the flow of blood to these tissues. The rupture of small blood vessels allows fluid to move from the vascular compartment into the tissues, resulting in edema formation.

Ohm's law, which correlates the effects of blood pressure and vascular resistance on blood flow through a vessel ($Q = \Delta P/R$), may also be applied to blood flow through the entire systemic circulation, or cardiac output:

$$\text{Cardiac Output} = \frac{\text{Mean Arterial Pressure}}{\text{Total Peripheral Resistance}}$$

This equation can be reorganized to determine MAP:

Mean arterial pressure = cardiac output × total peripheral resistance

Total peripheral resistance (TPR) is the resistance to blood flow offered by all systemic vessels taken together, especially by the arterioles, which are the primary resistance vessels. Therefore, MAP is regulated by cardiac activity and vascular smooth muscle tone. Any change in CO or TPR causes a change in MAP. The major factors that affect CO, TPR, and therefore MAP, are summarized in Figure 15.3, as well as in Table 15.1. These factors may be organized into several categories and will be discussed as such:

- Autonomic nervous system (ANS)
- Vasoactive substances
- Venous return
- Local metabolic activity

15.6 Autonomic nervous system

The effects of the *autonomic nervous system* on MAP are summarized in Figure 15.4. The *parasympathetic system* innervates the SA node and the AV node of the heart. The major cardiovascular effect of parasympathetic stimulation, by way of the vagus nerves, is to decrease HR, which decreases CO and MAP.

The *sympathetic system* innervates most tissues in the heart including the SA node, AV node, and ventricular muscle. Sympathetic stimulation causes an increase in HR as well as an increase in ventricular contractility, which

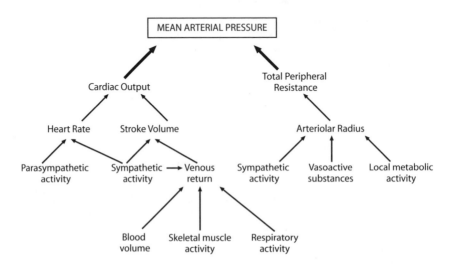

Figure 15.3 Factors that affect mean arterial pressure. Mean arterial pressure is determined by cardiac output and total peripheral resistance. Important factors that influence these two variables are summarized in this figure.

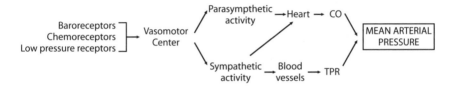

Figure 15.4 Effects of the autonomic nervous system on mean arterial pressure. The baroreceptors, chemoreceptors, and low-pressure receptors provide neural input to the vasomotor center in the brainstem. The vasomotor center integrates this input and determines the degree of discharge by the sympathetic and para-sympathetic nervous systems to the cardiovascular system. Cardiac output and total peripheral resistance are adjusted so as to maintain mean arterial pressure within the normal range.

enhances stroke volume (SV). The increases in HR and SV cause an increase in CO and therefore MAP (Figure 15.5).

The sympathetic system also innervates vascular smooth muscle and regulates the radius of the blood vessels. All types of blood vessels except capillaries are innervated; however, the most densely innervated vessels include arterioles and veins. An increase in sympathetic stimulation of vascular smooth muscle causes vasoconstriction and a decrease in stimulation causes vasodilation. Constriction of arterioles causes an increase in TPR and therefore MAP. Constriction of veins causes an increase in venous return (VR) which increases end-diastolic volume (EDV), SV (Frank–Starling law of the heart), CO, and MAP.

Sympathetic nerves are distributed to most vascular beds. They are most abundant in the renal, gastrointestinal, splenic, and cutaneous circulations. Recall that these tissues receive an abundant blood flow, more than is necessary simply to maintain metabolism. Therefore, when blood is needed by other parts of the body, such as working skeletal muscles, sympathetic vasoconstrictor activity reduces flow to the tissues receiving excess blood so that it may be redirected to the muscles. Interestingly, there is no sympathetic innervation to cerebral blood vessels. In fact, these vessels do not have α_1-adrenergic receptors, so they cannot be affected by circulating catecholamines. No physiological circumstance exists in which blood should be directed away from the brain.

Vasomotor center. Autonomic nervous activity to the cardiovascular system is regulated by the *vasomotor center* (see Figure 15.4). Located in the lower pons and the medulla of the brainstem, the vasomotor center is an integrating center for blood pressure regulation. It receives several sources of input, processes this information, and then adjusts sympathetic and parasympathetic discharge to the heart and blood vessels accordingly.

Sympathetic nerves going to the arterioles are tonically active. In other words, these nerves discharge continuously, causing *vasomotor tone*. As a result, under resting conditions, arterioles are partially constricted. This vasomotor tone is important because it helps to maintain MAP in the range

Table 15.1 Summary of Major Cardiovascular Principles

$$CO = VR$$

$$CO = HR \times SV$$

$$SV = EDV - ESV$$

$$Q = \frac{\Delta P}{R}$$

$$R \alpha \frac{1}{r^4}$$

$$Pulse\ Pressure = P_{systolic} - P_{diastolic}$$

$$MAP = P_{diastolic} + \frac{1}{3}\ (Pulse\ Pressure)$$

$$MAP = CO \times TPR$$

$$VR = \frac{P_v - P_{RA}}{R_v}$$

Notes: *CO*: cardiac output; *VR*: venous return; *HR*: heart rate; *SV*: stroke volume; *EDV*: end-diastolic volume; *ESV*: end-systolic volume; *Q*: blood flow; ΔP: pressure gradient; *R*: resistance; *r*: vessel radius; $P_{systolic}$: systolic pressure; $P_{diastolic}$: diastolic pressure; *MAP*: mean arterial pressure; *TPR*: total peripheral resistance, P_v: venous pressure; P_{RA}: right atrial pressure; R_v: venous resistance.

of 90 to 100 mmHg. Without this partial vasoconstriction of the arterioles, MAP would fall precipitously and blood flow to vital organs would be compromised. Another physiological advantage of vasomotor tone is that the degree of vasoconstriction can be increased or decreased. In this way, blood flow to the tissue can be increased or decreased. Without tone, the vessels could only constrict and blood flow to the tissue could only decrease.

Other regions of the vasomotor center transmit impulses to the heart via sympathetic nerves or the vagus nerves. An increase in sympathetic activity to the heart typically occurs concurrently with an increase in sympathetic activity to blood vessels and a decrease in vagal stimulation of the heart. Therefore, the resulting increases in CO and TPR work together to elevate MAP more effectively. Conversely, an increase in vagal stimulation of the heart typically occurs concurrently with a decrease in sympathetic activity to the heart and blood vessels. Therefore, decreases in CO and TPR work together to decrease MAP more effectively. The vasomotor center receives input from multiple sources (summarized in Table 15.2) including:

- Baroreceptors
- Chemoreceptors
- Low-pressure receptors

Table 15.2 Cardiovascular Receptors and Their Stimuli

Baroreceptors	Blood pressure
Chemoreceptors	Blood gases ($\downarrow O_2$, $\uparrow CO_2$, $\downarrow pH$)
Low-pressure receptors	Blood volume

Baroreceptors. The *baroreceptors* provide the most important source of input to the vasomotor center; these receptors monitor *blood pressure* in the systemic circulatory system. They are found in two locations: the arch of the aorta and the carotid sinuses. As the aorta exits the left ventricle, it curves over the top of the heart, forming an arch, and then descends through the thoracic and abdominal cavities. The coronary arteries, which supply the cardiac muscle, branch off the aorta in this most proximal portion of the aorta. The left and right common carotid arteries also branch off the aortic arch and ascend through the neck toward the head. Each common carotid artery bifurcates, or divides, forming an external carotid artery, which supplies the scalp, and an internal carotid artery, which supplies the brain. The carotid sinus is located at the bifurcation of each common carotid artery. Because blood flow to a tissue is dependent in large part upon blood pressure, baroreceptors are ideally located to monitor blood pressure in regions of the circulatory system responsible for delivering blood to the heart and brain, the two most vital organs in the body.

Because baroreceptors respond to stretch or distension of the blood vessel walls, they are also referred to as *stretch receptors*. A change in blood pressure will elicit the *baroreceptor reflex*, which involves *negative feedback responses* that return blood pressure to normal (see Figure 15.6). For example, an increase in blood pressure causes distension of the aorta and carotid arteries, thus stimulating the baroreceptors. As a result, the number of afferent nerve impulses transmitted to the vasomotor center increases. The vasomotor center processes this information and adjusts the activity of the autonomic nervous system accordingly. Sympathetic stimulation of vascular smooth muscle and the heart is decreased and parasympathetic stimulation of the heart is increased. As a result, venous return, CO, and TPR decrease so that MAP is decreased back toward its normal value.

On the other hand, a decrease in blood pressure causes less than normal distension or stretch of the aorta and carotid arteries and a decrease in baroreceptor stimulation. Therefore, fewer afferent nerve impulses are transmitted to the vasomotor center. The vasomotor center then alters autonomic nervous system activity so that sympathetic stimulation of vascular smooth muscle and the heart is increased and parasympathetic stimulation of the heart is decreased. As a result, venous return, CO, and TPR increase so that MAP is increased back toward its normal value. The effects are summarized in Figure 15.5.

It is important to note that the baroreceptor reflex is elicited whether blood pressure increases or decreases. Furthermore, these receptors are

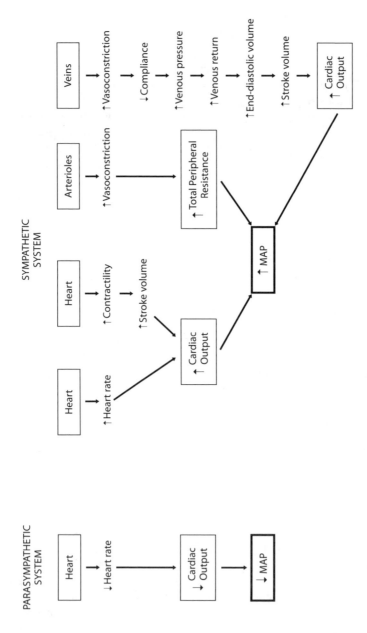

Figure 15.5 Effects of sympathetic and parasympathetic nervous activity on mean arterial pressure. The parasympathetic nervous system innervates the heart and therefore influences heart rate and cardiac output. The sympathetic nervous system innervates the heart and veins and thus influences cardiac output. This system also innervates the arterioles and therefore influences total peripheral resistance. The resulting changes in cardiac output and total peripheral resistance regulate mean arterial pressure.

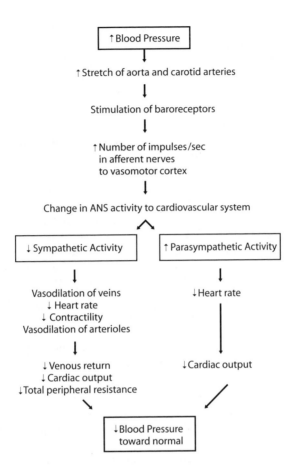

Figure 15.6 The baroreceptor reflex. Baroreceptors are the most important source of input to the vasomotor center. The reflex elicited by these receptors is essential in maintenance of normal blood pressure.

most sensitive in the normal range of blood pressures, so even a small change in MAP will alter baroreceptor, vasomotor center, and autonomic nervous system activity. As such, the baroreceptor reflex plays an important role in the short-term regulation of blood pressure. Without this reflex, changes in blood pressure in response to changes in posture, hydration (blood volume), cardiac output, regional vascular resistance, and emotional state would be far more pronounced. The baroreceptor reflex helps to minimize unintentional changes in MAP and maintain adequate blood flow to the tissues.

Chemoreceptors. The *peripheral chemoreceptors* include the *carotid bodies*, located at the bifurcation of the common carotid arteries, and the *aortic bodies*, located in the aortic arch. These receptors are stimulated by a decrease in arterial oxygen (*hypoxia*), an increase in arterial carbon dioxide (*hypercapnia*), and a decrease in arterial pH (acidosis). Therefore, as one might expect, chemoreceptors are primarily concerned with regulation of ventilation. A secondary function of these receptors is to influence MAP by providing input to the vasomotor center. A decrease in blood pressure causes a decrease in blood flow to the carotid and aortic bodies.

Assuming a constant rate of metabolism in these tissues (constant oxygen consumption as well as carbon dioxide and hydrogen ion production), then a decrease in blood flow results in hypoxia, hypercapnia, and a decrease in local pH. These conditions stimulate the chemoreceptors and cause an increase in the number of nerve impulses transmitted to the vasomotor center. The vasomotor center processes this input and adjusts activity of the autonomic nervous system accordingly. Sympathetic discharge to the cardiovascular system is increased; the predominant effect is an increase in TPR. As a result of this negative feedback mechanism, MAP is increased and blood flow to the chemoreceptors is increased toward its normal value. Interestingly, the chemoreceptor reflex does not affect the cardiovascular system until MAP decreases below 80 mmHg. Therefore, unlike the baroreceptor reflex, this reflex does not help to minimize the daily variations in MAP. Instead, it supplements activity of the baroreceptor reflex at lower pressures only.

Low-pressure receptors. The *low-pressure receptors* are located in the walls of the atria and the pulmonary arteries. Similar to baroreceptors, low-pressure receptors are also stretch receptors; however, stimulation of these receptors is caused by changes in blood volume in these low-pressure areas. An overall increase in blood volume results in an increase in venous return; an increase in the blood volume in the atria and the pulmonary arteries; and stimulation of the low-pressure receptors. These receptors then elicit reflexes by way of the vasomotor center that parallel those of baroreceptors. Because an increase in blood volume will initially increase MAP, sympathetic discharge decreases and parasympathetic discharge increases so that MAP decreases toward its normal value. The simultaneous activity of baroreceptors and low-pressure receptors makes the total reflex system more effective in the control of MAP.

15.7 Vasoactive substances

Substances released from many cells and tissues in the body, including the endothelium lining blood vessels, endocrine glands, and myocytes in the heart, may affect vascular smooth muscle tone. These substances may stimulate this muscle to cause vasoconstriction or inhibit it to cause vasodilation. As expected, vasoconstriction will increase TPR (and therefore MAP) and vasodilation will decrease TPR (and therefore MAP).

Vasoconstrictors. Many substances produced in the human body cause vasoconstriction under physiological and pathophysiological conditions. *Vasoconstrictors* of particular importance include:

- Catecholamines
- Angiotensin II
- Vasopressin
- Endothelin
- Thromboxane A_2

The major circulating hormones that influence vascular smooth muscle tone are the *catecholamines*: epinephrine and norepinephrine. These hormones are released from the adrenal medulla in response to sympathetic nervous stimulation. In humans, 80% of catecholamine secretion is epinephrine and 20% is norepinephrine. Stimulation of α_1-adrenergic receptors causes vasoconstriction. The selective α_1-adrenergic receptor antagonist, prazosin, is effective in management of hypertension because it causes arterial and venous smooth muscle to relax.

Angiotensin II (AgII) is a circulating peptide with powerful vasoconstrictor properties. The formation of Ag II is initiated by the enzyme renin, which converts the plasma-borne precursor angiotensinogen into angiotensin I. Angiotensin-converting enzyme (ACE) then converts angiotensin I into the active molecule, Ag II. The location of ACE is ideal for this function because it is found on the surface of endothelial cells in the lungs, which are exposed to the entire cardiac output. The release of renin from specialized cells in the kidneys occurs in response to sympathetic stimulation and when there is a decrease in renal blood flow.

Angiotensin II causes vasoconstriction by direct stimulation of AT_1 receptors on the vascular smooth muscle. It also enhances release of the neurotransmitter norepinephrine from the sympathetic nerve fibers present in the blood vessels. The vasopressor effects of Ag II may be inhibited pharmacologically in order to decrease TPR and treat hypertension. An important class of orally active drugs is the ACE inhibitors, including captopril and enalopril, which prevent formation of Ag II. More recently, angiotensin receptor antagonists have been developed that act at the vascular smooth muscle. These drugs, which include losartin and valsartan, are also orally active.

Vasopressin (antidiuretic hormone) is a peptide synthesized in the hypothalamus and secreted from the neurohypophysis of the pituitary gland. This substance plays an important role in the long-term regulation of blood pressure through its action on the kidney to increase reabsorption of water. The major stimulus for release of vasopressin is an increase in plasma osmolarity. The resulting reabsorption of water dilutes the plasma toward its normal value of 290 mOsM. This activity is discussed in more detail in Chapter 10 (the endocrine system) and Chapter 19 (the renal system).

Vasopressin also plays an important role in short-term regulation of blood pressure through its action on vascular smooth muscle. This hormone is the most potent known endogenous vasoconstrictor. Two types of vasopressin receptors have been identified: V_1 receptors mediate vasoconstriction and V_2 receptors mediate the antidiuretic effects of this hormone. Specific V_1 receptor antagonists of the vasoconstrictor activity of vasopressin are under development.

The vascular endothelium produces a number of substances that are released basally into the blood vessel wall to alter vascular smooth muscle tone. One such substance is *endothelin (ET-1)*. Endothelin exerts its effects throughout the body, causing vasoconstriction as well as positive inotropic and chronotropic effects on the heart. The resulting increases in TPR and CO contribute to an increase in MAP. Synthesis of endothelin appears to be enhanced by many stimuli, including Ag II, vasopressin, and the mechanical stress of blood flow on the endothelium. Synthesis is inhibited by vasodilator substances such as prostacyclin, nitric oxide, and atrial natriuretic peptide. There is evidence that endothelin is involved with the pathophysiology of many cardiovascular diseases, including hypertension, heart failure, and myocardial infarction. Endothelin receptor antagonists are currently available for research use only.

Another vasoactive substance produced by the endothelium is *thromboxane A_2 (TxA₂)*. Normally, small amounts of TxA_2 are released continuously; however, increased synthesis appears to be associated with some cardiac diseases. Synthesized from arachidonic acid, a plasma membrane phospholipid, TxA_2 is a potent vasoconstrictor. Furthermore, this substance stimulates platelet aggregation, suggesting that it plays a role in thrombotic events such as myocardial infarction (heart attack). Nonsteroidal anti-inflammatory drugs such as aspirin and ibuprofen block formation of TxA_2 and reduce formation of blood clots.

Pharmacy application: antihypertensive drugs

Hypertension is the most common cardiovascular disease; in fact, nearly 25% of adults in the U.S. are considered hypertensive. Hypertension is defined as a consistent elevation in blood pressure such that systolic/diastolic pressures are ≥140/90 mmHg. Over time, chronic hypertension can cause pathological changes in the vasculature and in the heart. As a result, hypertensive patients are at increased risk for atherosclerosis, aneurysm, stroke, myocardial infarction, heart failure, and kidney failure. There are several categories of antihypertensive agents:

- Diuretics. The primary mechanism by which diuretics reduce blood pressure is to decrease plasma volume. Acting at the kidney, diuretics increase sodium loss and, due to the osmotic effects of sodium, increase water loss. The decrease in plasma volume results in a decrease in VR, CO, and MAP.

- Sympatholytics. Sympathetic stimulation of the cardiovascular system may be altered by several mechanisms. Centrally acting agents exert their effects at the vasomotor center in the brainstem and inhibit sympathetic discharge. Reduced sympathetic stimulation of the heart and, especially, the vascular smooth muscle results in some decrease in CO and a marked decrease in TPR. Beta-adrenergic receptor antagonists reduce myocardial contractility and CO. These agents also inhibit the release of renin from the kidney. The resulting decrease in production of angiotensin II leads to vasodilation and a decrease in TPR. Alpha-adrenergic receptor antagonists reduce vascular resistance, therefore reducing blood pressure.
- Vasodilators. Hydralazine causes direct relaxation of arteriolar smooth muscle. An important consequence of this vasodilation, however, is reflex tachycardia ($\uparrow$ CO). It may also cause sodium retention ($\uparrow$ plasma volume). The resulting increase in CO tends to offset effects of the vasodilator. Therefore, these drugs are most effective when administered along with sympathetic agents such as β-adrenergic receptor antagonists, which prevent unwanted compensatory responses by the heart.
- Ca^{++}-channel blockers. Verapamil has powerful effects on the heart, decreasing heart rate and myocardial contractility ($\downarrow$ CO) and causing some vasodilation. On the other hand, nifedipine is a more potent vasodilator ($\downarrow$ TPR) with weaker myocardial effects. The effects of diltiazem are somewhat intermediate, in that this drug has moderate inhibitory effects on the myocardium and vascular smooth muscle.
- Angiotensin-converting enzyme (ACE) inhibitors. ACE inhibitors not only cause vasodilation ($\downarrow$ TPR), but also inhibit the aldosterone response to net sodium loss. Normally, aldosterone, which enhances reabsorption of sodium in the kidney, would oppose diuretic-induced sodium loss. Therefore, coadministration of ACE inhibitors would enhance the efficacy of diuretic drugs.
- Angiotensin II receptor antagonists. These agents promote vasodilation ($\downarrow$ TPR), increase sodium and water excretion, and, therefore, decrease plasma volume ($\downarrow$ CO).

Drug classification	Generic agents	CO	TPR	PV
Diuretics		↔	↓	↓
Thiazides	Hydrochlorothiazide			
Loop diuretics	Furosemide			
K⁺-sparing diuretics	Amiloride			
Sympatholytics				
Central acting	Methyldopa	↓	↓	↔
β-Antagonist	Propranolol	↓	↓	↔
α-Antagonist	Prazosin	↔	↓	↔
Vasodilators		↑	↓	↑
Arterial	Hydralazine			
Arterial and venous	Nitroprusside			
Ca⁺⁺-channel blockers				
	Verapamil	↓	↓	↔
	Nifedipine	↔	↓	↔
	Diltiazem	↓	↓	↔
ACE inhibitors	Captopril	↔	↓	↔
AgII-antagonists	Losartin	↔	↓	↔

Vasodilators. Many substances produced in the human body cause vasodilation under physiological and pathophysiological conditions. *Vasodilators* of particular importance include:

- Prostacyclin
- Nitric oxide
- Atrial natriuretic peptide

Another metabolite of arachidonic acid is *prostacyclin* (PGI_2). As with TxA_2, PGI_2 is produced continuously. Synthesized by vascular smooth muscle and endothelial cells, with the endothelium as the predominant source, PGI_2 mediates effects that are opposite to those of TxA_2. Prostacyclin causes vasodilation and inhibits platelet aggregation and, as a result, makes an important contribution to the antithrombogenic nature of the vascular wall.

First described in the 1980s as "endothelium-derived relaxing factor," *nitric oxide* (*NO*) is a vasodilator believed to play a role in regulation of blood pressure under physiologic and pathophysiological conditions. For example, inhibition of NO synthesis under normal conditions and during septic shock results in a significant elevation of blood pressure.

Pharmacy application: nitroglycerin and angina

Angina pectoris (chest pain) is the most common symptom of chronic ischemic heart disease. Angina is caused by an imbalance between the oxygen supply and oxygen demand of the cardiac muscle. Myocardial oxygen demand increases during exertion, exercise, and emotional stress. If coronary blood flow does not increase proportionately to meet this demand, then the affected tissue becomes ischemic and pain develops. This ischemia and pain may be treated pharmacologically with nitroglycerin, a drug that causes vasodilation and an increase in blood flow. However, this effect occurs not only in the coronary arteries, but also in blood vessels throughout the body. Therefore, in addition to improving coronary blood flow, administration of nitroglycerin may decrease systemic blood pressure. The mechanism of action of nitroglycerin involves release of NO in the vascular smooth muscle. Most frequently, this drug is administered in the sublingual form and its effects are apparent within 1 to 3 minutes.

Atrial natriuretic peptide (ANP) is produced by specialized myocytes in the atria of the heart. Secretion is stimulated by increased filling and stretch of the atria in response to plasma volume expansion. The effects of ANP include vasodilation, diuresis (increased urine production), and increased sodium excretion. Taken together, these effects decrease blood volume and blood pressure toward normal.

15.8 Venous return

Vessels of the circulatory system have varying degrees of *distensibility*, a feature that allows them to accommodate changes in blood volume. For example, the abrupt addition of the stroke volume to the aorta and large arteries during systole causes these vessels to expand and actually "store" a portion of the blood pumped by the heart. The subsequent elastic recoil of the arteries forces the stored blood forward during diastole. Therefore, the slight distensibility of arteries results in maintenance of blood flow to the tissues throughout the cardiac cycle.

The most distensible vessels in the circulatory system are the veins. As with arteries, this feature of the veins also has important physiological implications because it allows them to serve as *blood reservoirs*. The veins are so distensible that they are capable of holding large volumes of blood at very low pressures. In fact, under resting conditions, 64% of the blood volume is contained within these vessels.

Compliance (C) in the circulatory system describes the relationship between vascular blood volume (V) and intravascular pressure (P):

$$C = \frac{V}{P}$$

In other words, it is a measure of the inherent distensibility of the blood vessels. The more compliant the vessel is, then the greater the volume of blood that it is capable of accommodating. As mentioned, all blood vessels are compliant. However, the marked difference in distensibility between arteries and veins is illustrated by the following:

Compliance of the systemic arteries at rest;

$$C = \frac{13\% \text{ of the blood volume}}{100 \text{ mmHg}}$$

Compliance of the systemic veins at rest;

$$C = \frac{64\% \text{ of the blood volume}}{8 \text{ mmHg}}$$

Due to the significant amount of elastic connective tissue and smooth muscle in their walls, arteries tend to recoil rather powerfully, which keeps the pressure within them high. In contrast, veins contain less elastic connective tissue and smooth muscle so the tendency to recoil is significantly less and the pressure remains low.

The venous system, in general, serves as a reservoir for the circulatory system; however, some tissues are particularly important in this respect. These *specific blood reservoirs* include the spleen, liver, large abdominal veins, and the venous plexus beneath the skin. Common features of the vascular beds within these tissues are that they are very extensive and very compliant. In this way, under normal, resting conditions these vascular beds can accommodate large volumes of blood. In fact, taken together, these tissues may hold up to 1 l of blood, or 20% of the blood volume. Under pathological conditions such as hemorrhage or dehydration, blood may be mobilized from these tissues, thus allowing the circulatory system to function relatively normally until blood volume is restored to normal.

In addition to serving as blood reservoirs, veins help to *regulate cardiac output* (CO) by way of changes in *venous return* (VR). Venous return is defined as the volume of blood that flows from the systemic veins into the right atrium per minute. As discussed in Chapter 14 (cardiac output), a healthy heart pumps all of the blood returned to it. Therefore, CO is equal to VR:

$$CO = VR$$

On the other hand, the heart can only pump whatever blood it receives. Therefore, in order to increase CO, VR must also increase. As with blood flow through a vessel, blood flow through the venous system is determined by Ohm's law ($Q = \Delta P / R$). In other words, it depends on the pressure gradient in the venous system and venous resistance. Ohm's law may be rewritten to calculate VR:

$$VR = \frac{P_V - P_{RA}}{R_V}$$

The pressure gradient, or the inflow pressure minus the outflow pressure, is determined by the pressure at the beginning of the venous system (P_V) and right atrial pressure (P_{RA}) at the end of the system. The smaller compliant veins offer very little resistance to blood flow; the slightly stiffer large veins offer a small degree of resistance (R_V).

Several factors influence VR, including:

- Blood volume
- Sympathetic stimulation of the veins
- Skeletal muscle activity
- Respiratory activity

Blood volume. *Blood volume* has a direct effect on blood pressure. It also has an important effect on VR. A decrease in blood volume resulting from hemorrhage or dehydration causes a decrease in venous pressure and in VR. An increase in blood volume following oral or venous rehydration or a transfusion causes an increase in venous pressure and in VR.

Sympathetic stimulation of veins. The smaller, more compliant veins that serve generally as blood reservoirs as well as specific blood reservoirs are densely innervated by the *sympathetic system*. Stimulation of the vascular smooth muscle in the walls of these vessels causes vasoconstriction and a decrease in venous compliance. Vasoconstriction increases venous pressure in the veins; the blood is squeezed out of the veins and, due to the presence of one-way valves, moves toward the heart so that VR increases. A decrease in sympathetic stimulation allows the veins to relax and distend. The vessels become more compliant and capable of holding large volumes of blood at low pressures. In this case, VR decreases.

The effect of sympathetic stimulation on venous resistance is minimal. As previously stated, it is the larger, less flexible veins that provide resistance to blood flow. However, these blood vessels are sparsely innervated; therefore, little change takes place in vessel radius and physiological effect on blood flow is relatively insignificant.

Skeletal muscle activity. In the extremities (arms and legs), many veins lie between the skeletal muscles. Contraction of these muscles causes compression of the veins and an increase in venous pressure. This external compression squeezes the blood out and forces it toward the heart, causing an increase in VR. This action is referred to as the *skeletal muscle pump*.

The effect of the skeletal muscle pump is essential during exercise. Although a mass sympathetic discharge and venous vasoconstriction enhance VR, this mechanism alone is insufficient to increase VR and, therefore, CO to meet the metabolic demands of strenuous exercise. The skeletal muscle pump mobilizes the blood stored in these tissues and keeps it flowing toward the heart. As the number of muscles involved in the exercise increases, so does the magnitude of the increase in VR and CO.

Respiratory activity. Pressures in the venous system are altered during *respiration*. Inspiration causes a decrease in thoracic pressure and therefore a decrease in pressure within the venae cavae and the right atrium. Furthermore, downward movement of the diaphragm causes an increase in abdominal pressure. Many large veins and specific blood reservoirs are located in the abdomen. Compression of these tissues by the diaphragm causes an increase in venous pressure in this region. Therefore, the overall effect of inspiration is to increase the pressure gradient between extrathoracic and intrathoracic veins, resulting in an increase in VR.

15.9 Effects of gravity on the circulatory system

Gravitational forces may have a profound influence on blood flow through the circulatory system. As a result, VR and CO may be affected. Imagine that the circulatory system is a column of blood that extends from the heart to the feet. As in any column of fluid, the pressure at the surface is equal to zero. Due to the weight of the fluid, the pressure increases incrementally below the surface. This pressure is referred to as the *hydrostatic pressure*.

In an upright adult, the hydrostatic pressure of the blood in the feet may be as high as 90 mmHg. When this pressure is added to pressure in the veins generated by the pumping activity of the heart, the total pressure in veins in the feet may be as high as 100 mmHg. The valves in the veins effectively prevent the backward flow of blood toward the feet. However, the valves have no effect on the build-up of pressure in the veins in the lower extremities. The capillaries in the feet are also subjected to the effects of gravity. Pressure in these vessels may be in the range of 135 mmHg. Increased hydrostatic pressures in the veins and capillaries have two very detrimental effects on the circulatory system:

* Pooling of blood
* Edema formation

Blood tends to pool in the highly distensible veins. Furthermore, the excessive filtration of fluid out of the capillaries and into the tissues that occurs causes *edema* or swelling of the ankles and feet. As a result, VR and therefore CO are decreased, leading to a decrease in MAP. This fall in MAP can cause a decrease in cerebral blood flow and, possibly, syncope (fainting).

Compensatory mechanisms in the circulatory system are needed to counteract the effects of gravity. Two important mechanisms include:

- Baroreceptor reflex
- Skeletal muscle activity

Baroreceptors are sensitive to changes in MAP. As VR, CO, and MAP decrease, baroreceptor excitation is diminished. Consequently, the frequency of nerve impulses transmitted from these receptors to the vasomotor center in the brainstem is reduced. This elicits a reflex that will increase HR, increase contractility of the heart, and cause vasoconstriction of arterioles and veins. The increase in CO and TPR effectively increases MAP and therefore cerebral blood flow. Constriction of the veins assists in forcing blood toward the heart and enhances venous return. *Skeletal muscle activity* associated with simply walking decreases venous pressure in the lower extremities significantly. Contraction of the skeletal muscles in the legs compresses the veins and blood is forced toward the heart.

15.10 Regulation of blood flow through tissues

Blood flow to most tissues in the body is determined by the metabolic needs of those tissues. Metabolically active tissues require enhanced delivery of oxygen and nutrients as well as enhanced removal of carbon dioxide and waste products. In general, as the metabolic activity of a tissue increases, its blood flow increases. An important feature of the circulatory system is that each tissue has the intrinsic ability to control its own local blood flow in proportion to its metabolic needs.

Active hyperemia. The increase in blood flow caused by enhanced tissue activity is referred to as *active hyperemia*. Assuming a constant blood pressure, then according to Ohm's law ($Q = \Delta P/R$), the increase in blood flow is the result of a decrease in local vascular resistance. Tissue metabolism causes several local chemical changes that can mediate this metabolic vasodilation. These include:

- Decreased oxygen
- Increased carbon dioxide
- Increased hydrogen ions
- Increased potassium ions
- Increased adenosine

As metabolism increases, *oxygen consumption* and *carbon dioxide production* are enhanced. The concentration of *hydrogen ions* is also enhanced as more carbonic acid (formed from carbon dioxide) and lactic acid are produced by the working tissue. Furthermore, the concentration of *potassium ions* in the interstitial fluid is increased. The rate of potassium release from the cells due to repeated action potentials exceeds the rate of potassium return to the cells by way of the Na^+–K^+ pump. Finally, the release of *adenosine* is also believed to play a role in regulation of resistance vessels, particularly in the heart and skeletal muscle.

Each of these chemical changes promotes *vasodilation of arterioles*. In addition, the increase in *tissue temperature* associated with increased metabolism further contributes to metabolic vasodilation. The resulting increase in local blood flow restores these substances to their resting values. More oxygen is delivered and excess carbon dioxide, hydrogen and potassium ions, and adenosine are removed.

Autoregulation. A different situation arises when the metabolic rate of a tissue remains constant, but the blood pressure changes. According to Ohm's law ($Q = \Delta P / R$), an increase in blood pressure would tend to increase blood flow to a tissue. However, if the metabolic activity of the tissue does not change, then an increase in blood flow is unnecessary. In fact, blood flow to the tissue returns most of the way back to normal rather rapidly. The maintenance of a relatively constant blood flow to a tissue, in spite of changes in blood pressure, is referred to as *autoregulation*. Once again, resistance changes in the arterioles are involved.

Arteriolar resistance changes that take place in order to maintain a constant blood flow are explained by the *myogenic mechanism*. According to this mechanism, vascular smooth muscle contracts in response to stretch. For example, consider a situation in which blood pressure is increased. The increase in pressure causes an initial increase in blood flow to the tissue. However, the increased blood flow is associated with increased stretch of the vessel wall, which leads to the opening of stretch-activated calcium channels in the vascular smooth muscle. The ensuing increase in intracellular calcium results in vasoconstriction and a decrease in blood flow to the tissue toward normal.

15.11 Effects of acute exercise on the circulatory system

The primary goal of the circulatory system during exercise is to *increase blood flow to the working muscles*. This is accomplished by *increasing MAP* and *decreasing local vascular resistance*:

$$\uparrow\uparrow Q = \frac{\uparrow MAP}{\downarrow R}$$

At the onset of exercise, signals from the cerebral cortex are transmitted to the vasomotor center in the medulla of the brainstem. This *central command* inhibits parasympathetic activity and also initiates the *mass sympathetic discharge* associated with exercise. Sympathetic activity (including release of catecholamines from the adrenal medulla) increases proportionally with the intensity of exercise.

Sympathetic stimulation of the heart results in:

- Increased HR
- Increased myocardial contractility → increased SV
- Therefore, *increased CO*

Sympathetic stimulation of the veins and other blood reservoirs results in:

- Increased P_v → increased VR → increased EDV → increased SV
- Therefore, *increased CO*

In other words, the increase in cardiac output occurs by extrinsic (sympathetic stimulation) and intrinsic (increased VR and the Frank–Starling law of the heart) mechanisms. Venous return is also markedly increased by the compression of blood vessels in the working muscles. The increase in CO causes an *increase in MAP,* and the increase in MAP contributes to an increase in muscle blood flow.

Sympathetic stimulation of the arterioles results in:

- Increased TPR

Most arterioles of the peripheral circulation are strongly constricted by direct sympathetic stimulation. This widespread vasoconstriction serves two purposes. First, it contributes to the increase in MAP. Second, it is an important factor in the *redirection of blood flow* away from inactive tissues and toward the working muscles.

Resistance in the arterioles of the working muscles is regulated locally. As discussed previously, active hyperemia results in production of several factors that cause *metabolic vasodilation.* Exercising muscles generate CO_2, H^+ and K^+ ions, heat, and adenosine. The vasodilator effect of these locally produced substances overrides the vasoconstrictor effect of the sympathetic system in the muscle. As a result, *local vascular resistance is decreased.* The combination of increased driving pressure and decreased local vascular resistance causes an increase in blood flow to the working muscles.

15.12 Capillary exchange

Capillaries are the *site of exchange* between blood and the interstitial fluid surrounding tissue cells. Tissues with a higher metabolic rate have a more extensive capillary network, that is, a greater number of capillaries per unit area. Because of extensive branching of these vessels, the cells of the body are typically within 20 μm of the nearest capillary. Consequently, the distance that substances must travel between blood and the cells is minimized. Capillaries are permeable to water and small water-soluble substances, such as glucose, amino acids, lactic acid, and urea, and impermeable to proteins.

The *velocity of blood flow* through capillaries is slow compared to the rest of the circulatory system because of the very large *total cross-sectional surface area* of the capillaries. Although each individual capillary has a diameter of only about 5 to 10 μm, when the cross-sectional areas of the billions of capillaries are combined, the total is well over 1000 times larger than that of the aorta. As the total cross-sectional area increases, the velocity of blood flow decreases. The physiological significance of this low velocity of blood flow is that it allows adequate time for exchange of materials between blood and the tissue cells.

Blood flow through individual capillaries is *intermittent*, or sporadic. At the beginning of each capillary, where it branches off the arteriole, is a ring of smooth muscle referred to as the *precapillary sphincter*. This sphincter alternately contracts and relaxes; when it contracts, blood flow through the capillary is interrupted and when it relaxes, blood flow resumes. This process of contraction and relaxation of the precapillary sphincter is referred to as *vasomotion*. It is regulated by the rate of metabolism in the tissue, or the oxygen demand of the tissue. As metabolism in the tissue and the tissue's need for oxygen increase, the rate of vasomotion increases and the periods of relaxation are longer. In this way, blood flow through the capillary is markedly increased and the metabolic needs of the tissue are met. At rest, approximately 10 to 20% of the body's capillaries are perfused at any given moment. During exercise, these changes in vasomotion allow blood to flow through all capillaries in the working muscles, thus contributing significantly to enhanced perfusion.

Substances are exchanged across the capillary wall by means of three primary mechanisms:

- Diffusion
- Transcytosis
- Bulk flow

The most important mechanism is *diffusion*. If a substance is permeable, it moves in or out of the capillary down its concentration gradient. *Lipid-soluble substances* can diffuse through the endothelial cells at any point along the capillary. These molecules, especially oxygen and carbon dioxide, can pass directly through the lipid bilayer. However, *water-soluble substances* move across the membrane only through water-filled pores in the endothelial cells. Small, water-soluble substances such as glucose, amino acids, and ions pass readily through the pores.

Large, non-lipid-soluble molecules may cross the capillary wall by *transcytosis*. This mechanism involves the transport of vesicles from one side of the capillary wall to the other. Many hormones, including the catecholamines and those derived from proteins, exit the capillaries and enter their target tissues by way of transcytosis.

The third mechanism of capillary exchange is *bulk flow*. In this case, water and dissolved solutes move across capillaries due to *hydrostatic pressure* and *osmotic pressure*. When the balance of these two forces causes fluid to move out of the capillary, it is referred to as *filtration*. When these forces cause fluid to move into the capillary, it is referred to as *reabsorption*.

An interesting phenomenon in the circulatory system is that, even though capillaries have numerous pores in their walls, all of the fluid does not leak out of them into the interstitial space. If a balloon filled with water had multiple pin pricks in it, all of the water would clearly leak out. What prevents this from happening in the capillaries? The *Starling Principle* describes the process by which plasma is held within the vascular compartment.

Four forces determine the movement of fluid into or out of the capillary (see Figure 15.7):

- Capillary hydrostatic pressure (P_c)
- Interstitial fluid hydrostatic pressure (P_i)
- Plasma colloid osmotic pressure (π_p)
- Interstitial fluid colloid osmotic pressure (π_i)

Capillary hydrostatic pressure forces fluid out of the capillary. This pressure is higher at the inflow end of the capillary (30 mmHg) than it is at the outflow end (10 mmHg). The *interstitial fluid hydrostatic pressure* would tend to force fluid into the capillary if it were positive. However, this pressure is usually negative and instead acts as a suction and pulls fluid out of the capillary. Although it varies depending upon the specific tissue, the average interstitial fluid hydrostatic pressure is about –3 mmHg.

Plasma colloid osmotic pressure is generated by proteins in the plasma that cannot cross the capillary wall. These proteins exert an osmotic force, pulling fluid into the capillary. In fact, the plasma colloid osmotic pressure, which is about 28 mmHg, is the only force holding fluid within the capillaries. *Interstitial fluid colloid osmotic pressure* is generated by the small amount of plasma proteins that leaks into the interstitial space. Because these proteins

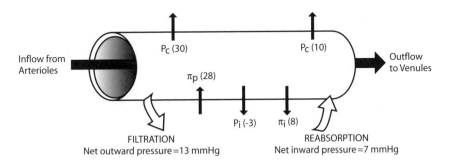

Figure 15.7 Starling principle; a summary of forces determining the bulk flow of fluid across the wall of a capillary. Hydrostatic forces include capillary pressure (P_c) and interstitial fluid pressure (P_i). Capillary pressure pushes fluid out of the capillary. Interstitial fluid pressure is negative and acts as a suction pulling fluid out of the capillary. Osmotic forces include plasma colloid osmotic pressure (π_p) and interstitial fluid colloid osmotic pressure (π_i). These forces are caused by proteins that pull fluid toward them. The sum of these four forces results in net filtration of fluid at the arteriolar end of the capillary (where P_c is high) and net reabsorption of fluid at the venular end of the capillary (where P_c is low).

are normally returned to the blood by way of the lymphatic system, protein concentration in the interstitial fluid is very low. The average interstitial fluid colloid osmotic pressure is 8 mmHg.

Note that, except for capillary hydrostatic pressure, the magnitude of these forces remains constant throughout the length of the capillary. The capillary hydrostatic pressure decreases steadily as blood flows from the arteriolar end to the venular end of the capillary. The steady decline in this pressure results in filtration of fluid at one end and reabsorption of fluid at the other end of the capillary.

At the *arteriolar end of the capillary,* the pressures forcing fluid out of the capillary include the following:

$$\text{Outward forces} = P_c + P_i + \pi_i$$

$$= 30 \text{ mmHg} + 3 \text{ mmHg} + 8 \text{ mmHg}$$

$$= 41 \text{ mmHg}$$

Although the interstitial fluid hydrostatic pressure is "negative," it causes fluid to be pulled out of the capillary, so this pressure is "added" to the other outward forces. The only force pulling fluid into the capillary is the plasma colloid osmotic pressure:

$$\text{Inward force} = \pi_p$$

$$= 28 \text{ mmHg}$$

The sum of the outward forces (41 mmHg) exceeds that of the inward force (28 mmHg) resulting in a *net filtration pressure* of 13 mmHg. In other words, net movement of fluid is out of the capillary at the arteriolar end.

At the *venular end of the capillary,* the sum of the pressures forcing fluid out of the capillary is decreased due to the fall in capillary hydrostatic pressure:

$$\text{Outward forces} = P_c + P_i + \pi_i$$

$$= 10 \text{ mmHg} + 3 \text{ mmHg} + 8 \text{ mmHg}$$

$$= 21 \text{ mmHg}$$

The plasma colloid osmotic pressure remains constant:

$$\text{Inward force} = \pi_p$$

$$= 28 \text{ mmHg}$$

Therefore, at the venular end of the capillary, the inward force (28 mmHg) exceeds the sum of the outward forces (21 mmHg) resulting in a *net reabsorption pressure* of 7 mmHg. In other words, net movement of fluid is into the capillary at the venular end.

Bulk flow plays only a minor role in the exchange of specific solutes between blood and tissue cells. A far more important function of bulk flow is to *regulate distribution of extracellular fluid* between the vascular compartment (plasma) and the interstitial space. Maintenance of an appropriate circulating volume of blood is an important factor in the maintenance of blood pressure. For example, dehydration and hemorrhage will cause a decrease in blood pressure leading to a decrease in capillary hydrostatic pressure. As a result, net filtration decreases and net reabsorption increases, causing movement, or bulk flow, of extracellular fluid from interstitial space into the vascular compartment. This fluid shift expands the plasma volume and compensates for the fall in blood pressure.

Over the course of a day, approximately 20 l of fluid are filtered from the capillaries and about 17 l of fluid are reabsorbed into the capillaries. The remaining 3 l is returned to the vascular compartment by way of the *lymphatic system*.

The *lymphatic capillaries* are close-ended vessels in close proximity to blood capillaries and, like blood capillaries, lymphatic capillaries are composed of a single layer of endothelial cells. However, large gaps in between these cells allow not only fluid, but also proteins and particulate matter to enter the lymphatic capillaries quite readily. Once the fluid has entered these capillaries, it is referred to as *lymph*. Not surprisingly, the composition of this fluid is similar to that of the interstitial fluid.

Lymphatic capillaries join together to form larger *lymphatic vessels* that have *valves* within them to ensure the one-way flow of lymph. The lymph is moved along by two mechanisms. Automatic, rhythmic waves of contraction of the smooth muscle in the walls of these vessels are the primary mechanism by which lymph is propelled through the system. Second, the contraction of skeletal muscles causes compression of lymphatic vessels. As in the veins, this pumping action of the surrounding skeletal muscles contributes to movement of the lymph. Ultimately, the lymph is returned to the blood when it empties into the subclavian and jugular veins near the heart.

Four general conditions can lead to *edema* formation, or excess fluid accumulation in the tissue:

- Increased capillary hydrostatic pressure
- Blockage of lymph vessels
- Increased capillary permeability
- Decreased concentration of plasma proteins

Increased capillary hydrostatic pressure promotes filtration and inhibits reabsorption. As a result, excess fluid is forced out of the capillary into the interstitial space. An increase in capillary pressure is generally caused by an increase in venous pressure. For example, under conditions of right-sided congestive heart failure, the heart cannot pump all of the blood returned to it. Consequently, blood becomes backed up in the venous system, thus increasing hydrostatic pressure of the veins and capillaries, particularly in the lower extremities. Left-sided congestive heart failure may cause pulmonary edema.

Another condition that can impair venous return is pregnancy. As the uterus enlarges during gestation, it may cause compression of the veins draining the lower extremities. Once again, venous and capillary pressures are increased. Filtration is enhanced, reabsorption is inhibited, and edema develops in the lower extremities.

Blockage of lymph vessels prevents the return of excess filtered fluid to the vascular compartment. Instead, this fluid remains within the tissue. Impaired lymph drainage may be caused by local inflammation, cancer, and parasites.

Increased capillary permeability may allow plasma proteins to leak into the interstitial spaces of a tissue. The presence of excess protein in these spaces causes an increase in interstitial fluid colloid osmotic pressure and pulls more fluid out of the capillaries. Mediators of inflammation such as histamine and bradykinin, which are active following tissue injury and during allergic reactions, increase capillary permeability and cause swelling.

A *decrease in the concentration of plasma proteins* causes a decrease in the plasma colloid osmotic pressure. As a result, filtration is increased, reabsorption is decreased, and fluid accumulates in the tissue. Most plasma proteins are made in the liver; therefore, a decrease in protein synthesis due to liver failure is an important cause of this condition. Malnutrition may also impair protein synthesis. Finally, kidney disease leading to proteinuria (protein loss in the urine) decreases the concentration of plasma proteins.

Bibliography

1. Benowitz, N.L., Antihypertensive agents, in *Basic and Clinical Pharmacology*, 8th ed., Katzung, B.G., Ed., Lange Medical Books/McGraw–Hill, New York, 2001, chap. 11.
2. Berne, R.M. and Levy, M.N., *Cardiovascular Physiology*, 8th ed., C.V. Mosby, St. Louis, 2001.
3. Campbell, W.B. and Halushka, P.V., Lipid-derived autacoids: eicosanoids and platelet-activating factor, in *Goodman and Gilman's: The Pharmacological Basis of Therapeutics*, 9th ed., Hardman, J.G. and Limbird, L.E., Eds., McGraw–Hill, New York, 1996, chap. 26.
4. Foegh, M.L. and Ramwell, P.W., The eicosanoids: prostaglandins, thromboxanes, leukotrienes and related compounds, in *Basic and Clinical Pharmacology*, 8th ed., Katzung, B.G., Ed., Lange Medical Books/McGraw–Hill, New York, 2001, chap. 18.
5. Guyton, A.C. and Hall, J.E., *Textbook of Medical Physiology*, 10th ed., W.B. Saunders, Philadelphia, 2000.

6. Hoffman, B.B., Adrenoceptor antagonist drugs, in *Basic and Clinical Pharmacology*, 8th ed., Katzung, B.G., Ed., Lange Medical Books/McGraw–Hill, New York, 2001, chap. 10.

7. Honig, C.R., *Modern Cardiovascular Physiology*, 2nd ed., Little, Brown, Boston/Toronto, 1988.

8. Jackson, E.K., Vasopressin and other agents affecting the renal conservation of water, in *Goodman and Gilman's: The Pharmacological Basis of Therapeutics*, 9th ed., Hardman, J.G. and Limbird, L.E., Eds., McGraw–Hill, New York, 1996, chap. 30.

9. Katzung, B.G. and Chatterjee, K., Vasodilators and the treatment of angina pectoris, in *Basic and Clinical Pharmacology*, 8th ed., Katzung, B.G., Ed., Lange Medical Books/McGraw–Hill, New York, 2001, chap. 12.

10. McCulloch, K.M. and McGrath, J.C., Neurohumoral regulation of vascular tone, in *An Introduction to Vascular Biology, from Physiology to Pathophysiology*, Halliday, A., Hunt, B.J., Poston, L., and Schachter, M., Eds., Cambridge University Press, Cambridge, U.K., 1998, chap. 5.

11. Oates, J.A., Antihypertensive agents and the drug therapy of hypertension, in *Goodman and Gilman's: The Pharmacological Basis of Therapeutics*, 9th ed., Hardman, J.G. and Limbird, L.E., Eds., McGraw–Hill, New York, 1996, chap. 33.

12. Reid, I.A., Vasoactive peptides, in *Basic and Clinical Pharmacology*, 8th ed., Katzung, B.G., Ed., Lange Medical Books/McGraw–Hill, New York, 2001, chap. 17.

13. Rhoades, R. and Pflanzer, R., *Human Physiology*, Thomson Learning, Pacific Grove, CA, 2003.

14. Robertson, R.M. and Robertson, D., Drugs used for the treatment of myocardial ischemia, in *Goodman and Gilman's: The Pharmacological Basis of Therapeutics*, 9th ed., Hardman, J.G. and Limbird, L.E., Eds., McGraw–Hill, New York, 1996, chap. 32.

15. Sherwood, L., *Human Physiology from Cells to Systems*, 4th ed., Brooks/Cole, Pacific Grove, CA, 2001.

16. Silverthorn, D.U., *Human Physiology: An Integrated Approach*, 2nd ed., Prentice-Hall, Upper Saddle River, NJ, 2001.

17. Zdanowicz, M.M., *Essentials of Pathophysiology for Pharmacy*, CRC Press, Boca Raton, FL, 2003.

chapter sixteen

Blood and hemostasis

Study objectives

- Discuss the major functions of plasma proteins
- Describe the morphological characteristics and the function of eryth-rocytes
- Explain how various blood types are determined and what blood types are compatible for transfusion
- Describe how the Rh factor may lead to hemolytic disease of the newborn
- Discuss the major functions of each of the five types of leukocytes: neutrophils, eosinophils, basophils, monocytes, and lymphocytes
- Describe the origin of thrombocytes
- Discuss the role of platelets in various aspects of hemostasis
- Describe the role of vascular constriction in hemostasis
- Explain how a platelet plug is formed
- Distinguish between the extrinsic and intrinsic mechanisms of blood coagulation
- Explain how blood clot growth is limited
- Explain how blood clots are dissolved

16.1 Introduction

Blood consists of cellular elements (red blood cells, white blood cells, and platelets) as well as plasma, the fluid in which the blood cells are suspended. Normally, total circulating blood volume is about 8% of body weight (about 5 l in women and 5.5 l in men). Adipose tissue is relatively avascular and therefore contains little blood compared to other tissues.

The cellular elements of the blood have a short life span and must be continuously replaced. The formation of red blood cells, white blood cells, and platelets, collectively, is referred to as *hematopoiesis*. This process takes place in the red bone marrow. In adults, red bone marrow is found in the pelvis, ribs, and sternum.

16.2 Plasma

The fluid portion of the blood, the *plasma*, accounts for 55 to 60% of total blood volume and is about 90% water. The remaining 10% contains proteins (8%) and other substances (2%) including hormones, enzymes, nutrient molecules, gases, electrolytes, and excretory products. All of these substances are dissolved in the plasma (e.g., oxygen) or are colloidal materials (dispersed solute materials that do not precipitate out, e.g., proteins). The three major plasma proteins include:

- Albumin
- Globulins
- Fibrinogen

Albumin is the most abundant (about 55%) of the plasma proteins. An important function of albumin is to bind with various molecules in the blood and serve as a *carrier protein*, transporting these substances throughout the circulation. Substances that bind with albumin include hormones; amino acids; fatty acids; bile salts; and vitamins. Albumin also serves as an *osmotic regulator*. Because capillary walls are impermeable to plasma proteins, these molecules exert a powerful osmotic force on water in the blood. In fact, the plasma colloid osmotic pressure exerted by plasma proteins is the only force that retains water within the vascular compartment and therefore maintains blood volume (see Chapter 15). Albumin is synthesized in the liver.

The *globulins* account for about 38% of plasma proteins. The three types of globulins are alpha (α), beta (β), and gamma (γ). The alpha and beta globulins are involved with several activities. They *transport substances* in the blood (hormones, cholesterol, iron), function as *clotting factors*, and serve as *precursor molecules* (angiotensinogen). The gamma globulins function as *antibodies*, which play an important role in the immune response. Alpha and beta globulins are synthesized in the liver; the gamma globulins are made by the lymphocytes (a type of white blood cell).

Fibrinogen also plays a role in the blood clotting process. It serves as a precursor for *fibrin*, which forms the *meshwork of a blood clot*. Fibrinogen is synthesized in the liver.

16.3 Erythrocytes

The most numerous of the cellular elements in the blood are the *erythrocytes* (*red blood cells*). On average, there are 5 million red blood cells per microliter (μl) of blood, or a total of about 25 to 30 trillion red blood cells in the adult human body. The percentage of the blood made up of red blood cells is referred to as *hematocrit*. An average hematocrit is about 45% (42% females, 47% males). As such, the *viscosity* of the blood is determined primarily by these elements.

Red blood cells are small biconcave discs. Each cell is approximately 7.5 μm in diameter and 2 μm thick. This shape maximizes the surface area of the cell and facilitates the diffusion of oxygen across the cell membrane. Furthermore, red blood cells are very flexible and easily change their shape. This feature allows them to squeeze through capillaries as narrow as 3 μm in diameter. However, as the red blood cells age, their membranes become quite fragile and the cells are prone to rupture. Aged cells are removed by the *spleen*. The average life span of a red blood cell is about 120 days. As such, red blood cells must be replaced at a rate of 2 to 3 million cells per second. Erythrocyte production is regulated by the hormone *erythropoietin*. Low levels of oxygen stimulate release of erythropoietin from the kidneys into the blood.

The primary function of red blood cells is to transport oxygen to the tissues. The red, oxygen-carrying molecule within the red blood cell is *hemoglobin*. This molecule has two components: the *globin portion* and the *heme portion*. There are one globin portion and four heme groups per molecule. Each heme group contains an *iron* atom that binds reversibly with oxygen. The average hemoglobin content in the blood is about 15 g/100 ml of blood, all of it within the red blood cells. In fact, because of their high hemoglobin content, each red blood cell has the capacity to transport more than 1 billion oxygen molecules. This hemoglobin/oxygen-carrying capacity of the red blood cell is facilitated by lack of a nucleus and any other membranous organelles within these cells.

16.4 Blood types

Erythrocytes are labeled with *cell surface antigens* that determine *blood type*. Two types of inherited antigens are found on red blood cells: A antigens and B antigens. Accordingly, four blood types are possible (see Table 16.1):

- Type A (A antigen)
- Type B (B antigen)
- Type AB (A and B antigens)
- Type O (neither A nor B antigens)

Antibodies are specialized molecules produced by the immune system to attack foreign antigens. Therefore, an individual with type A blood produces

Table 16.1 Summary of ABO Blood Type System

Blood Type	Possible genotypes	Antibodies produced	Possible transfusions	Frequency in U.S.
A	AA, AO	anti-B	A, O	41%
B	BB, BO	anti-A	B, O	10%
AB	AB	none	A, B, AB, O	4%
O	OO	anti-A, anti-B	O	45%

anti-B antibodies, which attack type B antigens. An individual with type B blood produces anti-A antibodies, which attack type A antigens. Consequently, mixing incompatible blood can cause red blood cell destruction. The antibodies produced against a foreign blood type may cause *agglutination* (clumping) or *hemolysis* (rupture) of the donated erythrocytes.

Type AB blood contains A and B antigens on the red blood cells. Therefore, individuals with this blood type produce neither anti-A nor anti-B antibodies and can receive a transfusion of any blood type. Individuals with type AB blood are referred to as *universal recipients*.

Type O blood contains no antigens on the cell surface. In this case, any antibodies that the transfusion recipient may produce (anti-A or anti-B antibodies) have no antigens to attack. Therefore, no immune response against this blood exists. Individuals with type O blood are referred to as *universal donors* because this blood is suitable for transfusion in all individuals.

Another type of cell surface antigen found on red blood cells is the *Rh factor*. Red blood cells that contain the Rh factor are referred to as *Rh-positive* and RBCs without this factor are referred to as *Rh-negative*. This antigen also stimulates antibody production. Therefore, Rh-negative individuals that produce anti-Rh antibodies should receive only Rh-negative blood. Rh-positive individuals that do not produce anti-Rh antibodies can receive Rh-negative or Rh-positive blood. Approximately 85% of Caucasians are Rh-positive and 15% are Rh-negative. Over 99% of Asians, 95% of American blacks, and 100% of African blacks are Rh-positive.

Rh incompatibility may occur when an Rh negative mother carries an Rh-positive fetus. At the time of delivery, a small amount of the baby's Rh-positive blood may gain access to the maternal circulation. In response, the immune system of the mother produces *anti-Rh antibodies*. During the subsequent pregnancy, the fetus is exposed to these antibodies as they cross the placenta. If this fetus is also Rh-positive, then the anti-Rh antibodies attack the fetal erythrocytes and cause *hemolytic disease of the newborn* (*erythroblastosis fetalis*). This may occur in about 3% of second Rh-positive babies and about 10% of third Rh-positive babies. The incidence continues to increase with subsequent pregnancies.

16.5 Leukocytes

There are normally 4000 to 11,000 *leukocytes* (*white blood cells*) per microliter of human blood. However, leukocytes act primarily within the tissues; those found in the blood are actually in transit. Leukocytes are also found in lymphoid tissues such as the thymus, spleen, and lymph nodes. These cells are referred to as "white" blood cells because they lack hemoglobin and are essentially colorless. Leukocytes are an important component of the immune system. General *inflammatory and immune functions* of these cells include:

- Destruction of invading microorganisms (bacteria and viruses)
- Identification and destruction of cancer cells

- Phagocytosis of tissue debris including dead and injured cells

Five types of leukocytes are classified as either granulocytes or agranu-locytes:

- Granulocytes:
  - Neutrophils
  - Eosinophils
  - Basophils
- Agranulocytes:
  - Monocytes
  - Lymphocytes

The *granulocytes* are *phagocytic cells*. Their nuclei tend to be segmented into multiple lobes and the cytoplasm of the cells contains numerous granules. These cells are identified by the staining properties of their granules.

Neutrophils are the most abundant of the leukocytes and account for about 60% of the total number of white blood cells. These cells are usually the first to arrive at a site of injury or inflammation. Their primary function is to attack and destroy invading bacteria. In fact, bacterial infection is typically associated with pronounced *neutrophilia* (an increase in the number of circulating neutrophils). These leukocytes are also involved in removal of tissue debris and therefore play a role in the healing process.

Neutrophils eliminate bacteria and tissue debris by way of *phagocytosis*. Small projections of the cell membrane extend outward and engulf the harmful organisms and particles. As a result, these materials are internalized within a cell membrane-bound vesicle. A lysosome — an organelle filled with hydrolytic enzymes — then fuses with the vesicle. In this way, the phagocytized material is degraded by these enzymes without any damage to the rest of the cell. Neutrophils have the capacity to phagocytize 5 to 25 bacteria before they also die.

Eosinophils, which constitute only 1 to 4% of the total number of white blood cells, are only weak phagocytes. These leukocytes are produced in large numbers in individuals with *internal parasitic infections*. The eosinophils attach to the parasites and secrete substances that kill them, including:

- Hydrolytic enzymes released from eosinophil granules (which are actually modified lysosomes)
- Highly reactive forms of oxygen that are particularly lethal
- Major basic protein — a larvacidal polypeptide also released from granules

Eosinophils also tend to accumulate at the sites of allergic reactions, particularly in the lungs and skin. The functions of the eosinophils in these areas include neutralization of inflammatory mediators released from mast cells as well as phagocytosis of allergen–antibody complexes. In this way, the spread of the inflammatory reaction is limited.

Basophils are the least abundant of the leukocytes and account for less than 1% of the total number of white blood cells. They are similar structurally and functionally to the *mast cells* found in connective tissues, especially in the lungs, skin, and gastrointestinal tract. Basophils and mast cells play an important role in allergic reactions. The granules of these cells contain many substances, including:

*   Heparin, which prevents blood coagulation
*   Histamine, which promotes bronchoconstriction as well as the vasodilation and increased capillary permeability that lead to inflammation

The leukocytes classified as *agranulocytes* contain very few granules in their cytoplasm. In further contrast to granulocytes, these cells have a single, large nonsegmented nucleus.

Monocytes account for about 5% of the total number of white blood cells in the blood. Immature in the blood, these leukocytes leave the vascular compartment and enter the tissues, within which they enlarge, mature, and develop into *macrophages*. Macrophages are large phagocytic cells that can ingest bacteria, necrotic tissue, and even dead neutrophils. These cells survive much longer than neutrophils and may ingest up to 100 bacteria. The life span of the macrophage may range from months to years until it is ultimately destroyed as a result of phagocytic activity.

Lymphocytes constitute about 30% of the total number of white blood cells. The two types of lymphocytes are:

*   B lymphocytes
*   T lymphocytes

The primary function of the *B lymphocytes* is to produce *antibodies*, which are molecules that identify and lead to the destruction of foreign substances such as bacteria. The B lymphocytes and the antibodies they produce are responsible for *humoral immunity*. *T lymphocytes* provide immunity against viruses and cancer cells. These lymphocytes directly attack and destroy their targets by forming holes in the target cell membrane, causing cell lysis. The T lymphocytes are responsible for *cell-mediated immunity*.

16.6 Platelets

The third of the cellular elements within the blood are the *platelets* (*thrombocytes*). Platelets are actually small, round or oval *cell fragments*. They are about 2 to 4 μm in diameter and have no nuclei. Platelets are formed in the red bone marrow as pinched-off portions of the very large *megakaryocytes*. Each megakaryocyte, which is confined to the bone marrow, can produce up to 1000 platelets. Normally, there are approximately 300,000 platelets per microliter of blood. They are replaced about once every 10 days.

Platelets are essential for many aspects of *hemostasis*, or the cessation of blood loss. Several substances are found within the cytoplasm of platelets that contribute to the arrest of bleeding as well as vessel repair:

- Actin and myosin molecules, and thrombosthenin, are contractile proteins that enable platelets to contract.
- Fragments of the endoplasmic reticulum and the golgi apparatus produce enzymes and store calcium.
- Mitochondria and enzyme systems form ATP and ADP.
- Enzyme systems produce prostaglandins; these are substances involved with formation of platelet plugs as well as limitation of clot growth.
- Fibrin-stabilizing factor is a protein involved with blood coagulation.
- Growth factor facilitates vascular endothelial cell, vascular smooth muscle cell, and fibroblast multiplication and growth, leading to repair of damaged blood vessels.

These substances are discussed more fully in the following section.

16.7 Hemostasis

The prevention of blood loss from a damaged blood vessel is referred to as *hemostasis*. Three inherent mechanisms contribute to hemostasis:

- Vascular constriction
- Formation of platelet plug
- Blood coagulation

Vascular constriction. The first mechanism to occur is *vascular constriction*. Immediately after a blood vessel is cut or severed, the vascular smooth muscle automatically constricts. This results in a decrease in the flow of blood through the vessel that helps to limit blood loss. The vasoconstriction is caused by several factors:

- Sympathetic nerve reflexes in response to pain
- Local myogenic vasospasm in response to injury
- Locally produced vasoconstrictors released from damaged tissue and from platelets

When the extent of the trauma to the vessel is increased, the degree of vascular constriction is increased. Accordingly, a sharply cut blood vessel bleeds far more profusely than a blood vessel damaged by a more crushing injury. The vasoconstriction may last for many minutes or hours, thus providing time for the two subsequent mechanisms to develop and get under way.

Formation of a platelet plug. The *formation of a platelet plug* physically blocks small holes in blood vessels. Normally, platelets are unable to adhere to the endothelial lining of the blood vessels. The surface of the platelets contains a coat of glycoproteins that repels the normal endothelium. Interestingly, these same glycoproteins enable the platelets to adhere to damaged vessels. When platelets come into contact with a damaged vascular surface, in particular collagen fibers in the vessel wall or damaged endothelial cells, the platelets become activated. These platelets become "sticky" and adhere to the damaged tissue. They also release ADP and thromboxane A_2, a prostaglandin metabolite, which enhance the stickiness of other platelets. Consequently, more and more platelets adhere to the damaged vessel, ultimately forming a plug. This process is also referred to as *agglutination*. Furthermore, thromboxane A_2, as well as serotonin (also released from the platelets), contributes to the initial mechanism of vasoconstriction.

Pharmacy application: antiplatelet drugs

Platelets play a role in each of the mechanisms of normal hemostasis: vasoconstriction, formation of the platelet plug, and blood coagulation. However, they are also involved in pathological processes that lead to atherosclerosis and thrombosis (formation of a blood clot within the vascular system). Antiplatelet drugs interfere with platelet function and are used to prevent the development of atherosclerosis and formation of arterial thrombi.

The prototype of antiplatelet drugs is aspirin, which inhibits cyclooxygenase, an enzyme involved in arachidonic acid metabolism. Inhibition of cyclooxygenase blocks the synthesis of thromboxane A_2, the platelet product that promotes vasoconstriction and platelet aggregation. Because platelets are simply cell fragments, they are incapable of synthesizing new proteins, including enzymes. Therefore, aspirin-induced inhibition of cyclooxygenase is permanent and lasts for the life of the platelet (7 to 10 days).

Aspirin is maximally effective as an antithrombotic agent at the comparatively low dose of 81 to 325 mg per day. (The antipyretic dose of aspirin in adults is 325 to 650 mg every 4 h.) Higher doses of aspirin are actually contraindicated in patients prone to thromboembolism. At higher doses, aspirin also reduces synthesis of prostacyclin, another arachidonic acid metabolite. Prostacyclin normally inhibits platelet aggregation. The prophylactic administration of low-dose aspirin has been shown to increase survival following myocardial infarction, decrease incidence of stroke, and assist in maintenance of patency of coronary bypass grafts.

Blood coagulation. The third major step in hemostasis is *coagulation*, or the formation of a blood clot. This complex process involves a series of reactions that result in formation of a protein fiber meshwork that stabilizes the platelet plug. Three essential steps lead to clotting (see Figure 16.1):

- Activation of factor X
- Conversion of prothrombin into thrombin
- Conversion of fibrinogen into fibrin

All together, 12 *clotting factors* are in the plasma. These factors, which are proteins synthesized in the liver, are normally found circulating in plasma

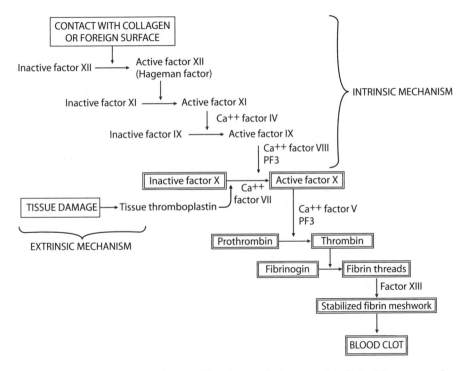

Figure 16.1 Coagulation pathways. Blood coagulation may be elicited by two mechanisms occurring independently or, more often, concurrently. The intrinsic mechanism begins when blood comes into contact with the collagen in a damaged vessel wall or with a foreign surface (e.g., test tube). This causes the activation of factor XII, or Hageman factor, followed by activation of other clotting factors and, finally, factor X. The extrinsic mechanism occurs when damaged tissue releases tissue thromboplastin; this mechanism activates factor X directly. Activation of factor X leads to the conversion of prothrombin into thrombin. Thrombin then leads to the conversion of fibrinogen into fibrin threads. The fibrin forms the stabilized meshwork that traps blood cells and forms the blood clot (PF3, platelet factor 3).

in their inactive forms. Activation of one of these factors leads to activation of another factor, and so on, resulting in a cascade of reactions culminating in fibrin formation.

Activated *factor X*, along with Ca^{++} ion, factor V, and PF3 (collectively referred to as the *prothrombin activator*), catalyzes the conversion of *prothrombin* into *thrombin*. Thrombin then catalyzes the conversion of *fibrinogen* into *fibrin*, an insoluble, thread-like polymer. The fibrin threads form a meshwork that traps blood cells, platelets, and plasma to form the blood clot. The clotting cascade may be elicited by means of two mechanisms (see Figure 16.1):

- Extrinsic mechanism
- Intrinsic mechanism

The *extrinsic mechanism* of blood coagulation begins when a blood vessel is ruptured and the surrounding tissues are damaged. The traumatized tissue releases a complex of substances referred to as *tissue thromboplastin*. The tissue thromboplastin further complexes with factor VII and Ca^{++} ions to activate factor X directly.

The *intrinsic mechanism* of blood coagulation causes the blood to clot within the vessel. It is activated when the blood is traumatized or when it comes into contact with the exposed collagen of a damaged vessel wall. This contact activates *factor XII (Hageman factor)* in the blood. Simultaneously, platelets are activated, so they begin adhering to the collagen in the vessel wall to form the platelet plug. In addition to ADP and thromboxane A_2, these aggregated platelets also release PF3. This substance plays a role in subsequent clotting reactions. (It is important to note at this point that platelets are involved in all three mechanisms of hemostasis: vascular constriction, formation of the platelet plugs, and blood coagulation.)

Activated factor XII leads to the activation of *factor XI*; in turn, activated factor XI, along with Ca^{++} ions and factor IV, leads to activation of *factor IX*. Activated factor IX, along with Ca^{++} ions, factor VIII, and PF3, leads to the activation of factor X. From the point of factor X activation, the extrinsic and intrinsic mechanisms follow the same pathway to fibrin formation.

The extrinsic and intrinsic mechanisms typically occur simultaneously. The extrinsic mechanism coagulates the blood that has escaped into the tissue prior to the sealing of the vessel. The intrinsic mechanism coagulates the blood within the damaged vessel. Another important difference involves the speed at which these two mechanisms cause coagulation. Because the extrinsic mechanism causes activation of factor X directly, clotting begins within seconds. The intrinsic mechanism is much slower, usually requiring 1 to 6 min to form a clot. However, the cascade of reactions characteristic of this mechanism allows for amplification. Each molecule of activated clotting factor may activate many molecules of the clotting factor in the next step of the cascade. Therefore, a few molecules of activated Hageman factor can lead to activation of hundreds of molecules of factor X and a very powerful coagulation response.

Once the clot is formed, the platelets trapped within it contract, shrinking the fibrin meshwork. This *clot retraction* pulls the edges of the damaged vessel closer together. Blood coagulation is limited to the site of damage. Once the blood clotting factors have carried out their activities, they are rapidly inactivated by enzymes present in plasma and surrounding tissue.

Positive feedback nature of clot formation. *Thrombin* promotes clot formation at several points in the coagulation cascade through *positive feedback*. Activities of thrombin include:

- Acts on prothrombin to make more thrombin, thus facilitating its own formation
- Accelerates the actions of several blood clotting factors (VIII, IX, X, XI, and XII)
- Enhances platelet adhesion and activation
- Activates factor XIII, which strengthens and stabilizes the fibrin meshwork of the clot

Clot dissolution. Once the blood vessel has been repaired, the clots must be removed in order to prevent permanent obstruction. *Plasmin* is a proteolytic enzyme that digests fibrin. It is synthesized from its precursor, *plasminogen*. The conversion of plasminogen into plasmin involves several substances, including factor XII (Hageman factor), that are also involved in the coagulation cascade. Within a few days after the blood has clotted, enough plasmin has been formed to dissolve the clot. The residue of the clot dissolution is removed by the phagocytic white blood cells (neutrophils and macrophages).

Prevention of blood clotting in the normal vascular system. Several factors contribute to the prevention of blood clotting in the normal vascular system:

- *Smoothness* of the endothelial lining prevents contact activation of the intrinsic mechanism.
- A layer of *glycocalyx* on the endothelium repels clotting factors and platelets.
- *Thrombomodulin* is a protein on the endothelium that (1) binds with thrombin, reducing its availability for the clotting process; and (2) activates protein C, which acts as an anticoagulant by inactivating factors V and VIII.
- *Tissue plasminogen activator* activates plasmin to dissolve the fibrin continuously made at low levels.

Pharmacy application: anticoagulant drugs

Anticoagulant drugs include heparin and warfarin (Couma-din®) —agents used to prevent deep vein thrombosis. They are also used to prevent formation of emboli due to atrial fibrillation, valvular heart disease, and other cardiac disorders. Heparin, which is not absorbed by the gastrointestinal tract, is available only by injection; its effect is immediate.

The most commonly used oral anticoagulant drug in the U.S. is warfarin. It acts by altering vitamin K so that it is unavailable to participate in synthesis of vitamin K-dependent coagulation factors in the liver (coagulation factors II, VII, IX, and X). Because of the presence of preformed clotting factors in the blood, the full antithrombotic effect of warfarin therapy may require 36 to 72 h.

The major adverse effect of warfarin is bleeding. (Ironically, this compound was originally introduced as a very effective ro-denticide. As the active ingredient in rodent poison, it causes death due to internal hemorrhaging.) Furthermore, because it readily crosses the placenta and can cause a hemorrhagic disorder in the fetus, it is contraindicated in pregnant women.

Bibliography

1. Ganong, W.F., *Review of Medical Physiology*, 19th ed., Appleton & Lange, Stam-ford, CT, 1999.

2. Gaspard, K.J., Blood cells and the hematopoietic system, in *Pathophysiology: Concepts of Altered Health States*, 5th ed., Porth, C.P., Ed., Lippincott, Philadel-phia, 1998.

3. Guyton, A.C. and Hall, J.E., *Textbook of Medical Physiology*, 10th ed., W.B. Saunders, Philadelphia, 2000.

4. Hambleton, J. and O'Reilly, R.A., Drugs used in disorders of coagulation, in *Basic and Clinical Pharmacology*, 8th ed., Katzung, B.G., Ed., Lange Medical Books/McGraw–Hill, New York, 2001, chap. 34.

5. Majerus, P.W., Broze, G.J., Miletich, J.P., and Tollefsen, D.M., Anticoagulant, thrombolytic, and antiplatelet drugs, in *Goodman and Gilman's: The Pharmaco-logical Basis of Therapeutics*, 9th ed., Hardman, J.G. and Limbird, L.E., Eds., McGraw–Hill, New York, 1996, chap. 54.

6. Sherwood, L., *Human Physiology from Cells to Systems*, 4th ed., Brooks/Cole, Pacific Grove, CA, 2001.

7. Silverthorn, D.U., *Human Physiology: An Integrated Approach*, 2nd ed., Prentice-Hall, Upper Saddle River, NJ, 2001.

chapter seventeen

The respiratory system

Study objectives

- Describe the blood–gas interface and explain why the lungs are ideally suited for gas exchange
- List components and functions of the conducting airways
- Distinguish between the various types of airways in terms of epithelium and cartilage
- Describe the forces and factors responsible for maintaining inflation of the lungs
- Explain how inspiration and expiration take place
- Distinguish among atmospheric pressure, alveolar pressure, intrapleural pressure, and transpulmonary pressure
- Define pulmonary compliance
- Describe the role of elastic connective tissues in elastic recoil of the lungs as well as in lung compliance
- Explain how surface tension affects the elastic behavior of the lungs
- Describe the functions of pulmonary surfactant
- Explain how interdependence promotes alveolar stability
- Describe factors that determine airway resistance
- Define tidal volume, residual volume, expiratory reserve volume, and inspiratory reserve volume
- Define functional residual capacity, inspiratory capacity, total lung capacity, and vital capacity
- Distinguish between total ventilation and alveolar ventilation
- Distinguish among anatomical dead space, alveolar dead space, and physiological dead space
- Explain how each factor in Fick's law of diffusion influences gas exchange
- List the partial pressures of oxygen and carbon dioxide in various regions of the respiratory and cardiovascular systems
- Explain how the PO_2 and PCO_2 of alveolar gas are determined

- Explain the effects of airway obstruction and obstructed blood flow on ventilation-perfusion matching
- Describe local control mechanisms that restore the V/Q ratio to one
- Explain how oxygen is transported in the blood
- Describe the physiological significance of the steep and plateau portions of the oxyhemoglobin dissociation curve
- Describe the effects of carbon dioxide, pH, temperature, 2,3-bisphosphoglycerate, anemia, and carbon monoxide poisoning on the transport of oxygen
- Explain how carbon dioxide is transported in the blood
- Compare and contrast functions of the dorsal and ventral respiratory groups in the medullary respiratory center
- List and describe sources of input to the medullary respiratory center
- Compare and contrast the function of the peripheral and central chemoreceptors

17.1 Introduction

The cells of the body require a continuous supply of oxygen to produce energy and carry out their metabolic functions. Furthermore, these aerobic metabolic processes produce carbon dioxide, which must be continuously eliminated. The primary functions of the respiratory system include:

- Obtaining oxygen from the external environment and supplying it to the body's cells
- Eliminating carbon dioxide produced by cellular metabolism from the body

The process by which oxygen is taken up by the lungs and carbon dioxide is eliminated from the lungs is referred to as *gas exchange.*

17.2 Blood–gas interface

Gas exchange takes place at the *blood–gas interface,* which exists where the alveoli and the pulmonary capillaries come together. The *alveoli* are the smallest airways in the lungs; the *pulmonary capillaries* are found in the walls of the alveoli. Inspired oxygen moves from the alveoli into the capillaries for eventual transport to tissues. Entering the lungs by way of the pulmonary circulation, carbon dioxide moves from the capillaries into the alveoli for elimination by expiration. Oxygen and carbon dioxide move across the blood–gas interface by way of *simple diffusion* from an area of high concentration to an area of low concentration.

According to *Fick's law of diffusion,* the amount of gas that moves across the blood–gas interface is proportional to the surface area of the interface and inversely proportional to thickness of the interface. In other words, gas exchange in the lungs is promoted when the *surface area* for diffusion is maximized and the *thickness of the barrier* to diffusion is minimized. In fact, anatomically, the lungs are ideally suited for the function of gas exchange. There are 300 million alveoli in the lungs. Furthermore, the walls of each alveolus are completely lined with capillaries. There are as many as 280 billion pulmonary capillaries or almost 1000 capillaries per alveolus, resulting in a vast surface area for gas exchange of approximately 70 m².

More specifically, the blood–gas interface consists of the alveolar epithelium, capillary endothelium, and interstitium. The alveolar wall is made up of a single layer of flattened *type I alveolar cells*. The capillaries surrounding the alveoli also consist of a single layer of cells — *endothelial cells*. In between the alveolar epithelium and capillary endothelium is a very small amount of *interstitium*. Taken together, only 0.5 µm separates the air in the alveoli from the blood in the capillaries. The extreme thinness of the blood–gas interface further facilitates gas exchange by way of diffusion.

17.3 Airways

The airways of the lungs consist of a series of branching tubes; each level of branching results in another generation of airways. As they branch, the airways become narrower, shorter, and more numerous. There are a total of 23 *generations of airways* with the alveoli comprising 23rd generation.

Air is carried to and from the lungs by the *trachea* extending toward the lungs from the larynx. The trachea divides into the *right* and *left main bronchi;* these *primary bronchi* each supply a lung. The primary bronchi branch and form the *secondary*, or *lobar, bronchi*, one for each lobe of lung. The left lung consists of two lobes and the right lung has three lobes. The lobar bronchi branch and form the *tertiary*, or *segmental, bronchi*, one for each of the functional segments within the lobes. These bronchi continue to branch and move outward toward the periphery of the lungs. The smallest airways without alveoli are the *terminal bronchioles*. Taken together, the airways from the trachea through and including the terminal bronchioles are referred to as *conducting airways*. This region, which consists of the first 16 generations of airways, contains no alveoli, so no gas exchange takes place in this area. Consequently, it is also referred to as *anatomical dead space*. The volume of the anatomical dead space is approximately 150 ml (or about 1 ml per pound of ideal body weight).

The conducting airways carry out two major functions. The first is to lead inspired air to the more distal gas-exchanging regions of the lungs. The second is to warm and humidify the inspired air as it flows through them. The alveoli are delicate structures and may be damaged by excessive exposure to cold, dry air.

Branching from the terminal bronchioles are the *respiratory bronchioles*. This is the first generation of airways to have alveoli in their walls. Finally, there are the *alveolar ducts* which are completely lined with *alveolar sacs*. This region, from the respiratory bronchioles through the alveoli, is referred to as the *respiratory zone*, which comprises most of the lungs and has a volume of about 3000 ml at the end of a normal expiration.

Epithelium. All of the conducting airways (trachea through terminal bronchioles) are lined with *pseudostratified ciliated columnar epithelium*. Interspersed among these epithelial cells are mucus-secreting *goblet cells*. Furthermore, *mucus glands* are found in the larger airways. Consequently, the surface of the conducting airways consists of a mucus-covered ciliated epithelium. The cilia beat upward at frequencies between 600 and 900 beats per minute. As a result, the cilia continuously move the mucus away from the respiratory zone and up toward the pharynx. This *mucociliary escalator* provides an important protective mechanism that removes inhaled particles from the lungs. Mucus that reaches the pharynx is usually swallowed or expectorated. Interestingly, the nicotine found in cigarette smoke paralyzes the cilia, impairing their ability to remove any toxic substances. The respiratory bronchioles are lined with *cuboidal epithelial cells* that gradually flatten and become squamous type cells. As mentioned previously, the alveoli are composed of large, flat *simple squamous epithelium*.

Cartilage. The trachea and primary bronchi contain *C-shaped cartilage rings* in their walls; the lobar bronchi contain *plates of cartilage* that completely encircle the airways. The cartilage in these large airways provides structural support and prevents collapse of the airways. As the bronchi continue to branch and move out toward the lung periphery, the cartilage diminishes progressively until it disappears in airways about 1 mm in diameter. Airways with no cartilage are referred to as *bronchioles*. As the cartilage becomes more sparse, it is replaced by *smooth muscle*. Therefore, the bronchioles, which have no cartilage to support them and smooth muscle capable of vigorous constriction, are susceptible to collapse under certain conditions, such as an asthmatic attack.

17.4 The pleura

Each lung is enclosed in a double-walled sac referred to as the *pleura*. The *visceral pleura* is the membrane adhered to the external surface of the lungs. The *parietal pleura* lines the walls of the thoracic cavity. The space in between the two layers, the *pleural space*, is very thin and completely closed. The pleural space is filled with *pleural fluid* that lubricates the membranes and reduces friction between the layers as they slide past each other during breathing. This fluid also plays a role in maintaining lung inflation. The surface tension between the molecules of the pleural fluid keeps the two layers of the pleura "adhered" to each other — a concept similar to the effect of water between two glass microscope slides. The water molecules pull tightly together and oppose the separation of the slides. In this way, the lungs are in contact with the thoracic wall, fill the thoracic cavity, and remain inflated. In other words, surface tension in the pleural space opposes the tendency of the lungs to collapse.

17.5 Mechanics of breathing

The mechanics of breathing involve volume and pressure changes occurring during ventilation that allow air to move in and out of the lungs. Air will move from an area of high pressure to an area of low pressure. Therefore, a pressure gradient between the atmosphere and the alveoli must be developed. This section will explain how changes in thoracic volume, lung volume, and pulmonary pressures occur in order to cause the pressure gradients responsible for inspiration and expiration.

Thoracic volume. The volume of the thoracic cavity increases during inspiration and decreases during expiration.

Inspiration. The most important muscle of inspiration is the *diaphragm*, a thin, dome-shaped muscle inserted into the lower ribs. A skeletal muscle, it is supplied by the *phrenic nerves*. When the diaphragm contracts, it flattens and pushes downward against the contents of the abdomen. Therefore, contraction of the diaphragm causes an increase in the vertical dimension of the thoracic cavity and an increase in thoracic volume. In fact, the diaphragm is responsible for 75% of the enlargement of the thoracic cavity during normal, quiet breathing.

Assisting the diaphragm with inspiration are the *external intercostal muscles*, which connect adjacent ribs. When the external intercostal muscles contract, the ribs are lifted upward and outward (much like a handle on a bucket). Therefore, contraction of these muscles causes an increase in the horizontal dimension of the thoracic cavity and a further increase in thoracic volume. The external intercostal muscles are supplied by the *intercostal nerves*.

Deeper inspirations are achieved by more forceful contraction of the diaphragm and external intercostal muscles. Furthermore, *accessory inspiratory muscles*, including the scalenus and sternocleidomastoid muscles, contribute to this process. Located mainly in the neck, these muscles raise the sternum and elevate the first two ribs. As a result, the upper portion of the thoracic cavity is enlarged.

Expiration. Expiration during normal, quiet breathing is *passive*. In other words, no active muscle contraction is required. When the diaphragm is no longer stimulated by the phrenic nerves to contract, it passively returns to its original preinspiration position under the ribs. Relaxation of the external intercostal muscles allows the rib cage to fall inward and downward, largely due to gravity. As a result, these movements cause a decrease in thoracic volume.

During exercise or voluntary hyperventilation, expiration becomes an *active* process. Under these conditions, a larger volume of air must be exhaled more rapidly. Therefore, two muscle groups are recruited to facilitate this process. The most important muscles of expiration are the *muscles of the abdominal wall*. Contraction of these muscles pushes inward on the abdominal contents and increases abdominal pressure. As a result, the diaphragm is pushed upward more rapidly and more forcefully toward its preinspiration position. Assisting the muscles of the abdominal wall are the *internal inter-costal muscles*. These muscles are also found between the ribs; however, they are oriented in a direction opposite to that of the external intercostal muscles. Contraction of these muscles pulls the ribs inward and downward.

Lung volume. No real physical attachments exist between the lungs and the thoracic wall. Instead, the lungs literally float in the thoracic cavity, surrounded by pleural fluid. Therefore, the question arises of how the volume of the lungs increases when the volume of the thoracic cavity increases. The mechanism involves the pleural fluid and the surface tension between the molecules of this fluid. As mentioned previously, the surface tension of the pleural fluid keeps the parietal pleura lining the thoracic cavity and the visceral pleura on the external surface of the lungs "adhered" to each other. In other words, the pleural fluid keeps the lungs in contact with the chest wall. Therefore, as the muscles of inspiration cause the chest wall to expand (thus increasing the thoracic volume), the lungs are pulled open as well. As a result, lung volume also increases.

Pulmonary pressures. Changes in thoracic volume and lung volume cause pressures within the airways and the pleural cavity to change. These pressure changes create the pressure gradients responsible for airflow in and out of the lungs. Four pressures must be considered (see Figure 17.1):

- Atmospheric
- Intrapleural
- Alveolar
- Transpulmonary

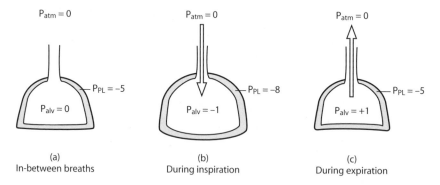

$P_{atm} = 0$ $P_{atm} = 0$ $P_{atm} = 0$

$P_{PL} = -5$ $P_{PL} = -8$ $P_{PL} = -5$

$P_{alv} = 0$ $P_{alv} = -1$ $P_{alv} = +1$

| (a) | (b) | (c) |
| In-between breaths | During inspiration | During expiration |

Figure 17.1 Pulmonary pressures. (a) In between breaths, alveolar pressure (P_{alv}) is equal to atmospheric pressure (P_{atm}), which is 0 cmH$_2$O. No air flows in or out of the lungs. (b) During inspiration, as lung volume increases, alveolar pressure decreases and becomes subatmospheric (−1 cmH$_2$O). The pressure gradient between the atmosphere and the alveoli allows air to flow into the lungs. (c) During expiration, the lungs recoil and lung volume decreases. Alveolar pressure increases and becomes greater (+1 cmH$_2$O) than atmospheric. The pressure gradient between atmosphere and alveoli forces air to flow out of the lungs.

As it does with all objects on the surface of the Earth, gravity exerts its effects on the molecules of the atmosphere. The weight generated by these molecules is referred to as *atmospheric*, or *barometric*, *pressure* (P_{atm}). At sea level, atmospheric pressure is 760 mmHg. In order to simplify this discussion, atmospheric pressure will be normalized to 0 mmHg (or 0 cmH$_2$O) and all other pressures are referenced to this.

Intrapleural pressure (P_{pl}) is the pressure within the pleural cavity. Under equilibrium conditions, the chest wall tends to pull outward and the elastic recoil of the lungs tends to pull them inward (like a collapsing balloon). These opposing forces create a subatmospheric or negative pressure within the pleural space. In between breaths, intrapleural pressure is –5 cmH$_2$O. During inspiration, the lungs follow the chest wall as it expands. However, the lung tissue resists being stretched, so the intrapleural pressure becomes even more negative and is –8 cmH$_2$0.

Alveolar pressure (P_{alv}) is the pressure within the alveoli. In between breaths, it is equal to 0 cmH$_2$O. Because no pressure gradient exists between the atmosphere and the alveoli, there is no airflow. However, in order for air to flow into the lungs, alveolar pressure must fall below atmospheric pressure. In other words, alveolar pressure becomes slightly negative. According to Boyle's law, at a constant temperature, the volume of a gas and its pressure are inversely related:

$$P \propto 1/V$$

Therefore, as lung volume increases during inspiration, the pressure within the alveoli decreases. Atmospheric pressure is now greater than alveolar pressure and air enters the lungs. Because the lungs are normally very compliant, or distensible, only a small pressure gradient is necessary for air to flow into the lungs. During inspiration, alveolar pressure is –1 cmH$_2$O. During expiration the opposite occurs. Lung volume decreases and pressure within the alveoli increases. Alveolar pressure is now greater than atmospheric pressure and air flows out of the lungs. Alveolar pressure during expiration is +1 cmH$_2$O.

Transpulmonary pressure (P_{tp}) is the pressure difference between the inside and outside of the lungs. In other words, it is the pressure difference between the alveoli and the pleural space:

$$P_{tp} = P_{alv} - P_{pl}$$

$$= 0 \text{ cmH}_2\text{O} - (-5 \text{ cmH}_2\text{O})$$

$$= + 5 \text{ cmH}_2\text{O}$$

In between breaths, the transpulmonary pressure is +5 cmH$_2$O. The transpulmonary pressure is also referred to as the *expanding pressure* of the lungs. A force of +5 cmH$_2$O expands, or pushes outward on, the lungs so that they fill the thoracic cavity. As might be expected, during inspiration, the transpulmonary pressure increases, causing greater expansion of the lungs:

$$P_{tp} = (-1 \text{ cmH}_2\text{O}) - (-8 \text{ cmH}_2\text{O})$$

$$= +7 \text{ cmH}_2\text{O}$$

The entry of air into the pleural cavity is referred to as a *pneumothorax*. This may occur spontaneously when a "leak" develops on the surface of the lung, allowing air to escape from the airways into pleural space. It may also result from a physical trauma that causes penetration of the chest wall so that air enters pleural space from the atmosphere. In either case, the pleural cavity is no longer a closed space and the pressure within it equilibrates with the atmospheric pressure (0 cmH$_2$O). As a result, the transpulmonary pressure is also equal to 0 cmH$_2$O and the lung collapses.

17.6 Elastic behavior of lungs

In a healthy individual, the lungs are very distensible; in other words, they can be inflated with minimal effort. Furthermore, during normal, quiet breathing, expiration is passive. The lungs inherently recoil to their preinspiratory position. These processes are attributed to the *elastic behavior* of the lungs. The elasticity of the lungs involves the following two interrelated properties:

- Elastic recoil
- Pulmonary compliance

The *elastic recoil* of the lungs refers to their ability to return to their original configuration following inspiration. It may also be used to describe the tendency of the lungs to oppose inflation. Conversely, *pulmonary compliance* describes how easily the lungs inflate. Compliance is defined as the change in lung volume divided by the change in transpulmonary pressure:

$$C = \frac{\Delta V}{\Delta P}$$

A highly compliant lung is one that requires only a small change in pressure for a given degree of inflation; a less compliant lung requires a larger change in pressure for the same degree of inflation. For example, during normal, quiet breathing, all adults inhale a tidal volume of about 500 ml per breath. In an individual with healthy, compliant lungs, the transpulmonary pressure gradient needed to be generated by the inspiratory muscles is very small (approximately 2 to 3 cmH$_2$O). The patient with less compliant, or "stiff," lungs must generate a larger transpulmonary pressure to inflate the lungs with the same 500 ml per breath. In other words, more vigorous contraction of the inspiratory muscles is required. Therefore, the *work of breathing* is increased. The elastic behavior of the lungs is determined by two factors:

- Elastic connective tissue in the lungs
- Alveolar surface tension

The *elastic connective tissue* in the lungs consists of *elastin* and *collagen* fibers found in the alveolar walls and around blood vessels and bronchi. When the lungs are inflated, the connective tissue fibers are stretched, or distorted. As a result, they have a tendency to return to their original shape and cause the elastic recoil of the lungs following inspiration. However, due to the interwoven mesh-like arrangement of these fibers, the lungs remain very compliant and readily distensible.

The alveoli are lined with fluid. At an air–water interface, the water molecules are much more strongly attracted to each other than to the air at their surface. This attraction produces a force at the surface of the fluid referred to as *surface tension (ST)*. Alveolar surface tension exerts two effects on the elastic behavior of the lungs. First, it decreases the compliance of the lungs. For example, inflation of the lung would increase its surface area and pull the water molecules lining the alveolus apart from each other. However, the attraction between these water molecules, or the surface tension, resists this expansion of the alveolus. Opposition to expansion causes a decrease in compliance; the alveolus is more difficult to inflate and the work of breathing is increased. The greater the surface tension, the less compliant are the lungs.

The second effect of surface tension is that it causes the alveolus to become as small as possible. As the water molecules pull toward each other, the alveolus forms a sphere, which is the smallest surface area for a given volume. This generates a pressure directed inward on the alveolus, or a *collapsing pressure*. The magnitude of this pressure is determined by the *Law of LaPlace*:

$$P = \frac{2ST}{r}$$

The collapsing pressure (*P*) is proportional to the alveolar surface tension (*ST*) and inversely proportional to the radius (*r*) of the alveolus. In other words, the greater the surface tension and the smaller the radius, the greater the collapsing pressure.

Due to this collapsing pressure, alveoli are inherently unstable. For example, if two alveoli of different sizes have the same surface tension, the smaller alveolus has a greater collapsing pressure and would tend to empty into the larger alveolus (see Figure 17.2, panel a). Air flows from an area of higher pressure to an area of lower pressure. As a result, the air within the smaller alveolus flows into the larger one and an area of *atelectasis* (airway collapse) develops. Therefore, if alveolar surface tension were to remain the same throughout the lungs, it would have the potential to cause widespread alveolar collapse.

Normal lungs, however, produce a chemical substance referred to as *pulmonary surfactant*. Made by *alveolar type II cells* within the alveoli, surfactant is a complex mixture of proteins (10 to 15%) and phospholipids (85 to 90%), including dipalmitoyl phosphatidyl choline, the predominant constituent. By interspersing throughout the fluid lining the alveoli, surfactant disrupts the cohesive forces between the water molecules. As a result, pulmonary surfactant has three major functions:

- Decreases surface tension
- Increases alveolar stability
- Prevents transudation of fluid

Pulmonary surfactant *decreases surface tension* of alveolar fluid. Reduced surface tension leads to a decrease in the collapsing pressure of the alveoli, an increase in pulmonary compliance (less elastic recoil), and a decrease in the work required to inflate the lungs with each breath. Also, pulmonary surfactant *promotes the stability of the alveoli*. Because the surface tension is reduced, the tendency for small alveoli to empty into larger ones is decreased (see Figure 17.2, panel b). Finally, surfactant *inhibits the transudation of fluid* out of the pulmonary capillaries into the alveoli. Excessive surface tension would tend to reduce the hydrostatic pressure in the tissue outside the capillaries. As a result, capillary filtration would be promoted. The movement of water out of the capillaries may result in interstitial edema formation and excess fluid in the alveoli.

Pharmacy application: infant respiratory distress syndrome

Infant respiratory distress syndrome (IRDS), also known as hyaline membrane disease, is one of the most common causes of respiratory disease in premature infants. In fact, it occurs in 30,000 to 50,000 newborns per year in the U.S. — most commonly in neonates born before week 25 of gestation. IRDS is characterized by areas of atelectasis, hemorrhagic edema, and the formation of hyaline membranes within the alveoli. IRDS is caused by a deficiency of pulmonary surfactant. Alveolar type II cells, which produce surfactant, do not begin to mature until weeks 25 to 28 of

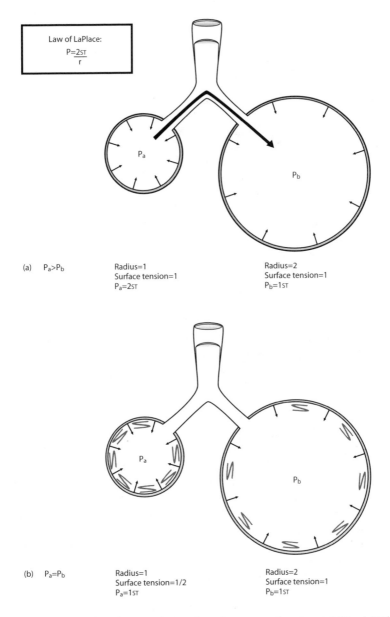

(a) $P_a > P_b$

Radius=1
Surface tension=1
$P_a = 2ST$

Radius=2
Surface tension=1
$P_b = 1ST$

(b) $P_a = P_b$

Radius=1
Surface tension=1/2
$P_a = 1ST$

Radius=2
Surface tension=1
$P_b = 1ST$

Figure 17.2 Effects of surface tension and surfactant on alveolar stability. (a) Effect of surface tension. According to the law of LaPlace ($P = 2ST/r$), if two alveoli have the same surface tension (*ST*), the alveolus with the smaller radius (*r*), and therefore a greater collapsing pressure (*P*), would tend to empty into the alveolus with the larger radius. (b) Effect of surfactant. Surfactant decreases the surface tension and thus the collapsing pressure in smaller alveoli to a greater extent than it does in larger alveoli. As a result, the collapsing pressures in all alveoli are equal. This prevents alveolar collapse and promotes alveolar stability.

gestation. Therefore, premature infants may have poorly functioning type II cells and insufficient surfactant production.

At birth, the first breath taken by the neonate requires high inspiratory pressures to cause the initial expansion of the lungs. Normally, the lungs will retain a portion of this first breath (40% of the residual volume), so subsequent breaths require much lower inspiratory pressures. In infants lacking surfactant, the lungs collapse between breaths and their airless portions become stiff and noncompliant. Therefore, every inspiration is as difficult as the first. In fact, a transpulmonary pressure of 25 to 30 mmHg is needed to maintain a patent airway (compared to the normal 5 mmHg). This results in a significant increase in the work of breathing and a decrease in ventilation. The inability of the neonate to ventilate adequately leads to progressive atelectasis, hypoxia, hypercarbia (increased carbon dioxide), and acidosis. Furthermore, formation of the hyaline membranes impairs gas exchange, which exacerbates these conditions.

The therapy for IRDS includes mechanical ventilation with continuous positive airway pressure. This maintains adequate ventilation and prevents airway collapse between breaths with the formation of atelectasis. Therapy also includes administration of exogenous pulmonary surfactant. Two types of surfactants are used to prevent and treat IRDS in the U.S. These include surfactants prepared from animal sources as well as synthetic surfactants. Exogenous pulmonary surfactants are administered as a suspension (in saline) through the endotracheal tube used for mechanical ventilation.

Many exogenous pulmonary surfactants are derived from bovine extracts. For example, Infasurf® contains the active ingredient calfactant, which is an unmodified calf lung extract that includes mostly phospholipids and hydrophobic surfactant-specific proteins. Other exogenous pulmonary surfactants derived from bovine lung extracts include Survanta® (active ingredient, beractant) and Bovactant® (active ingredient, alveofact). Exosurf® is a synthetic surfactant. It contains colfosceril palmitate, which is a phospholipid and an important constituent of natural and many synthetic pulmonary surfactant compounds.

17.7 Interdependence

Another important factor in maintaining alveolar stability is *interdependence*. Each alveolus in the lungs is surrounded by other alveoli (see Figure 17.3, panel a) and all of these alveoli are interconnected with each other by connective tissue. Because of these interconnections, any tendency for an alveolus to collapse is opposed by the surrounding alveoli. As the central

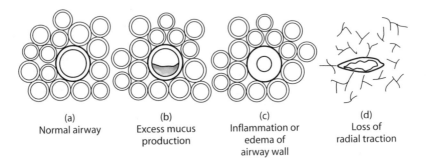

(a)
Normal airway

(b)
Excess mucus
production

(c)
Inflammation or
edema of
airway wall

(d)
Loss of
radial traction

Figure 17.3 Airway obstruction. (a) Normal, patent airway with radial traction offered to it by surrounding airways. Resistance in this airway is low and air flows through it freely. (b) The airway is obstructed by the presence of excess mucus and airway resistance is increased. Airflow is reduced. (c) Thickening of the airway wall due to inflammation or edema narrows the lumen of the airway. The decrease in airway radius increases airway resistance and decreases airflow. (d) Destruction of surrounding airways results in the loss of interdependence, or radial traction. Without the structural support offered by surrounding airways, the central airway collapses and airflow through it is reduced.

alveolus collapses, it pulls inward on the surrounding alveoli, stretching them and distorting their shape. In response, the distorted alveoli pull back in the opposite direction to regain their normal shape. In other words, they exert *radial traction* on the central alveolus. As a result, the alveolus is pulled open and collapse is prevented.

17.8 Airway resistance

The factors determining the flow of air through the airways are analogous to those determining flow of blood through the vessels and are described by Ohm's law:

$$\text{Airflow} = \frac{\Delta P}{R}$$

Airflow through the airways is proportional to the gradient between atmospheric pressure and alveolar pressure (ΔP) and inversely proportional to the *airway resistance* (R).

Factors determining resistance to airflow are also analogous to those determining the resistance to blood flow and include viscosity, length of the airway, and airway radius. Under normal conditions, the viscosity of the air is fairly constant and the length of the airway is fixed. Therefore, airway radius is the critically important physiological factor determining airway resistance:

$$R \alpha \frac{1}{r^4}$$

Airway resistance is inversely proportional to the *radius* (*r*) of the airway to the fourth power. In other words, when the radius is reduced by a factor of two (50%), the airway resistance increases 16-fold. Several factors determine airway resistance, including:

- Lung volume
- Airway obstruction
- Bronchial smooth muscle tone

Lung volume. As *lung volume* increases, airway resistance decreases, that is, as the lungs inflate, the airways expand and become larger. The increase in airway radius decreases airway resistance. Conversely, as lung volume decreases, airway resistance increases. In fact, at very low lung volumes, the small airways may close completely. This is a problem, especially at the base of the lungs, where, due to the weight of the lungs, the airways are less well expanded.

Airway obstruction. *Airway obstruction* may be caused by several factors including:

- Excess mucus production
- Inflammation and edema of the airway wall
- Airway collapse

Asthma and chronic bronchitis are characterized by *overproduction of a thick, viscous mucus* (see Figure 17.3, panel b). This mucus blocks the airways and, in effect, reduces the radius of the airways and increases airway resistance. A severe asthmatic attack may be accompanied by formation of mucus plugs, which completely obstruct airflow. Asthma and chronic bronchitis, which are considered chronic inflammatory conditions, are also characterized by *inflammation and edema of the airway walls* (see Figure 17.3, panel c). This thickening of the airway wall narrows the lumen of the airway and increases airway resistance. Increase in airway resistance due to excess mucus production and inflammation is reversible pharmacologically. The pathophysiology of emphysema involves the breakdown, or destruction, of alveoli. This results in the loss of interdependence, or the effect of radial traction, on airways and leads to *airway collapse* (see Figure 17.3, panel d). Increase in airway resistance due to this form of lung obstruction is irreversible.

Bronchial smooth muscle tone. Changes in *bronchial smooth muscle tone* are particularly important in the bronchioles compared to the bronchi. Recall that the walls of the bronchioles consist almost entirely of smooth muscle. Contraction and relaxation of this muscle has a marked effect on the internal radius of the airway. An increase in bronchial smooth muscle tone, or *bronchoconstriction*, narrows the lumen of the airway and increases resistance to airflow. The activation of irritant receptors in the trachea and large bronchi by airborne pollutants, smoke, and noxious chemicals elicits reflex bronchoconstriction. This reflex is mediated by the *parasympathetic nervous system*, specifically, by the vagus nerve. Acetylcholine released from the vagus nerve stimulates muscarinic receptors on the bronchial smooth muscle to cause bronchoconstriction. This parasympathetic reflex is meant to be a protective response, limiting the penetration of toxic substances deep into the lungs. Parasympathetic stimulation of the lungs also enhances mucus production in an effort to trap inhaled particles.

Bronchoconstriction is also elicited by several endogenous chemicals released from mast cells during an allergy or asthmatic attack. These substances, including histamine and the leukotrienes, may also promote the inflammatory response and edema formation.

A decrease in bronchial smooth muscle tone, or *bronchodilation*, widens the lumen of the airway and decreases the resistance to airflow. *Sympathetic nervous stimulation* causes bronchodilation. The adrenergic receptors found on the airway smooth muscle are β_2-adrenergic receptors. Recall that norepinephrine has a very low affinity for these receptors. Therefore, direct sympathetic stimulation of the airways has little effect. Epinephrine released from the adrenal medulla causes most of this bronchodilation. Epinephrine has a strong affinity for β_2-adrenergic receptors. Therefore, during a mass sympathetic discharge, as occurs during exercise or the "fight-or-flight" response, epinephrine-induced bronchodilation minimizes airway resistance and maximizes airflow.

Pharmacy application: pharmacological treatment of asthma

Bronchial asthma is defined as a chronic inflammatory disease of the lungs; it affects an estimated 9 to 12 million individuals in the U.S. Furthermore, its prevalence has been increasing in recent years. Asthma is characterized by reversible airway obstruction (in particular, bronchospasm), airway inflammation, and increased airway responsiveness to a variety of bronchoactive stimuli. Many factors may induce an asthmatic attack, including allergens; respiratory infections; hyperventilation; cold air; exercise; various drugs and chemicals; emotional upset; and airborne pollutants (smog, cigarette smoke).

The desired outcome in the pharmacological treatment of asthma is to prevent or relieve the reversible airway obstruction and airway hyperresponsiveness caused by the inflammatory process. Therefore, categories of medications include bronchodilators and anti-inflammatory drugs.

A commonly prescribed class of bronchodilators is the β_2-adrenergic receptor agonists (e.g., albuterol, metaproterenol) that cause relaxation of bronchial smooth muscle and relieve the congestion of bronchial mucosa. Beta two-adrenergic receptor agonists are useful during an acute asthmatic attack and are effective when taken prior to exercise in individuals with exercise-induced asthma. These drugs are usually administered by inhalation or by a nebulizer. Another bronchodilator is ipratropium, an anticholinergic drug that blocks muscarinic receptors on the airway smooth muscle. This results in bronchodilation, particularly in large airways. This agent has no effect on the composition or viscosity of bronchial mucus. Also used to treat acute asthmatic attacks, ipratropium is administered by inhalation.

Corticosteroids (e.g., beclomethazone, flunisolide, triamcinolone) have anti-inflammatory and immunosuppressant actions. These drugs are used prophylactically to prevent the occurrence of asthma in patients with frequent attacks. Because they are not useful during an acute attack, corticosteroids are prescribed along with maintenance bronchodilators. These drugs are also administered by inhalation. Cromolyn is another anti-inflammatory agent used prophylactically to prevent an asthmatic attack. The exact mechanism of action of cromolyn is not fully understood; however, it is likely to involve the stabilization of mast cells. This prevents the release of the inflammatory mast cell mediators involved in inducing an asthmatic attack. Cromolyn has proven effective in patients with exercise-induced asthma.

17.9 Ventilation

Ventilation is the exchange of air between the external atmosphere and the alveoli. It is typically defined as the volume of air entering the alveoli per minute. A complete understanding of ventilation requires the consideration of lung volumes.

Standard lung volumes. The size of the lungs and therefore the lung volumes depend upon an individual's height, weight or body surface area, age, and gender. This discussion will include the typical values for a 70-kg adult. The *four standard lung volumes* are (see Figure 17.4):

- Tidal volume
- Residual volume
- Expiratory reserve volume
- Inspiratory reserve volume

The *tidal volume* (V_T) is the volume of air that enters the lungs per breath. During normal, quiet breathing, tidal volume is 500 ml per breath. This volume increases significantly during exercise. The *residual volume* (RV) is the volume of air remaining in the lungs following a maximal forced expiration. Dynamic compression of the airways causes collapse and trapping

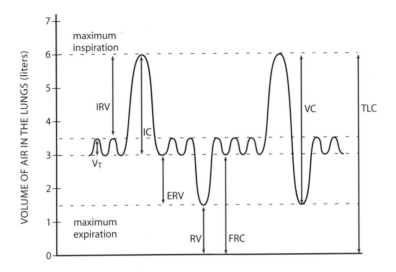

Figure 17.4 Standard lung volumes and lung capacities (typical values for 70-kg adult). Tidal volume (V$_T$) is 500 ml during normal, quiet breathing. Inspiratory reserve volume (IRV) is obtained with a maximal inspiration and is 2.5 l. Tidal volume and IRV together determine the inspiratory capacity (IC), which is 3.0 l. Expiratory reserve volume (ERV) is obtained with maximal expiration and is 1.5 l. The volume of air remaining in the lungs following maximal expiration is the residual volume (RV), which is 1.5 l. The functional residual capacity (FRC) is the volume of air remaining in the lungs following a normal expiration and is 3.0 l. Vital capacity (VC) is obtained with deepest inspiration and most forceful expiration and is 4.5 l. The maximum volume to which the lungs can be expanded is the total lung capacity (TLC) and is approximately 6.0 l in adult males and 5.0 l in adult females.

of air in the alveoli. Residual volume is normally 1.5 l. It can be much greater in patients with emphysema because of the increased tendency for airway collapse. *Expiratory reserve volume (ERV)* is the volume of air expelled from the lungs during a maximal forced expiration beginning at the end of a normal expiration. The ERV is normally about 1.5 l. The *inspiratory reserve volume (IRV)* is the volume of air inhaled into the lungs during a maximal forced inspiration beginning at the end of a normal inspiration. The IRV is normally about 2.5 l and is determined by the strength of contraction of the inspiratory muscles and the inward elastic recoil of the lungs.

The *four standard lung capacities* consist of two or more lung volumes in combination (see Figure 17.4):

- Functional residual capacity
- Inspiratory capacity
- Total lung capacity
- Vital capacity

The *functional residual capacity* (FRC) is the volume of air remaining in the lungs at the end of a normal expiration. The FRC consists of the residual volume and the expiratory reserve volume and is equal to 3 l. The *inspiratory capacity* (IC) is the volume of air that enters the lungs during a maximal forced inspiration beginning at the end of a normal expiration (FRC). The IC consists of the tidal volume and the inspiratory reserve volume and is equal to 3 l. The *total lung capacity* (TLC) is the volume of air in the lungs following a maximal forced inspiration. In other words, it is the maximum volume to which the lungs can be expanded. It is determined by the strength of contraction of the inspiratory muscles and the inward elastic recoil of the lungs. The TLC consists of all four lung volumes and is equal to about 6 l in a healthy adult male and about 5 l in a healthy adult female. The *vital capacity* (VC) is the volume of air expelled from the lungs during a maximal forced expiration following a maximal forced inspiration. In others words, it consists of the tidal volume as well as the inspiratory and expiratory reserve volumes. Vital capacity is approximately 4.5 l.

Total ventilation. The total ventilation (*minute volume*) is the volume of air that enters the lungs per minute. It is determined by tidal volume and breathing frequency:

$$\text{Total ventilation} = \text{tidal volume} \times \text{breathing frequency}$$

$$= 500 \text{ ml/breath} \times 12 \text{ breaths/min}$$

$$= 6000 \text{ ml/min}$$

With an average tidal volume of 500 ml/breath and breathing frequency of 12 breaths/min, 6000 ml or 6 l of air move in and out of the lungs per minute. These values apply to conditions of normal, quiet breathing; tidal volume and breathing frequency increase substantially during exercise.

Alveolar ventilation. Alveolar ventilation is less than the total ventilation because the last portion of each tidal volume remains in the conducting airways; therefore, that air does not participate in gas exchange. As mentioned at the beginning of the chapter, the volume of the conducting airways is referred to as anatomical dead space. The calculation of alveolar ventilation includes the tidal volume adjusted for anatomical dead space and includes only air that actually reaches the respiratory zone:

Alveolar ventilation

$$= (\text{tidal volume} - \text{anatomical dead space}) \times \text{breathing frequency}$$

$$= (500 \text{ ml/breath} - 150 \text{ ml dead space}) \times 12 \text{ breaths/min}$$

$$= 4200 \text{ ml/min}$$

During exercise, the working muscles need to obtain more oxygen and eliminate more carbon dioxide. Alveolar ventilation is increased accordingly. Interestingly, the increase in tidal volume is greater than the increase in breathing frequency. This is the most efficient mechanism by which to enhance alveolar ventilation. Using the preceding values, a twofold increase in breathing frequency, from 12 breaths/min to 24 breaths/min, results in an alveolar ventilation of 8400 ml/min. In other words, alveolar ventilation also increases by a factor of two. However, a twofold increase in tidal volume, from 500 ml/breath to 1000 ml/breath, results in an alveolar ventilation of 10,200 ml/min. Alveolar ventilation is enhanced more in this case because a greater percentage of the tidal volume reaches the alveoli. At a tidal volume of 500 ml/breath and an anatomical dead space of 150 ml, 30% of the inspired air is wasted because it does not reach the alveoli to participate in gas exchange. However, when the tidal volume is 1000 ml/breath, only 15% of the inspired air remains in the anatomical dead space.

Dead space. *Anatomical dead space* is equal to the volume of the conducting airways. This is determined by the physical characteristics of the lungs because, by definition, these airways do not contain alveoli to participate in gas exchange. *Alveolar dead space* is the volume of air that enters unperfused alveoli. In other words, these alveoli receive airflow but no blood flow; with no blood flow to the alveoli, gas exchange cannot take place. Therefore, alveolar dead space is based on functional considerations rather than anatomical factors. Healthy lungs have little or no alveolar dead space. Various pathological conditions, such as low cardiac output, may result in alveolar dead space. The anatomical dead space combined with the alveolar dead space is referred to as *physiological dead space*:

Physiological dead space = anatomical dead space + alveolar dead space

Physiological dead space is determined by measuring the amount of carbon dioxide in the expired air. Therefore, it is based on the functional characteristics of the lungs because only perfused alveoli can participate in gas exchange and eliminate carbon dioxide.

Pharmacy application: drug-induced hypoventilation

Hypoventilation is defined as a reduction in the rate and depth of breathing. Inadequate ventilation results in hypoxemia, or a decrease in the concentration of oxygen in the arterial blood. Hypoventilation may be induced inadvertently by various pharmacological agents, including opioid analgesics such as morphine. These medications cause hypoventilation by way of their effects on the respiratory centers in the brainstem. Doses of morphine too small to alter a patient's consciousness may cause discernible respiratory depression. This inhibitory effect on the respiratory drive increases progressively as the dose of morphine is increased. In fact, in humans, death due to morphine poisoning is almost always due to respiratory arrest. Although therapeutic doses of morphine decrease tidal volume, the decrease in breathing frequency is the primary cause of decreased minute volume.

17.10 Diffusion

Oxygen and carbon dioxide cross the blood–gas interface by way of *diffusion*. The factors that determine the rate of diffusion of each gas are described by *Fick's law of diffusion*:

$$V_{gas} \alpha \frac{A \times D \times (\Delta P)}{T}$$

Diffusion is proportional to the surface area of the blood–gas interface (A); the diffusion constant (D); and the partial pressure gradient of the gas (ΔP). Diffusion is inversely proportional to the thickness of the blood–gas interface (T).

The *surface area* of the blood–gas interface is about 70 m^2 in a healthy adult at rest. Specifically, 70 m^2 of the potential surface area for gas exchange in the lungs is ventilated and perfused. The amount of this surface area may be altered under various conditions. For example, during exercise, an increased number of pulmonary capillaries are perfused (due to increased cardiac output, and therefore blood flow, through the lungs). As a result, a larger percentage of the alveoli are ventilated and perfused, which increases the surface area for gas exchange. Conversely, a fall in the cardiac output reduces the number of perfused capillaries, thus reducing the surface area for gas exchange. Another pathological condition affecting surface area is emphysema. This pulmonary disease, usually associated with cigarette smoking, causes destruction of alveoli.

The *diffusion constant* for a gas is proportional to the solubility of the gas and inversely proportional to the square root of the molecular weight of the gas:

$$D \alpha \frac{solubility}{\sqrt{MW}}$$

Oxygen and carbon dioxide are small molecules with low molecular weights; however, carbon dioxide is 20 times more soluble than oxygen. Therefore, the value of the diffusion constant for carbon dioxide is larger than that of oxygen, which facilitates the exchange of carbon dioxide across the blood–gas interface.

The *thickness* of the blood–gas interface is normally less than 0.5 μm. This extremely thin barrier promotes the diffusion of gases. The thickness may increase, however, under conditions of interstitial fibrosis, interstitial edema, and pneumonia. Fibrosis involves the excess production of collagen fibers by fibroblasts in the interstitial space. Edema is the movement of fluid from the capillaries into the interstitial space. Pneumonia causes inflammation and alveolar flooding. In each case, the thickness of the barrier between the air and the blood is increased and diffusion is impaired.

The diffusion of oxygen and carbon dioxide also depends on their *partial pressure gradients*. Oxygen diffuses from an area of high partial pressure in the alveoli to an area of low partial pressure in the pulmonary capillary blood. Conversely, carbon dioxide diffuses down its partial pressure gradient from the pulmonary capillary blood into the alveoli.

According to *Dalton's law*, the partial pressure of a gas (P_{gas}) is equal to its fractional concentration (% total gas) multiplied by the total pressure (P_{tot}) of all gases in a mixture:

$$P_{gas} = \% \text{ total gas} \times P_{tot}$$

The atmosphere is a mixture of gases containing 21% oxygen and 79% nitrogen. Due to the effects of gravity, this mixture exerts a total atmospheric pressure (barometric pressure) of 760 mmHg at sea level. Using these values of fractional concentration and total pressure, the partial pressures for oxygen (PO_2) and nitrogen (PN_2) can be calculated:

$$PO_2 = 0.21 \times 760 \text{ mmHg} = 160 \text{ mmHg}$$

$$PN_2 = 0.79 \times 760 \text{ mmHg} = 600 \text{ mmHg}$$

The PO_2 of the atmosphere at sea level is 160 mmHg and the PN_2 is 600 mmHg. The total pressure (760 mmHg) is equal to the sum of the partial pressures.

Under normal, physiological conditions, the partial pressure gradient for oxygen between the alveoli and the pulmonary capillary blood is quite substantial. However, this gradient may be diminished under certain conditions, such as ascent to altitude and hypoventilation. Altitude has no effect on the concentration of oxygen in the atmosphere. However, the effects of gravity on barometric pressure progressively decrease as elevation increases. For example, at an elevation of 17,000 ft, which is the height of Pike's Peak, the barometric pressure is only 380 mmHg. Therefore, the PO_2 of the atmosphere at this altitude is 80 mmHg ($PO_2 = 0.21 \times 380 \text{ mmHg} = 80 \text{ mmHg}$). This results in a marked decrease in the partial pressure gradient between the alveoli and the pulmonary capillary blood. Consequently, diffusion is impaired. Hypoventilation decreases the rate of oxygen uptake into the alveoli; once again, the partial pressure gradient and the rate of diffusion

Table 17.1 Partial Pressures of Oxygen and Carbon Dioxide

Location	PO_2 (mmHg)	PCO_2 (mmHg)
Atmosphere	160	0
Conducting airways (inspired)	150	0
Alveolar gas	100	40
Arterial blood	100	40
Tissues	40	45
Mixed venous blood	40	45

are reduced. Conditions resulting in impaired diffusion lead to the development of *hypoxemia*, or decreased oxygen in the arterial blood.

17.11 Partial pressures of oxygen and carbon dioxide

As explained in the previous section, the PO_2 of the atmosphere is 160 mmHg. The partial pressure of carbon dioxide (PCO_2) is negligible (see Table 17.1). As air is inspired, it is warmed and humidified as it flows through the conducting airways. Therefore, water vapor is added to the gas mixture. This is accounted for in the calculation of PO_2 in the conducting airways:

$$PO_2 \text{ inspired air} = 0.21 \times (760 \text{ mmHg} - 47 \text{ mmHg})$$

$$= 150 \text{ mmHg}$$

The partial pressure of the water vapor is 47 mmHg and, as a result, the PO_2 is slightly decreased to 150 mmHg. The PCO_2 remains at 0 mmHg. By the time the air reaches the alveoli, the PO_2 has decreased to about 100 mmHg. The PO_2 of the alveolar gas is determined by two processes:

- Rate of replenishment of oxygen by ventilation
- Rate of removal of oxygen by the pulmonary capillary blood

The primary determinant of alveolar PO_2 is the rate of replenishment of oxygen by ventilation. As mentioned previously, hypoventilation causes a decrease in alveolar PO_2. The rate of removal of oxygen by the pulmonary capillary blood is determined largely by the oxygen consumption of the tissues. As metabolic activity and oxygen consumption increase, the PO_2 of the mixed venous blood decreases. As a result, the partial pressure gradient for oxygen between the alveoli and the blood is increased and the diffusion of oxygen is enhanced.

The PCO_2 of the alveoli is about 40 mmHg and is also determined by two processes:

- Rate of delivery of carbon dioxide to the lungs from the tissues
- Rate of elimination of carbon dioxide by ventilation

As cellular metabolism increases, the rate of production of carbon dioxide also increases. Typically, increased activity is associated with an increase in ventilation so that the increased amounts of carbon dioxide delivered to the lungs are eliminated. Hypoventilation impairs the elimination of carbon dioxide and causes an increase in alveolar PCO_2.

Assuming that oxygen diffuses down its partial pressure gradient from the alveoli into the pulmonary capillary blood until equilibration is reached, the PO_2 of this blood reaches 100 mmHg. This blood flows back to the left side of the heart and into the systemic circulation. Therefore, the PO_2 of the arterial blood is 100 mmHg. Likewise, assuming that carbon dioxide diffuses down its partial pressure gradient from the pulmonary capillary blood into the alveoli until equilibration is reached, the PCO_2 of the blood leaving these capillaries should be 40 mmHg. Therefore, the PCO_2 of the arterial blood is 40 mmHg.

The arterial blood, which is high in oxygen and low in carbon dioxide, is delivered to the tissues. Within the tissues, oxygen is consumed by metabolism and carbon dioxide is produced. Under typical resting conditions, the PO_2 of the tissues is 40 mmHg. Therefore, oxygen diffuses down its concentration gradient from the systemic capillary blood into the cells of the tissues until equilibration is reached. The PO_2 of the venous blood leaving the tissues is also 40 mmHg. The PCO_2 of the tissues is 45 mmHg. Therefore, carbon dioxide diffuses down its concentration gradient from the tissues into the blood until equilibration is reached. The PCO_2 of the venous blood leaving the tissues is 45 mmHg.

The mixed venous blood, which is low in oxygen and high in carbon dioxide, flows back to the lungs to obtain oxygen and eliminate carbon dioxide. Note that the partial pressure gradient for oxygen between the alveoli (100 mmHg) and the mixed venous blood (40 mmHg) is 60 mmHg. The partial pressure gradient for carbon dioxide between the mixed venous blood (45 mmHg) and the alveoli (40 mmHg) is 5 mmHg. According to Fick's law of diffusion, the small partial pressure gradient for carbon dioxide would tend to reduce the exchange of this gas; however, its relatively high solubility and diffusion constant allow it to diffuse quite readily across the blood–gas interface.

17.12 Ventilation–perfusion matching

In order to optimize gas exchange, the uptake of oxygen from the alveolar gas into the pulmonary blood, and the elimination of carbon dioxide from the pulmonary blood into the alveolar gas, a given lung unit must be equally well ventilated and perfused. In other words, the air and blood must be brought together for the exchange gases. This is referred to as *ventilation–perfusion (V/Q) matching*. The most effective conditions for gas exchange occur when the V/Q ratio is equal to one, or when the amount of ventilation in a lung unit is balanced, or matched, by the amount of perfusion. In this region, the mixed venous blood entering the pulmonary capillaries has a PO_2 of 40

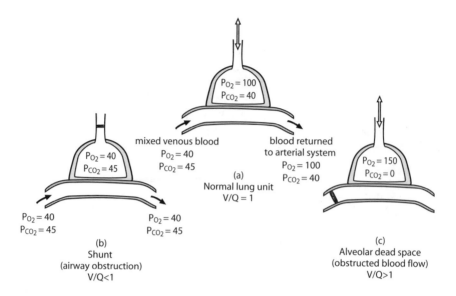

Figure 17.5 Ventilation–perfusion matching. (a) Normal lung unit. Ventilation and perfusion are matched so that the V/Q ratio is equal to one and gas exchange is optimized. Mixed venous blood low in oxygen and high in carbon dioxide enters the pulmonary capillaries. As the blood flows through these capillaries in the walls of the alveoli, oxygen is obtained and carbon dioxide is eliminated. Blood returning to the heart and the arterial system is high in oxygen and low in carbon dioxide. (b) Shunt. Airway obstruction with normal perfusion can lead to shunt (V/Q < 1). Blood flows through the lungs without obtaining oxygen or eliminating carbon dioxide. This V/Q mismatch causes hypoxemia. (c) Alveolar dead space. Obstructed blood flow with normal ventilation causes development of alveolar dead space (V/Q > 1). The partial pressures of oxygen and carbon dioxide in the alveoli are similar to those of conducting airways. This ventilation is wasted because it does not participate in gas exchange.

mmHg and a PCO_2 of 45 mmHg. The alveolar gas has a PO_2 of 100 mmHg and a PCO_2 of 40 mmHg. Ventilation–perfusion matching results in efficient gas exchange, a PO_2 of 100 mmHg and a PCO_2 of 40 mmHg in the blood, leaving the capillaries and returning to the heart (see Figure 17.5, panel a).

Airway obstruction leads to a reduction in the V/Q ratio to a value less than one. In this lung unit, perfusion is greater than ventilation (see Figure 17.5, panel b). Complete airway obstruction leads to *shunt*, which refers to blood that enters the arterial system without passing through a region of ventilated lung. In other words, mixed venous blood travels through the pulmonary circulation without participating in gas exchange. This blood enters the pulmonary capillaries with a PO_2 of 40 mmHg and a PCO_2 of 45 mmHg. If the lung unit is not ventilated, then this blood exits the capillaries and returns to the heart with the partial pressures of oxygen and carbon dioxide unchanged. The addition of blood low in oxygen to the rest of the blood returning from the lungs causes *hypoxemia*. The degree of hypoxemia is determined by the magnitude of the shunt. As airway obstruction increases throughout the lungs, this widespread decrease in the V/Q ratio results in a greater volume of poorly oxygenated blood returning to the heart and a greater degree of hypoxemia. As discussed, airway obstruction may be caused by many factors, including bronchoconstriction, excess mucus production, airway collapse, and alveolar flooding.

Obstructed blood flow leads to an increase in the V/Q ratio to a value greater than one and, in this lung unit, ventilation is greater than perfusion (see Figure 17.5, panel c). Complete loss of blood flow leads to *alveolar dead space*. In this lung unit, the air enters the alveoli with partial pressures of oxygen and carbon dioxide equal to those of the conducting airways (PO_2 of 150 mmHg and PCO_2 of 0 mmHg). With no perfusion, oxygen is not taken up from this mixture, nor is carbon dioxide added to the mixture to be eliminated. Alveolar dead space may be caused by pulmonary thromboembolism, which is when a pulmonary blood vessel is occluded by a blood clot. Alveolar dead space may also occur when alveolar pressure is greater than pulmonary capillary pressure. This leads to compression of the capillaries and a loss of perfusion. Alveolar pressure may be increased by positive pressure mechanical ventilation. Pulmonary capillary pressure may be decreased by hemorrhage and a decrease in cardiac output.

Ventilation–perfusion mismatch leads to hypoxemia. Reduced ventilation caused by obstructed airflow or reduced perfusion caused by obstructed blood flow leads to impaired gas exchange. Interestingly, each of these conditions is minimized by *local control mechanisms* that attempt to match airflow and blood flow in a given lung unit.

Bronchiolar smooth muscle is sensitive to changes in carbon dioxide levels. Excess carbon dioxide causes bronchodilation and reduced carbon dioxide causes bronchoconstriction. Pulmonary vascular smooth muscle is sensitive to changes in oxygen levels; excess oxygen causes vasodilation and insufficient oxygen (hypoxia) causes vasoconstriction. The changes in bronchiolar and vascular smooth muscle tone alter the amount of ventilation and perfusion in a lung unit to return the V/Q ratio to one.

In a lung unit with high blood flow and low ventilation (airway obstruction), the level of carbon dioxide is increased and the level of oxygen is decreased. The excess carbon dioxide causes bronchodilation and an increase in ventilation. The reduced oxygen causes vasoconstriction and a decrease in perfusion. In this way, the V/Q ratio is brought closer to one and gas exchange is improved.

In a lung unit with low blood flow and high ventilation (alveolar dead space), the level of carbon dioxide is decreased and the level of oxygen is increased. The reduced carbon dioxide causes bronchoconstriction and a decrease in ventilation. The excess oxygen causes vasodilation and an increase in perfusion and, once again, the V/Q ratio is brought closer to one and gas exchange is improved.

17.13 Gas transport in blood

Once the oxygen has diffused from the alveoli into pulmonary circulation, it must be carried, or transported, in the blood to cells and tissues that need it. Furthermore, once the carbon dioxide has diffused from the tissues into the systemic circulation, it must be transported to the lungs, where it can be eliminated. This section considers mechanisms by which these gases are transported.

Transport of oxygen. Oxygen is carried in the blood in two forms:

- Physically dissolved
- Chemically combined with hemoglobin

Oxygen is poorly soluble in plasma. At a PO_2 of 100 mmHg, only 3 ml of oxygen is *physically dissolved* in 1 l of blood. Assuming a blood volume of 5 l, a total of 15 ml of oxygen is in the dissolved form. A normal rate of oxygen consumption at rest is about 250 ml/min. During exercise, oxygen consumption may increase to 3.5 to 5.5 l/min. Therefore, the amount of dissolved oxygen is clearly insufficient to meet the needs of the tissues. Most of the oxygen in the blood (98.5%) is transported *chemically combined with hemoglobin.* A large complex molecule, hemoglobin consists of four polypeptide chains (globin portion), each of which contains a ferrous iron atom (heme portion). Each iron atom can bind reversibly with an oxygen molecule:

$$O_2 + Hb \leftrightarrow HbO_2$$

The binding of oxygen to hemoglobin follows the *law of mass action* so that, as the PO_2 increases (as it does in the lungs), more will combine with hemoglobin. When the PO_2 decreases, as it does in the tissues consuming it, the reaction moves to the left and the hemoglobin releases the oxygen. Each gram of hemoglobin can combine with up to 1.34 ml of oxygen. In a healthy individual, there are 15 g of hemoglobin per 100 ml of blood. Therefore, the oxygen content of the blood is 20.1 ml O_2/100 ml blood:

$$\frac{15 \text{ g Hb}}{100 \text{ ml blood}} \times \frac{1.34 \text{ ml } O_2}{\text{g Hb}} = \frac{20.1 \text{ ml } O_2}{100 \text{ ml blood}}$$

It is important to note that oxygen bound to hemoglobin has no effect on the PO_2 of the blood. The amount of oxygen bound to hemoglobin determines *oxygen content* of the blood. The PO_2 of the blood is determined by the amount of oxygen dissolved in the plasma.

The PO_2 of blood is the major factor determining the amount of oxygen chemically combined with hemoglobin, or the *percent of hemoglobin saturation.* The relationship between these two variables is illustrated graphically by the *oxyhemoglobin dissociation curve* (see Figure 17.6). This relationship is not

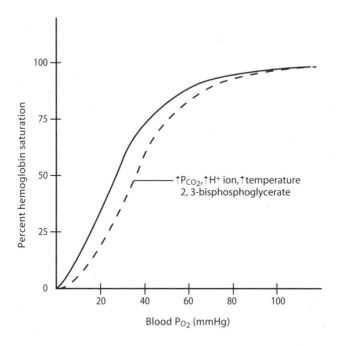

Figure 17.6 Oxyhemoglobin dissociation curve. The percent of hemoglobin saturation depends upon the PO_2 of the blood, which in pulmonary capillaries is 100 mmHg. Consequently, in the lungs the hemoglobin loads up with oxygen and becomes 97.5% saturated. The average PO_2 of the blood in systemic capillaries is 40 mmHg. Therefore, in the tissues, hemoglobin releases oxygen and saturation falls to 75%. Increased PCO_2, H^+ ion concentration, temperature and 2,3-bisphosphoglycerate shifts the oxyhemoglobin dissociation curve to the right. As a result, at any given PO_2, the hemoglobin releases more oxygen to the tissue.

linear. The amount of oxygen carried by hemoglobin increases steeply up to a PO_2 of about 60 mmHg. Beyond this point, the curve becomes much flatter, so little change occurs in the percent of hemoglobin saturation as PO_2 continues to increase. At a PO_2 of 100 mmHg, which is the normal PO_2 of the alveoli, and therefore the arterial blood, the hemoglobin is 97.5% saturated with oxygen.

Each region of the curve (the steep and flat plateau portions) has important physiological significance. The *steep portion of the curve*, between 0 and 60 mmHg, is the PO_2 range found in the cells and tissues. On average, the PO_2 of the tissues and therefore the mixed venous blood is about 40 mmHg at rest. At a PO_2 of 40 mmHg, the hemoglobin is 75% saturated with oxygen. In other words, as the blood flows through the systemic capillaries, the hemoglobin releases 22.5% of its oxygen to the tissues. An increase in the metabolic activity of a tissue, and thus an increase in oxygen consumption, will decrease the PO_2 in that tissue. The fall in PO_2 in this region of the oxyhemoglobin dissociation curve has a profound effect on the percent of hemoglobin saturation. At a PO_2 of 15 mmHg, the hemoglobin is only 25% saturated with oxygen; in this case, the hemoglobin has released 72.5% of its oxygen to the tissue. Therefore, a small drop in PO_2 (from 40 to 15 mmHg) results in a marked increase in the unloading of oxygen (more than three times as much oxygen has been released to the tissue that needs it).

The *plateau portion of the curve*, between 60 and 100 mmHg, is the PO_2 range found in the alveoli. As the mixed venous blood flows through the pulmonary capillaries in the walls of the alveoli, the hemoglobin loads up with oxygen. As mentioned earlier, at a normal alveolar PO_2 of 100 mmHg, the hemoglobin becomes almost fully saturated with oxygen (97.5%). Interestingly, at a PO_2 of 60 mmHg, the hemoglobin still becomes 90% saturated with oxygen. In other words, the hemoglobin remains quite saturated with oxygen even with a marked fall in PO_2 (40 mmHg). This provides a good margin of safety for the oxygen-carrying capacity of blood. Therefore, if an individual ascends to some altitude above sea level or has pulmonary disease such that the alveolar PO_2 falls, the oxygen content of the blood remains high.

Factors affecting transport of oxygen. Several factors affect the transport of oxygen, including:

- PCO_2, pH, and temperature
- 2,3-Bisphosphoglycerate
- Anemia
- Carbon monoxide

An *increase in* PCO_2, a *decrease in pH*, and an *increase in temperature* shift the oxyhemoglobin dissociation curve to the right. As a result, at any given PO_2, the hemoglobin releases more oxygen to the tissue (see Figure 17.6). Carbon dioxide and hydrogen ion can bind to hemoglobin; the binding of these substances changes the conformation of the hemoglobin and reduces its affinity for oxygen. An increase in temperature also reduces the affinity of hemoglobin for oxygen. This effect benefits a metabolically active tissue. As the rate of metabolism increases, as it does during exercise, oxygen consumption, and therefore the demand for oxygen, increases. In addition, the carbon dioxide, hydrogen ions, and heat produced by the tissue are increased. These products of metabolism facilitate the release of oxygen from the hemoglobin to the tissue that needs it.

2,3-Bisphosphoglycerate (2,3-BPG) is produced by red blood cells. This substance binds to hemoglobin, shifting the oxyhemoglobin dissociation curve to the right. Once again, the rightward shift of the curve reduces the affinity of hemoglobin for oxygen so that more oxygen is released to the tissues. Levels of 2,3-BPG are increased when the hemoglobin in the arterial blood is chronically undersaturated or, in other words, during *hypoxemia*. Decreased arterial PO_2 may occur at altitude or as the result of various cardiovascular or pulmonary diseases. The rightward shift of the curve is beneficial at the level of the tissues because more of the oxygen bound to the hemoglobin is released to the tissues. However, the shift of the curve may be detrimental in the lungs because loading of hemoglobin may be impaired. Levels of 2,3-BPG may be decreased in blood stored in a blood bank for as little as 1 week. A decrease in 2,3-BPG shifts the oxyhemoglobin dissociation curve to the left. In this case, at any given PO_2, unloading of oxygen to the tissues is decreased. The progressive depletion of 2,3-BPG can be minimized by storing the blood with citrate–phosphate–dextrose.

Anemia decreases the oxygen content of the blood and therefore the supply of oxygen to tissues. It is characterized by a low hematocrit that may be caused by a number of pathological conditions, such as a decreased rate of erythropoiesis (red blood cell production), excessive loss of erythrocytes, or a deficiency of normal hemoglobin in the erythrocytes. Although the oxygen content of the blood decreases, it is important to note that anemia has no effect on the PO_2 of the blood or on the oxyhemoglobin dissociation curve (see Figure 17.7). Arterial PO_2 is determined only by the amount of oxygen dissolved in the blood, which is unaffected. Furthermore, the affinity of hemoglobin for oxygen has not changed; what has changed is the amount of hemoglobin in the blood. If less hemoglobin is available to bind with oxygen, then less oxygen is in the blood.

Carbon monoxide interferes with the transport of oxygen to the tissues by way of two mechanisms:

- Formation of carboxyhemoglobin
- Leftward shift of the oxyhemoglobin dissociation curve

Carbon monoxide has a much greater affinity (240 times) for hemoglobin than does oxygen, so *carboxyhemoglobin* is readily formed. Therefore, even small amounts of carbon monoxide can tie up the hemoglobin and prevent loading of oxygen. Furthermore, formation of carboxyhemoglobin causes a *leftward shift of the oxyhemoglobin dissociation curve* (see Figure 17.7). As a result, at any given PO_2, unloading of oxygen to the tissues is impaired. Therefore, the hemoglobin not only carries less oxygen, but also does not release this oxygen to the tissues that need it. The concentration of hemoglobin in the blood and the PO_2 of the blood are normal.

Carbon monoxide poisoning is particularly insidious. An individual exposed to carbon monoxide is usually unaware of it because this gas is odorless, colorless, and tasteless. Furthermore, it does not elicit any irritant reflexes that result in sneezing, coughing, or feelings of dyspnea (difficulty in breathing). Finally, carbon monoxide does not stimulate ventilation. As will be discussed in a subsequent section, the peripheral chemoreceptors are sensitive to decreases in PO_2, not oxygen content.

Transport of carbon dioxide. Carbon dioxide is carried in the blood in three forms:

- Physically dissolved
- Carbamino hemoglobin
- Bicarbonate ions

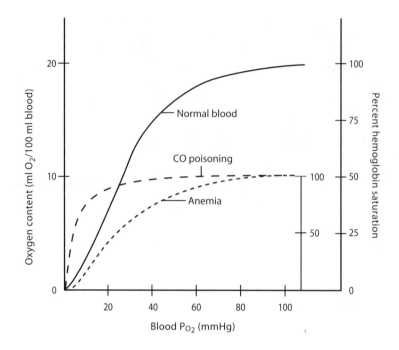

Figure 17.7 Effect of anemia and carbon monoxide poisoning on oxygen transport. Anemia results from a deficiency of normal hemoglobin. The PO_2 of the blood and the percent of hemoglobin saturation remain normal. However, because less hemoglobin is present to transport oxygen, oxygen content of the blood is decreased. Carbon monoxide impairs transport of oxygen to the tissues by two mechanisms. First, it binds preferentially with hemoglobin and prevents it from binding with oxygen. As a result, the hemoglobin remains fully saturated (although with carbon monoxide instead of oxygen) and the oxygen content of the blood is decreased. Second, it shifts the oxyhemoglobin dissociation curve to the left and inhibits the release of oxygen from the hemoglobin. As with anemia, the PO_2 of the blood is unaffected.

As with oxygen, the amount of carbon dioxide *physically dissolved* in the plasma is proportional to its partial pressure. However, carbon dioxide is 20 times more soluble in plasma than is oxygen. Therefore, approximately 10% of carbon dioxide in blood is transported in the dissolved form.

Carbon dioxide can combine chemically with the terminal amine groups (NH_2) in blood proteins. The most important of these proteins for this process is hemoglobin. The combination of carbon dioxide and hemoglobin forms *carbamino hemoglobin*:

$$Hb \cdot NH_2 + CO_2 \leftrightarrow Hb \cdot NH \cdot COOH$$

Deoxyhemoglobin can bind more carbon dioxide than oxygenated hemoglobin. Therefore, unloading of oxygen in the tissues facilitates loading of carbon dioxide for transport to the lungs. Approximately 30% of carbon dioxide in the blood is transported in this form.

The remaining 60% of carbon dioxide is transported in the blood in the form of *bicarbonate ions*. This mechanism is made possible by the following reaction:

$$H_2O + CO_2 \xleftarrow{\quad CA \quad} H_2CO_3 \leftrightarrow H^+ + HCO_3^-$$

The carbon dioxide produced during cellular metabolism diffuses out of the cells and into the plasma. It then continues to diffuse down its concentration gradient into the red blood cells. Within these cells, the enzyme *carbonic anhydrase* (CA) facilitates combination of carbon dioxide and water to form *carbonic acid* (H_2CO_3). The carbonic acid then dissociates into hydrogen ion (H^+) and bicarbonate ion (HCO_3^-).

As the bicarbonate ions are formed, they diffuse down their concentration gradient out of the red blood cell and into the plasma. This process is beneficial because bicarbonate ion is far more soluble in the plasma than carbon dioxide. As the negatively charged bicarbonate ions exit the red blood cell, chloride ions, the most abundant anions in the plasma, enter the cells by way of HCO_3^-–Cl^- carrier proteins. This process, referred to as the *chloride shift*, maintains electrical neutrality. Many of the hydrogen ions bind with hemoglobin. As with carbon dioxide, deoxyhemoglobin can bind more readily with hydrogen ions than oxygenated hemoglobin.

This entire reaction is reversed when the blood reaches the lungs. Because carbon dioxide is eliminated by ventilation, the reaction is pulled to the left. Bicarbonate ions diffuse back into the red blood cells. The hemoglobin releases the hydrogen ions and is now available to load up with oxygen. The bicarbonate ions combine with the hydrogen ions to form carbonic acid, which then dissociates into carbon dioxide and water. The carbon dioxide diffuses down its concentration gradient from the blood into the alveoli and is exhaled. A summary of the three mechanisms by which carbon dioxide is transported in the blood is illustrated in Figure 17.8.

17.14 Regulation of ventilation

The rate and depth of breathing are perfectly adjusted to meet the metabolic needs of the tissues and to maintain a PO_2 of 100 mmHg, a PCO_2 of 40 mmHg, and a pH of 7.4 in the arterial blood. Breathing is initiated spontaneously by the central nervous system and occurs in a continuous cyclical pattern of inspiration and expiration. The three major components of the regulatory system for ventilation are:

- Medullary respiratory center
- Receptors and other sources of input
- Effector tissues (respiratory muscles)

a) In the tissues

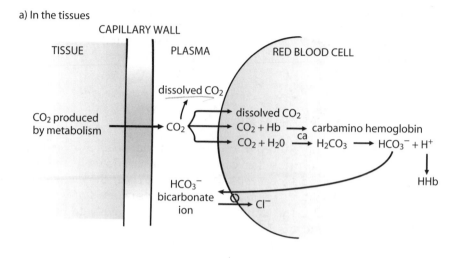

b) In the lungs

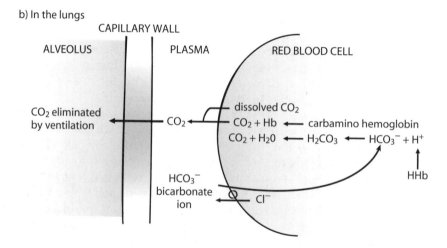

Figure 17.8 Transport of carbon dioxide in the blood. Carbon dioxide (CO_2) is transported in the blood in three forms: dissolved, bound with hemoglobin, and as bicarbonate ion (HCO_3^-). The carbon dioxide produced by the tissues diffuses down its concentration gradient into the plasma and red blood cells. A small amount of CO_2 remains in the dissolved form. Second, within the red blood cell, carbon dioxide can bind with reduced hemoglobin to form carbamino hemoglobin. Third, due to the presence of the enzyme carbonic anhydrase (CA), carbon dioxide can also combine with water to form carbonic acid (H_2CO_3). Carbonic acid then dissociates into bicarbonate ion and hydrogen ion (H^+). The hydrogen ion is picked up by the reduced hemoglobin (HHb). The bicarbonate ion diffuses down its concentration gradient into the plasma. In order to maintain electrical neutrality, as the bicarbonate ion exits the cell, a chloride ion (Cl^-) enters the cell, a process referred to as the chloride shift. In the lungs, these reactions reverse direction and carbon dioxide is eliminated by ventilation.

Aggregates of cell bodies within the medulla of the brainstem form the *medullary respiratory center,* which has two distinct functional areas:

- Dorsal respiratory group
- Ventral respiratory group

The aggregate of cell bodies in the dorsal region of the medulla is the *dorsal respiratory group (DRG).* The DRG consists primarily of *inspiratory neurons.* These neurons are self-excitable and repetitively generate action potentials to cause inspiration. The inspiratory neurons descend to the spinal cord where they stimulate neurons that supply the inspiratory muscles, including those of the phrenic nerves and the intercostal nerves. These nerves then stimulate the diaphragm and the external intercostal muscles to contract and cause inspiration. When the inspiratory neurons are electrically inactive, expiration takes place. Therefore, this cyclical electrical activity of the DRG is responsible for the basic rhythm of breathing. Furthermore, the DRG is likely the site of integration of the various sources of input that alter the spontaneous pattern of inspiration and expiration.

The aggregate of cell bodies in the ventral region of the medulla is the *ventral respiratory group (VRG).* The VRG consists of expiratory and inspiratory neurons. This region is inactive during normal, quiet breathing. (Recall that expiration at this time is a passive process.) However, the VRG is active when the demands for ventilation are increased, such as during exercise. Under these conditions, action potentials in the *expiratory neurons* cause forced, or active, expiration. These neurons descend to the spinal cord where they stimulate the neurons that supply the expiratory muscles, including those that innervate the muscles of the abdominal wall and the internal intercostal muscles. Contractions of these muscles cause a more rapid and more forceful expiration.

Inspiratory neurons of the VRG augment inspiratory activity. These neurons descend to the spinal cord where they stimulate neurons that supply the accessory muscles of inspiration including those that innervate the scalenus and sternocleidomastoid muscles. Contractions of these muscles cause a more forceful inspiration.

In summary, the regulation of ventilation by the medullary respiratory center determines the:

- Interval between the successive groups of action potentials of the inspiratory neurons, which determines the rate or *frequency of breathing* (as the interval shortens, the breathing rate increases)
- Frequency of action potential generation and duration of this electrical activity to the motor neurons, and therefore the muscles of inspiration and expiration, which determines the depth of breathing, or the *tidal volume* (as the frequency and duration of stimulation increase, the tidal volume increases)

The medullary respiratory center receives excitatory and inhibitory inputs from many areas of the brain and peripheral nervous system, including:

- Lung receptors
- Proprioceptors
- Pain receptors
- Limbic system
- Chemoreceptors

Pulmonary stretch receptors are responsible for initiating the *Hering–Breuer reflex*. These stretch receptors are located within the smooth muscle of large and small airways. They are stimulated when the tidal volume exceeds 1 l. Nerve impulses are transmitted by the vagus nerve to the medullary respiratory center and inhibit the inspiratory neurons. The primary function of these receptors and the Hering–Breuer reflex is to prevent overinflation of the lungs.

Irritant receptors are located throughout the respiratory system in the nasal mucosa, upper airways, tracheobronchial tree, and possibly the alveoli. Mechanical or chemical stimulation of these receptors can cause a reflex cough or sneeze. In either case, a deep inspiration is followed by a forced expiration against a closed glottis, which causes a marked increase in intrapulmonary pressure. The glottis then opens suddenly, resulting in an explosive expiration. The ensuing high airflow rate is meant to eliminate the irritant from the respiratory tract. In a cough, expiration occurs by way of the mouth; in a sneeze, expiration is through the nose. Stimulation of irritant receptors also causes hyperpnea (increased ventilation) and bronchoconstriction.

Proprioceptors are located in muscles, tendons, and joints; their stimulation causes an increase in ventilation. These receptors are believed to play a role in initiating and maintaining the elevated ventilation associated with exercise.

Pain receptors also influence the medullary respiratory center. Pain may cause a reflex increase in ventilation in the form of a "gasp." Somatic pain typically causes hyperpnea and visceral pain typically causes apnea, or decreased ventilation.

Breathing is modified during the expression of various emotional states. For example, the normal cyclical pattern of breathing is interrupted during laughing, crying, sighing, or moaning. The modifications in ventilation associated with these activities are elicited by input from the *limbic system* to the medullary respiratory center.

Chemoreceptors provide the most important input to the medullary respiratory center in terms of regulating ventilation to meet the metabolic requirements of the body. Chemoreceptors are sensitive to changes in PO_2, PCO_2, and pH. The two types of chemoreceptors are:

- Peripheral chemoreceptors
- Central chemoreceptors

The *peripheral chemoreceptors* include the carotid and aortic bodies. The *carotid bodies*, which are more important in humans, are located near the bifurcation of the common carotid arteries. The *aortic bodies* are located in the arch of the aorta. The peripheral chemoreceptors respond to a decrease in PO_2, an increase in PCO_2, and a decrease in pH (increase in H^+ ion concentration) of the arterial blood.

The *central chemoreceptors* are located near the ventral surface of the medulla in close proximity to the respiratory center. These receptors are surrounded by the extracellular fluid (ECF) of the brain and respond to changes in H^+ ion concentration. The composition of the ECF surrounding the central chemoreceptors is determined by the cerebrospinal fluid (CSF), local blood flow, and local metabolism.

A summary of the responses of the peripheral and the central chemoreceptors to reduced arterial oxygen, increased arterial carbon dioxide, and increased arterial hydrogen ion concentration is found in Table 17.2.

Chemoreceptor response to decreased arterial PO_2. Hypoxia has a direct depressant effect on central chemoreceptors as well as on the medullary respiratory center. In fact, hypoxia tends to inhibit activity in all regions of the brain. Therefore, the ventilatory response to hypoxemia is elicited only by the peripheral chemoreceptors.

A decrease in arterial PO_2 causes stimulation of the peripheral chemoreceptors. The ensuing elevation in ventilation increases the uptake of oxygen and returns PO_2 to its normal value of 100 mmHg. However, this stimulatory effect does not occur until the arterial PO_2 falls below 60 mmHg. The physiological explanation for this delayed response to hypoxemia is provided by the shape of the oxyhemoglobin dissociation curve (see Figure 17.6). The plateau portion of the curve illustrates that hemoglobin remains quite saturated (90%) at a PO_2 of 60 mmHg. Therefore, when the PO_2 of arterial blood is between 60 and 100 mmHg, the oxygen content of the blood is still very high. An increase in ventilation at this point is not critical. However, below a PO_2 of 60 mmHg, the saturation of hemoglobin, and therefore the oxygen content of the blood, decreases rapidly. Stimulation of the peripheral chemoreceptors in order to increase ventilation and enhance uptake of oxygen is now essential to meet the metabolic needs of the body. Let it be clear, however, that this ventilatory response to hypoxemia is due to the change in PO_2, not oxygen content. For example, as discussed previously, anemia,

Table 17.2 Chemoreceptor Responses to Changes in Arterial PO_2, PCO_2, and $H^\pm$ Ion Concentration

Change in arterial blood	Effect on peripheral chemoreceptors	Effect on central chemoreceptors
↓ Arterial PO_2	Stimulates (PO_2 < 60 mmHg)	Depresses
↑ Arterial PCO_2	Weakly stimulates	Strongly stimulates
↑ Arterial H^+ ion	Stimulates	No effect

which decreases oxygen content but not PO_2, does not cause an increase in ventilation.

It is important to note that a decrease in PO_2 is not the primary factor in the minute-to-minute regulation of ventilation. This is because the peripheral chemoreceptors are not stimulated until the PO_2 falls to life-threatening levels. A decrease of this magnitude would likely be associated with abnormal conditions, such as pulmonary disease, hypoventilation, or ascent to extreme altitude.

Chemoreceptor response to increased arterial PCO_2. An increase in arterial PCO_2 causes weak stimulation of the peripheral chemoreceptors. The ensuing mild increase in ventilation contributes to elimination of carbon dioxide and decrease in PCO_2 to its normal value of 40 mmHg. The response of the peripheral chemoreceptors to changes in arterial PCO_2 is much less important than that of the central chemoreceptors. In fact, less than 20% of the ventilatory response to an increase in arterial PCO_2 is elicited by the peripheral chemoreceptors.

An increase in arterial PCO_2 results in marked stimulation of the central chemoreceptors. In fact, this is the most important factor in regulation of ventilation. It is well known that it is impossible to hold one's breath indefinitely. As carbon dioxide accumulates in the arterial blood, the excitatory input to the respiratory center from the central chemoreceptors overrides the voluntary inhibitory input and breathing resumes. Furthermore, this occurs well before the arterial PO_2 falls low enough to stimulate the peripheral chemoreceptors.

Interestingly, the central chemoreceptors are insensitive to carbon dioxide, although they are very sensitive to changes in the H^+ ion concentration in the ECF surrounding them. How does an increase in arterial PCO_2 cause an increase in H^+ ion concentration in the brain? Carbon dioxide crosses the blood–brain barrier readily. As the arterial PCO_2 increases, carbon dioxide diffuses down its concentration gradient into the ECF of the brain from the cerebral blood vessels. Due to the presence of the enzyme carbonic anhydrase, the following reaction takes place in the ECF of the brain:

$$CO_2 + H_2O \xleftrightarrow{\text{CA}} H_2CO_3 \longleftrightarrow H^+ + HCO3^-$$

Carbonic anhydrase (CA) facilitates the formation of carbonic acid (H_2CO_3) from carbon dioxide and water. The carbonic acid then dissociates to liberate hydrogen ion (H^+) and bicarbonate ion ($HCO3^-$). The hydrogen ions strongly stimulate the central chemoreceptors to increase ventilation. The ensuing elimination of excess carbon dioxide from the arterial blood returns the PCO_2 to its normal value.

Conversely, a decrease in the arterial PCO_2 due to hyperventilation results in a decrease in the H^+ ion concentration in the ECF of the brain. Decreased stimulation of the central chemoreceptors (and therefore a decrease in the excitatory input to the medullary respiratory center) causes a decrease in ventilation. Continued metabolism allows carbon dioxide to accumulate in the blood such that the PCO_2 returns to its normal value.

Chemoreceptor response to increased arterial hydrogen ion concentration. An increase in arterial hydrogen ion concentration, or a decrease in arterial pH, stimulates the peripheral chemoreceptors and enhances ventilation. This response is important in maintaining acid-base balance. For example, under conditions of *metabolic acidosis*, caused by the accumulation of acids in the blood, the enhanced ventilation eliminates carbon dioxide and thus reduces the concentration of H^+ ions in the blood. Metabolic acidosis may occur in patients with uncontrolled diabetes mellitus or when tissues become hypoxic and produce lactic acid. An increase in arterial hydrogen ion concentration has no effect on the central chemoreceptors. Hydrogen ions are unable to cross the blood–brain barrier.

17.15 Ventilatory response to exercise

Exercise results in an increase in oxygen consumption and in carbon dioxide production by the working muscles. In order to meet the metabolic demands of these tissues, ventilation increases accordingly. Minute ventilation increases linearly in response to oxygen consumption and carbon dioxide production up to a level of approximately 60% of an individual's work capacity. During this period of mild to moderate exercise, mean arterial PO_2 and PCO_2 remain relatively constant at their normal values. In fact, the partial pressures of these gases may even improve (arterial PO_2 is increased; arterial PCO_2 is decreased). Therefore, it does not appear that hypoxic or hypercapnic stimulation of the peripheral chemoreceptors plays a role in ventilatory response to mild to moderate exercise.

Beyond this point, during more severe exercise associated with anaerobic metabolism, minute ventilation increases faster than the rate of oxygen consumption, but proportionally to the increase in carbon dioxide production. The mechanism of the ventilatory response to severe exercise involves metabolic acidosis caused by anaerobic metabolism. The lactic acid produced under these conditions liberates an H^+ ion that effectively stimulates the peripheral chemoreceptors to increase ventilation.

During exercise, the increase in minute ventilation results from increases in tidal volume and breathing frequency. Initially, the increase in tidal volume is greater than the increase in breathing frequency. As discussed earlier in this chapter, increases in tidal volume increase alveolar ventilation more effectively. Subsequently, however, as metabolic acidosis develops, the increase in breathing frequency predominates.

The mechanisms involved with the ventilatory response to exercise remain quite unclear. No single factor, or combination of factors, can fully account for the increase in ventilation during exercise. Therefore, much of this response remains unexplained. Factors that appear to play a role include:

- Impulses from the cerebral cortex
- Impulses from proprioceptors
- Body temperature
- Epinephrine

At the beginning of exercise, ventilation immediately increases. This increase is thought to be caused by two mechanisms involving the cerebral cortex. Neurons of the primary motor cortex stimulate alpha motor neurons in the spinal cord to cause skeletal muscle contraction. In addition, *impulses from the motor cortex*, transmitted through collateral interconnections to the medullary respiratory center, stimulate ventilation. The motor cortex is also involved in stimulation of the cardiovascular system during exercise. These adjustments, which occur before any homeostatic factors (e.g., blood gases) have changed, are referred to as *anticipatory adjustments*. The immediate increase in ventilation may account for as much as 50% of the total ventilatory response to exercise. A *conditioned reflex*, or a learned response to exercise, may also be involved. Once again, impulses from the cerebral cortex provide input to the medullary respiratory center.

Proprioceptors originating in muscles and joints of the exercising limbs provide substantial input to the medullary respiratory center. In fact, even passive movement of the limbs causes an increase in ventilation. Therefore, the mechanical aspects of exercise also contribute to the ventilatory response. The increased metabolism associated with exercise increases *body temperature*, which further contributes to the increase in ventilation during exercise. (Not surprisingly, ventilation is also enhanced in response to a fever.) Exercise is associated with a mass sympathetic discharge. As a result, *epinephrine* release from the adrenal medulla is markedly increased. Epinephrine is believed to stimulate ventilation.

Bibliography

1. Levitsky, M.G., *Pulmonary Physiology*, 5th ed., McGraw–Hill, New York, 1999.
2. Porth, C.M., *Pathophysiology: Concepts of Altered Health States*, 4th ed., J.B. Lippincott Company, Philadelphia, 1998.
3. Reisine, T. and Pasternak, G., Opioid analgesics and antagonists, in *Goodman and Gilman's: The Pharmacological Basis of Therapeutics*, 9th ed., Hardman, J.G. and Limbird, L.E., Eds., McGraw–Hill, New York, 1996, chap. 23.
4. Robergs, R.A. and Roberts, S.O., *Exercise Physiology, Exercise, Performance, and Clinical Applications*, C.V. Mosby, St. Louis, 1997.
5. Schmann, L., Obstructive pulmonary disorders, in *Perspectives on Pathophysiology*, Copstead, L.-E.C., Ed., W.B. Saunders, Philadelphia, 1995, chap. 20.
6. Schmann, L., Ventilation and respiratory failure, in *Perspectives on Pathophysiology*, Copstead, L.-E.C., Ed., W.B. Saunders, Philadelphia, 1995, chap. 22.
7. Sherwood, L., *Human Physiology from Cells to Systems*, 4th ed., Brooks/Cole, Pacific Grove, CA, 2001.
8. Silverthorn, D.U., *Human Physiology: An Integrated Approach*, 2nd ed., Prentice-Hall, Upper Saddle River, NJ, 2001.

9. *Taber's Cyclopedic Medical Dictionary*, 19th ed., F.A. Davis Co., Philadelphia, PA, 2001.

10. Ward, J.P.T., Ward, J., Wiener, C.M., and Leach, R.M., *The Respiratory System at a Glance*, Blackwell Science Ltd., Oxford, 2002.

11. West, J.B., *Pulmonary Physiology and Pathophysiology, an Integrated, Case-Based Approach*, Lippincott/Williams & Wilkins, Philadelphia, 2001.

chapter eighteen

The digestive system

Study objectives

- Describe the anatomical and functional characteristics of each of the four layers of the digestive tract wall: mucosa, submucosa, muscularis externa, and serosa
- Distinguish between the two types of gastrointestinal motility: segmentation and peristalsis
- Explain how each of the three types of sensory receptors within the digestive tract is stimulated: chemoreceptors, osmoreceptors, and mechanoreceptors
- Explain how the following mechanisms regulate activity of the digestive system: intrinsic nerve plexuses, extrinsic autonomic nerves, and gastrointestinal hormones
- List the components of saliva and their functions
- Describe how salivary secretion is regulated
- Explain how swallowing takes place
- For the esophagus, stomach, small intestine, and large intestine, describe:
  - Specialized anatomical modifications
  - Type of motility and how it is regulated
  - Types of secretions and how they are regulated
  - Digestive processes that take place
  - Absorptive processes that take place

18.1 Introduction

The function of the digestive system is to make ingested food available to the cells of the body. Most ingested food is in the form of very large molecules that must be broken down by mechanical and biochemical processes into their smaller components (see Table 18.1). These smaller units are then absorbed across the wall of the digestive tract and distributed throughout the body. Not all ingested materials may be completely

Table 18.1 Ingested and Absorbable Molecules for Three Major Nutrient Categories

Ingested Form of Nutrient Molecules	Absorbable Form of Nutrient Molecules
Carbohydrates	Monosaccharides
• Polysaccharides (starch)	• Glucose
• Disaccharides	• Galactose
• Sucrose (table sugar)	• Fructose
• Lactose (milk sugar)	
Proteins	Amino acids
Fats	Monoglycerides
• Triglycerides	Free fatty acids

digested and absorbed by the human gastrointestinal tract. For example, cellulose, the fibrous form of plant carbohydrates, is indigestible by humans. Normally, about 95% of ingested food materials are made available for use by the body. Interestingly, as long as food remains within the digestive tract, it is technically outside the body. Not until the materials have crossed the epithelium that lines the tract are they considered to have "entered" the body.

The digestive system consists of:

• Gastrointestinal tract
• Accessory digestive organs

The *gastrointestinal tract* is essentially a tube that runs through the center of the body from the mouth to the anus. This tube consists of the following organs:

• Mouth
• Pharynx
• Esophagus
• Stomach
• Small intestine
• Large intestine

Although these organs are continuous with one another, each has important anatomical modifications that allow it to carry out its specific functions.

The *accessory digestive organs* exist outside the gastrointestinal tract; however, each of these organs empties secretions into the tract that contribute to the process of digestion. These accessory digestive organs include:

• Salivary glands
• Liver
• Gallbladder
• Pancreas

18.2 Digestive tract wall

The digestive tract wall has the same basic structure from the esophagus through and including the colon. The four major layers within the wall are:

- Mucosa
- Submucosa
- Muscularis externa
- Serosa

Mucosa. The innermost layer of the wall is the *mucosa*, which consists of a mucous membrane, the lamina propria, and the muscularis mucosa. The *mucous membrane* provides important protective and absorptive functions for the digestive tract. The nature of the epithelial cells lining the tract varies from one region to the next. Rapidly dividing stem cells continually produce new cells to replace worn out epithelial cells. The average life span of these epithelial cells is only a few days. The *lamina propria* is a thin middle layer of connective tissue. This region contains the capillaries and small lymphatic vessels that take up the digested nutrient molecules. The *muscularis mucosa* is a thin layer of smooth muscle. Contraction of this muscle may alter the effective surface area for absorption in the lumen.

Submucosa. The *submucosa* is a thick middle layer of connective tissue. This tissue provides the digestive tract wall with its distensibility and elasticity as nutrient materials move through the system.

Muscularis externa. The outer layer of the wall is the *muscularis externa*. In most regions of the tract, it consists of two layers of muscle: an inner circular layer and an outer longitudinal layer. Contraction of the circular layer narrows the lumen of the tube. Contraction of the longitudinal layer causes the tube to shorten.

The muscle of the digestive tract consists of *single-unit smooth muscle*. Within each layer, the muscle cells are connected by gap junctions forming a syncytium. Action potentials generated at a given site travel along the muscle layer. Furthermore, this muscle is self-excitable; it undergoes slow but continuous electrical activity producing rhythmic contractions of the digestive tract wall. The cycles of depolarization and repolarization in the smooth muscle are referred to as *slow-wave potentials*. These potentials do not reach threshold during each cycle, so contraction does not necessarily occur with each depolarization. Smooth muscle contraction will take place only when the slow wave actually depolarizes all the way to threshold. At this point, voltage-gated Ca^{++} channels open, Ca^{++} ions enter the cell and one or more action potentials are generated. These action potentials result in *phasic contractions*. The force and duration of muscle contraction is determined by the number of action potentials generated. Typically, phasic contractions last only a few seconds.

Muscular activity, or *gastrointestinal motility*, is enhanced by stretching the muscle, as occurs with the presence of food materials and distension of the digestive tract wall. It is also enhanced by parasympathetic nervous stimulation and by several specific gastrointestinal hormones. Motility is inhibited by sympathetic nervous stimulation and by circulating epinephrine. The two basic forms of gastrointestinal motility are:

- Segmentation
- Peristalsis

The contents of the digestive tract must be constantly churned and mixed so that materials are exposed to digestive enzymes and come into contact with the wall of the tract for absorption. This mixing is carried out by *segmentation*, or stationary muscular contractions. This form of motility divides some portion of the tract into alternating constricted and unconstricted regions. Segmentation contractions move back and forth so that a previously constricted region relaxes and a previously relaxed region contracts. This activity results in thorough mixing of the contents with digestive enzymes and other secretions. This is the more important form of motility in the small intestine, where most digestion and absorption take place.

The contents of the tract must also be continually moved along so that it can be acted upon by the sequential regions of the tract. *Peristalsis* is a muscular contraction that produces a ring of contraction that moves along the length of the tract. This wave-like contraction causes propulsion and forces the contents forward. Peristalsis is more important in the esophagus and stomach.

Gastrointestinal sphincters are formed where the circular layer of smooth muscle is thickened. Sphincters occur at several points along the tract. Their function is to limit the movement of food materials from one region to another. For example, the pyloric sphincter found between the stomach and duodenum of the small intestine plays an important role in limiting the rate of gastric emptying. Sphincters undergo *tonic contractions* that may be sustained for minutes or hours.

Serosa. The connective tissue membrane that surrounds the wall of the digestive tract is the *serosa*. This membrane secretes a watery fluid that provides lubrication and prevents friction between the digestive organs as they move about in the abdomen. The serosa is continuous with the *peritoneum*, which is the serous membrane lining the abdominal cavity. The peritoneum also forms sheets of tissue, or *mesentery*, that suspend the digestive organs from the wall of the abdomen. The mesentery acts as a sling that, while offering structural support for the organs, also provides for the range of movement needed during the digestive process.

18.3 Regulation of gastrointestinal function

The digestive tract contains three types of sensory receptors that are sensitive to chemical or mechanical changes within the system. These include:

- Chemoreceptors
- Osmoreceptors
- Mechanoreceptors

Chemoreceptors respond to various chemical components within the gastrointestinal lumen. For example, in the duodenum of the small intestine, chemoreceptors are stimulated by excessive amounts of hydrogen ion secreted by the stomach. *Osmoreceptors* are sensitive to the osmolarity of the contents within the lumen. As the digestive process progresses, large nutrient molecules are split into their smaller components. This increases the number of molecules and therefore the osmolarity of material being processed. Excessive osmolarity may suggest that absorption is not keeping pace with digestion. *Mechanoreceptors* respond to stretch or distension of the gastrointestinal tract wall.

Receptor stimulation may lead to activation of any or all of the following regulatory mechanisms within the tract:

- Intrinsic nerve plexuses
- Extrinsic autonomic nerves
- Gastrointestinal hormones

Intrinsic nerve plexuses. The *intrinsic nerve plexuses* are interconnecting networks of nerve cells located entirely within the gastrointestinal tract and are responsible for *intratract reflexes*. The stimulation of a receptor in one region of the tract neurally influences activity of another region of the tract. These reflexes occur directly, independent of the central nervous system. Intratract reflexes provide a mechanism for self-regulation of the tract and help to coordinate the activity of the organs within it. An example of such a reflex is the *enterogastric reflex*, in which receptor stimulation in the duodenum of the small intestine elicits neural activity that regulates muscle contraction and glandular secretion in the stomach.

Extrinsic autonomic nerves. Gastrointestinal activity is also modified by *extrinsic autonomic nerves*. The tract is innervated by the sympathetic and parasympathetic divisions of the autonomic nervous system. The effects of these two divisions tend to oppose each other: the parasympathetic system stimulates most digestive activities while the sympathetic system inhibits them. Interestingly, the autonomic nerves to the digestive system, especially the vagus nerve of the parasympathetic system, can be discretely activated. In this way, digestive activity can be modified without affecting tissue function in other regions of the body.

Gastrointestinal hormones. A third factor contributing to regulation of digestive activity is the secretion of *gastrointestinal hormones*. These hormones may be released in one region of the tract, travel in the circulatory system to other regions of the tract, and influence the activity of effector cells in that region. A summary of the source, stimulus for release, and actions of several important hormones is found in Table 18.2.

Table 18.2 Digestive Hormones

Hormone	Source	Stimulus for Release	Hormone actions
Gastrin	G cells in pyloric region of the stomach	Protein in stomach; vagal stimulation	Stimulates parietal cells (HCl) and chief cells (pepsinogen) in stomach; enhances gastric motility
Secretin	Endocrine cells in mucosa of duodenum	Acid in duodenum	Inhibits gastric emptying and gastric secretion; stimulates secretion of bicarbonate from pancreas; stimulates secretion of bicarbonate-rich bile from liver
Cholecystokinin	Endocrine cells in mucosa of duodenum	Breakdown products of lipid and, to a small extent, protein digestion in duodenum	Inhibits gastric emptying and gastric secretion; stimulates contraction of gallbladder; stimulates secretion of digestive enzymes from pancreas
Gastric inhibitory peptide	Endocrine cells in mucosa of duodenum	Lipids, acid, and hyperosmotic chyme in duodenum; distension of duodenum	Inhibits gastric emptying and gastric secretion; stimulates secretion of insulin from pancreas

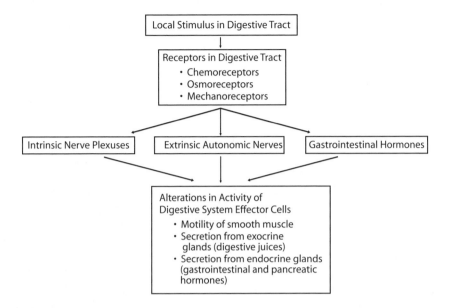

Figure 18.1 Summary of the regulatory mechanisms influencing gastrointestinal function.

A summary of these three mechanisms that regulate the activity of the digestive system is illustrated in Figure 18.1. A local change in the tract may lead to stimulation of one or more of the three types of receptors present in the tract wall. Receptor stimulation may then activate any or all of the three regulatory mechanisms. These mechanisms then alter the activity of the effector tissues within the digestive system, including smooth muscle, and exocrine and endocrine glands.

The following sections will discuss each region of the digestive system separately. Where appropriate, the basic digestive processes — motility, secretion, digestion, and absorption — will be considered.

18.4 Mouth

The *mouth* is the region from the lips to the pharynx. The first step in the digestive process is chewing, or *mastication*, which is an initial mechanical breakdown of the food that facilitates its movement to the stomach. The mouth is lined with *stratified squamous epithelium* that provides extra protection from injury by coarse food materials. Three pairs of salivary glands secrete saliva into the oral cavity:

- Parotid glands located between the angle of the jaw and the ear
- Sublingual glands located below the tongue
- Submandibular glands located below the jaw

Saliva contains:

- Water
- Mucus
- Lysozyme
- Salivary amylase
- Lingual lipase

Approximately 99.5% of saliva is *water*. Swallowing is facilitated by the moistening of food materials; furthermore, it serves as a solvent for molecules that stimulate the taste buds. The presence of *mucus*, which is thick and slippery, lubricates the mouth and the food and assists in swallowing. *Lysozyme* is an enzyme that lyses or kills many types of bacteria that may be ingested.

Saliva begins the process of chemical digestion with *salivary amylase*. This enzyme splits starch molecules into fragments. Specifically, polysaccharides, or starches, are broken down into maltose, a disaccharide consisting of two glucose molecules. Salivary amylase may account for up to 75% of starch digestion before it is denatured by gastric acid in the stomach.

A small amount of *lingual lipase* is also present and plays a role in the breakdown of dietary lipid. This enzyme is optimally active at an acidic pH and therefore remains active through the stomach and into the intestine.

Due to parasympathetic stimulation of the salivary glands, saliva is secreted continuously at a basal rate of approximately 0.5 ml/min. Secretion may be enhanced by two types of reflexes:

- Simple or unconditioned salivary reflex
- Acquired or conditioned salivary reflex

The *simple or unconditioned salivary reflex* occurs when food is present within the oral cavity and causes stimulation of chemoreceptors and pressure receptors. These receptors then transmit impulses to the *salivary center* in the medulla of the brainstem. Parasympathetic efferent impulses are transmitted back to the salivary glands and secretion is enhanced.

The *acquired or conditioned salivary reflex* is elicited in response to the thought, sight, smell, or sound of food. As demonstrated with Pavlov's dog, these stimuli result in a learned response. Another stimulus that enhances salivation is nausea. Salivary secretion is inhibited by fatigue, sleep, fear, and dehydration. Overall, 1 to 2 l of saliva may be produced per day.

Pharmacy application: effects of anticholinergic drugs on the digestive system

In addition to their therapeutic actions, many drugs have undesirable side effects that may influence the digestive system. An example of such a drug is scopolamine, one of the most effective agents used for prevention of motion sickness. This drug may be administered transdermally in a multilayered adhesive unit, or "patch" form. Its mechanism of action likely involves inhibition of muscarinic receptors in the vestibular apparatus of the inner ear. This interrupts transmission of nerve impulses from the inner ear to the emetic center in the medulla of the brainstem. As a result, vomiting in response to motion is inhibited. However, the salivary glands are also quite sensitive to the activity of muscarinic receptor antagonists. In fact, scopolamine and other anticholinergic agents may severely inhibit the copious, watery secretion of the salivary glands. In this case, the mouth becomes dry and swallowing and speaking may become difficult. Other anticholinergic agents may be used to: (1) reduce muscle rigidity and muscle tremor in Parkinson's disease (benztropine mesylate); (2) reduce bronchospasm and airway mucus secretion in asthma and chronic obstructive pulmonary disease (COPD) (ipratropium); and (3) reduce accumulation of secretions in the trachea and the possibility of laryngospasm prior to administration of general anesthesia. In each case, these medications also inhibit salivary secretion and cause "dry mouth."

18.5 Pharynx

The *pharynx* is the cavity at the rear of the throat and links the mouth with the esophagus. It serves as a common passageway for the respiratory and digestive systems. The *swallowing reflex* takes place largely in the pharynx. This is an example of an all-or-none reflex in which, once the process has begun, it cannot stop. Swallowing may be initiated voluntarily when the tongue pushes a bolus of food toward the back of the mouth and into the pharynx. The stimulation of pressure receptors in the pharynx results in transmission of nerve impulses to the *swallowing center* in the medulla of the brainstem. This elicits a coordinated involuntary reflex that involves contraction of muscles in the appropriate sequence. A wave of contraction sweeps down the constrictor muscles of the pharynx. The epiglottis moves downward over the larynx to seal off the trachea and the upper esophageal sphincter relaxes, allowing the bolus of food to enter the esophagus. Once the food bolus enters the esophagus, the upper esophageal sphincter closes in order to prevent the swallowing of air. This phase of the swallowing reflex is referred to as the *pharyngeal stage* and lasts approximately 1 sec.

18.6 Esophagus

Located behind the trachea, the *esophagus* is a muscular tube connecting the pharynx and the stomach and lined with *stratified squamous epithelium*. The only substance secreted by the esophagus is *mucus*. The protective mucus provides lubrication for the passage of food and helps to prevent damage to the esophageal wall by coarse food materials. The esophagus is sealed off by two sphincters, one at either end of the tube: the *upper esophageal sphincter* (*UES*) and the *lower esophageal sphincter* (*LES*). Each is normally closed except during the process of swallowing. The normal function of the respiratory system creates a subatmospheric pressure in the thoracic cavity. If, indeed, the esophagus were open to the atmosphere, this pressure gradient would pull air into the esophagus and stomach during each inspiration. Therefore, the closure of these sphincters prevents large volumes of air from entering the digestive tract.

The *esophageal stage* of the swallowing reflex involves a *primary peristaltic wave* of contraction initiated by the swallowing center and mediated by the vagus nerve. This wave begins at the UES and moves slowly down the esophagus at a rate of 2 to 6 cm/sec until it reaches the LES. Some particularly large or sticky food particles may remain in the esophagus after the primary peristaltic wave. The distension of the esophagus by the presence of these particles elicits *secondary peristaltic waves* that do not involve the swallowing center. The smooth muscle of the LES relaxes immediately prior to the arrival of the peristaltic contraction to allow for movement of food into the stomach.

18.7 Stomach

The *stomach*, located on the left side of the abdominal cavity just below the diaphragm, lies between the esophagus and small intestine. As with the esophagus, it has a sphincter at either end: the previously mentioned LES at the entrance to the stomach and the *pyloric sphincter* at the exit of the stomach into the duodenum of the small intestine. The LES is normally closed except during swallowing. The pyloric sphincter is subject to tonic contraction, which keeps it almost, but not completely, closed so that fluids may easily pass through it. The movement of food materials through this sphincter requires strong gastric contractions. Even then, only a few milliliters are pushed through at a time. Gastric contractions mash the food materials and thoroughly mix them with gastric secretions. This produces a thick, semifluid mixture referred to as *chyme*.

Three regions make up the stomach:

- *Fundus*: uppermost region of the stomach located above the junction with the esophagus
- *Body*: middle or main portion of the stomach
- *Antrum*: terminal region of the stomach leading to the gastroduodenal junction

The stomach performs several important functions:

- Stores ingested food until it can be processed by the remainder of the digestive tract
- Mechanically mashes ingested food and mixes it with gastric secretions
- Begins the process of protein digestion

Food is stored in the body of the stomach, which may expand to hold as much as 1 l of chyme. As food enters the stomach, it undergoes a reflex relaxation referred to as *receptive relaxation*. It enhances the ability of the stomach to accommodate an increase in volume with only a small increase in stomach pressure. The fundus does not typically store food because it is located above the esophageal opening into the stomach. Instead, it usually contains a pocket of gas.

Gastric motility. In addition to the circular and longitudinal layers of smooth muscle, the stomach contains an extra layer of smooth muscle. Beginning at the UES, the *oblique layer* of smooth muscle fans out across the anterior and posterior surfaces of the stomach and fuses with the circular layer in the lower region. This extra layer of muscle enhances gastric motility and therefore mixing and mashing of food.

Contraction of gastric smooth muscle occurs in the form of *peristalsis*. Peristaltic contractions begin in the body of the stomach and proceed in a wave-like fashion toward the duodenum. These contractions are weak in the upper portion of the stomach where the muscle layers are relatively thin. The contractions become much stronger in the lower portion of the stomach as the muscle layers become thicker. As the wave of contraction sweeps through the antrum, a small amount of chyme is pushed through the partially open pyloric sphincter. When the peristaltic contraction actually reaches the pyloric sphincter, it closes and the rest of the chyme in this region is forced back toward the body of the stomach where more mixing and mashing takes place.

It may take many hours for the contents of the stomach to be processed and moved into the small intestine. Several factors influence gastric motility and therefore the rate of gastric emptying. These include:

- Volume of chyme in the stomach
- Fluidity of chyme
- Volume and chemical composition of chyme in the duodenum

The major gastric factor that affects motility and the rate of emptying is the *volume of chyme in the stomach*. As the volume of chyme increases, the wall of the stomach becomes distended and mechanoreceptors are stimulated. This elicits reflexes that enhance gastric motility by way of the intrinsic and vagus nerves. The release of the hormone gastrin from the antral region of the stomach further contributes to enhanced motility.

The degree of *fluidity of chyme* also affects the rate of gastric emptying. Ingested liquids move through the pyloric sphincter and begin to empty almost immediately. Ingested solids must first be converted into a semifluid mixture of uniformly small particles. The faster the necessary degree of fluidity is achieved, the more rapidly the contents of the stomach may empty into the duodenum.

The most important factors that regulate gastric motility and the rate of emptying of the stomach involve the *volume and chemical composition of chyme in the duodenum*. Receptors in the duodenum are sensitive to:

- Distension
- Lipids
- Acid
- Chyme osmolarity

The ultimate goal of these duodenal factors is to maintain a rate of gastric emptying consistent with the proper digestion and absorption of nutrient molecules in the small intestine. In other words, emptying must be regulated so that the duodenum has adequate opportunity to process the chyme that it already contains before it receives more from the stomach. Regulation occurs by way of the *enterogastric reflex*, which inhibits gastric motility, increases contraction of the pyloric sphincter, and therefore decreases rate of gastric emptying. This reflex is mediated through the intrinsic and vagus nerves. Regulation also occurs by way of a *hormonal response* that involves the release of the *enterogastrones* from the duodenum. These hormones, *secretin, cholecystokinin* and *gastric inhibitory peptide*, travel in the blood to the stomach where they inhibit gastric contractions.

As the volume of the chyme in the duodenum increases, it causes *distension* of the duodenal wall and stimulation of *mechanoreceptors*. This receptor stimulation elicits reflex inhibition of gastric motility mediated through the intrinsic and vagus nerves. Distension also causes release of gastric inhibitory peptide from the duodenum, which contributes to inhibition of gastric contractions.

Duodenal receptors are also sensitive to the chemical composition of chyme and are able to detect the presence of lipids, excess hydrogen ion, and hyperosmotic chyme. These conditions also elicit the enterogastric reflex and release of the enterogastrones in order to decrease the rate of gastric emptying.

Of the three major categories of nutrients, *lipids* are the slowest to be digested and absorbed. Furthermore, these processes take place only in the small intestine, so in order to ensure complete lipid digestion and absorption, the rate of movement of lipid from the stomach to the duodenum must be carefully regulated. The presence of lipid in the duodenum stimulates intestinal chemoreceptors. This receptor stimulation elicits reflex inhibition of gastric motility and slows the addition of more lipid from the stomach. Lipid also causes the release of cholecystokinin and gastric inhibitory peptide from the duodenum. These hormones contribute to inhibition of gastric contractions. The significance of the inhibitory effect of lipid is illustrated by the comparison between a high-fat meal (up to 6 h for gastric emptying) and a meal consisting of carbohydrates and protein (3 h for gastric emptying). Therefore, a fatty meal is "more filling" than a low-fat meal due its effect on gastric motility.

An important gastric secretion is the *hydrochloric acid* that performs a number of functions in the stomach. This stomach acid is neutralized by pancreatic bicarbonate ion in the duodenum. Excess acid in the chyme stimulates chemoreceptors in the duodenum. This receptor stimulation elicits reflex inhibition of gastric motility. Excess acid also causes the release of secretin and gastric inhibitory peptide from the duodenum. These hormones contribute to inhibition of gastric contractions so that the neutralization process may be completed before additional acid arrives in chyme from the stomach.

Chyme within the duodenum has, by this point, undergone some degree of carbohydrate and protein digestion. Salivary amylase has fragmented starch molecules and, as will be discussed, pepsin from the stomach has fragmented proteins. Therefore, the number of disaccharides and small peptides has increased, which leads to an increase in the *osmolarity of the chyme*. The rate of absorption of these smaller molecules must keep pace with the rate of digestion of the larger molecules. If not, the stimulation of *osmoreceptors* in the duodenum by the hyperosmotic chyme will inhibit gastric motility and gastric emptying. This effect is mediated through reflex inhibition as well as the release of gastric inhibitory peptide from the duodenum.

Gastric secretion. The human stomach secretes 1 to 2 l of gastric juice per day. The gastric mucosa, which produces these secretions, is divided into two functional regions:

- Oxyntic gland area
- Pyloric gland area

The *oxyntic gland area* is located in the proximal 80% of the stomach. These glands consist of three types of cells:

- Mucous neck cells
- Parietal cells
- Chief cells

The *pyloric gland area* is located in the remaining distal 20% of the stomach. Secretions of the stomach include:

- Hydrochloric acid
- Pepsinogen
- Mucus
- Intrinsic factor
- Gastrin

Hydrochloric acid (HCl), a strong acid that dissociates into an H^+ and a Cl^- ion, is produced by the *parietal cells*. These ions are actively transported into the lumen of the stomach by the *proton pump*. Functions of HCl include:

- Activation of pepsinogen, the precursor for the pepsin enzyme
- Assisting in breakdown of connective tissue and muscle fibers within ingested food
- Killing of most types of microorganisms ingested with food

Pepsinogen is produced by the *chief cells*. Within the lumen of the stomach, this precursor molecule is split by HCl to form the active enzyme *pepsin*. Optimally active at an acidic pH (pH = 2), pepsin begins protein digestion by fragmenting proteins into smaller peptide chains.

Mucus is produced by the *mucus neck cells* and by the *surface epithelial cells* of the stomach wall. A thick layer of mucus adheres to the wall of the stomach, forming the *gastric mucosal barrier*. The function of this barrier is to protect the gastric mucosa from injury — specifically, from the corrosive actions of HCl and pepsin. Together with bicarbonate ion released into the lumen of the stomach, mucus neutralizes the acid and maintains the mucosal surface at a nearly neutral pH.

Pharmacy application: drug-induced gastric disease

In addition to their beneficial effects, some medications may actually cause cellular injury and disease. An example of this phenomenon involves nonsteroidal anti-inflammatory drugs (NSAIDS). These drugs include aspirin (a derivative of salicylic acid), ibuprofen (arylpropionic acid, Advil®), and acetaminophen (para-aminophenol derivative, Tylenol®). Because of their benefi-cial pharmacological effects, consumption of these agents has increased significantly in recent years. NSAIDS have the ability to treat fever, pain, acute inflammation, and chronic inflammatory diseases such as arthritis. They are also used prophylactically to prevent heart disease, stroke, and colon cancer.

Unfortunately, frequent exposure to NSAIDS may also cause two detrimental effects. These agents inhibit the activity of cyc-lo-oxygenase, an important enzyme in synthesis of gastroprotec-tive prostaglandins. More importantly, NSAIDS may cause breaks in the gastric mucosal barrier. The normal gastric mucosa is relatively impermeable to H^+ ion. When the gastric mucosal barrier is weakened or damaged, H^+ ion leaks into the mucosa in exchange for Na^+ ion. As H^+ ion accumulates in the mucosa, intracellular buffer systems become saturated, the pH decreases, and cell injury and cell death occur. These damaged cells then secrete more HCl, which causes more injury, and so on, resulting in a positive feedback cycle. An ulcer may form when injury from the gastric secretions, HCl and pepsin, overwhelms the ability of the mucosa to protect itself and replace damaged cells. Local capillaries are also damaged, causing bleeding or hemorrhage into the gastric lumen.

Intrinsic factor is produced by the *parietal cells*. Within the stomach, it combines with *vitamin B_{12}* to form a complex necessary for absorption of this vitamin in the ileum of the small intestine. Vitamin B_{12} is an essential factor in the formation of red blood cells. Individuals unable to produce intrinsic factor cannot absorb vitamin B_{12} and red blood cell production is impaired. This condition, referred to as *Pernicious anemia*, occurs as a result of an autoimmune disorder involving destruction of parietal cells.

Gastrin is a hormone produced by gastric endocrine tissue — specifically, the *G cells* in the pyloric gland area. It is released into the blood and carried back to the stomach. The major function of gastrin is to enhance acid secretion by directly stimulating parietal cells (HCl) and chief cells (pepsinogen). Gastrin also stimulates the local release of histamine from *enterochromaffin-like cells* in the wall of the stomach. *Histamine* stimulates parietal cells to release HCl.

The three major phases of gastric secretion are:

- Cephalic phase: 20 to 30% of gastric secretory response to a meal
- Gastric phase: 60 to 70% of gastric secretory response to a meal
- Intestinal phase: approximately 10% of gastric secretory response to a meal

The *cephalic phase* of gastric secretion occurs before food even enters the stomach. Thoughts of food; sensory stimuli such as the smell, sight, or taste of food; and activities such as chewing and swallowing enhance gastric secretion. The cephalic phase is mediated by the vagus nerve and gastrin, which is released in response to vagal stimulation. These mechanisms promote secretion of HCl and pepsinogen.

The *gastric phase* is elicited by the presence of food in the stomach. Distension of the stomach wall, as well as the presence of protein, caffeine, and alcohol, enhances gastric secretion. This phase is mediated by the intrinsic nerves, the vagus nerve, and gastrin. Each of these mechanisms promotes secretion of HCl and pepsinogen.

Pharmacy application: pharmacological treatment of gastric ulcers

The pharmacological treatment of ulcers involves the inhibition of gastric acid secretion. However, more than one approach may be used to accomplish this goal: H_2-receptor antagonists and proton pump inhibitors. Histamine does not play a role in normal acid production; however, it may stimulate release of HCl under pathological conditions. In the case of an ulcer, when H^+ ion enters the gastric mucosa, it stimulates the release of histamine from local mast cells. The histamine then stimulates H_2-receptors on the parietal cells to release more HCl. Therefore, excess acid release may be prevented with the administration of H_2-receptor antagonists such as cimetidine (Tagamet®) and famotidine (Pepcid®). However, the inhibition of histamine-induced acid secretion is not adequate in all patients. More recently, proton pump inhibitors, such as omeprazole (Prilosec®) and lansoprazole (Prevacid®) have been used to treat ulcers and gastroesophageal reflux disease (GERD). These drugs bind irreversibly to the proton pump (H^+, K^+–ATPase), which is found only in the parietal cell. This causes permanent inhibition of enzyme activity and, as a result, the secretion of H^+ ions into the lumen of the stomach is inhibited. The secretion of acid resumes only after new molecules of H^+, K^+–ATPase are inserted into the gastric mucosa.

The *intestinal phase* has two components that influence gastric secretion:

- Excitatory
- Inhibitory

The *excitatory component* involves the release of *intestinal gastrin* that occurs in response to the presence of products of protein digestion in the duodenum. Intestinal gastrin travels in the blood to the stomach, where it enhances the secretion of HCl and pepsinogen. The magnitude of this effect is very small, however, because it accounts only for approximately 10% of the acid secretory response to a meal. In contrast to the excitatory component, the *inhibitory component* of the intestinal phase has a very strong influence on gastric secretion. As with gastric motility, the volume and composition of the chyme in the duodenum affect gastric secretion. Distension of the duodenal wall, as well as the presence of lipids, acid, and hyperosmotic chyme, inhibits secretion by way of the enterogastric reflex and the release of enterogastrones.

18.8 Liver

The *liver* is the largest internal organ, weighing about 1.5 kg (3.3 lb) in the adult. The blood flow to the liver is 1350 ml/min (27% of the cardiac output) on average and comes from two sources:

- Hepatic artery
- Hepatic portal vein

The *hepatic artery* supplies the liver with 300 ml/min of oxygenated blood from the aorta. The remaining 1050 ml/min of blood flow is delivered by the *hepatic portal vein*. This blood comes directly from the digestive tract. It is low in oxygen but contains a high concentration of nutrients absorbed from the intestines.

The liver performs many important functions, including:

- Storage of blood
- Filtration of blood
- Storage of vitamins and iron
- Formation of blood coagulation factors
- Metabolism and excretion of certain drugs, bilirubin, and hormones
- Metabolism of carbohydrates, proteins, and lipids
- Formation of bile

The liver is a large and distensible organ. As such, large quantities of blood may be stored in its blood vessels providing a *blood reservoir* function. Under normal physiological conditions, the hepatic veins and hepatic sinuses contain approximately 450 ml of blood, or almost 10% of blood volume. When needed, this blood may be mobilized to increase venous return and cardiac output.

Blood flowing from the intestines to the liver through the hepatic portal vein often contains bacteria. *Filtration of this blood* is a protective function provided by the liver. Large phagocytic macrophages, referred to as *Kupffer cells*, line the hepatic venous sinuses. As the blood flows through these sinuses, bacteria are rapidly taken up and digested by the Kupffer cells. This system is very efficient and removes more than 99% of the bacteria from the hepatic portal blood.

The liver serves as an important *storage site for vitamins and iron*. Sufficient quantities of several vitamins may be stored so as to prevent vitamin deficiency for some period of time:

- Vitamin A: up to 10 months
- Vitamin D: 3 to 4 months
- Vitamin B_{12}: at least 1 year

Iron is stored in the liver in the form of *ferritin*. When the level of circulating iron becomes low, ferritin releases iron into the blood.

Several substances that contribute to the *blood coagulation* process are formed in the liver. These include fibrinogen, prothrombin, and several of the blood clotting factors (II, VII, IX, and X). Deficiency in any of these substances leads to impaired blood coagulation.

The liver is capable of *detoxifying or excreting into the bile many drugs*, such as sulfonamides (antibacterial drugs), penicillin, ampicillin, and erythromycin. *Bilirubin*, the major end-product of hemoglobin degradation, is also excreted in the bile. In addition, several *hormones* are metabolized by the liver, including thyroid hormone and all of the steroid hormones, such as estrogen, cortisol, and aldosterone.

In terms of nutrients, the liver is the most important metabolic organ in the body. It receives a large volume of nutrient-rich blood directly from the digestive tract, which provides an abundant amount of substrates for metabolism. *Metabolic processes involving carbohydrates* include:

- Storage of a significant amount of glycogen
- Conversion of galactose and fructose into glucose
- Gluconeogenesis

Metabolic processes involving proteins include the following:

- Deamination of amino acids
- Formation of urea (for removal of ammonia from body fluids)
- Formation of plasma proteins
- Conversion of amino acids into other amino acids and essential compounds

Most cells in the body metabolize lipids; however, some processes of *fat metabolism* occur mainly in the liver. These include:

- Oxidation of fatty acids to supply energy for other body functions
- Synthesis of cholesterol, phospholipids, and lipoproteins
- Synthesis of fat from proteins and carbohydrates

Another important product of liver metabolism is the *bile* necessary for digestion and absorption of dietary lipids. Bile is an aqueous, alkaline fluid consisting of a complex mixture of organic and inorganic components. The major organic constituents of bile are the *bile salts*, which account for approximately 50% of the solid components. Derived from cholesterol, bile salts are *amphipathic molecules*; in other words, these molecules have a hydrophilic region and a hydrophobic region. Inorganic ions are also present in the bile and include Na^+, K^+, Ca^{++}, Cl^-, and $HCO3^-$ ions. The total number of cations exceeds the total number of anions.

Bile is produced continuously by the liver; bile salts are secreted by the hepatocytes; and the water, sodium bicarbonate, and other inorganic salts are added by the cells of the bile ducts within the liver. The bile is then transported by way of the *common bile duct* to the duodenum. Bile facilitates fat digestion and absorption throughout the length of the small intestine. In the terminal region of the ileum, the final segment of the small intestine, the bile salts are actively reabsorbed into the blood, returned to the liver by way of the hepatic portal system, and resecreted into the bile. This recycling of the bile salts from the small intestine back to the liver is referred to as *enterohepatic circulation*.

Bile secretion by the liver is stimulated by:

- Bile salts
- Secretin
- Parasympathetic stimulation

The return of the *bile salts* to the liver from the small intestine is the most potent stimulus of bile secretion. In fact, these bile salts may cycle two to five times during each meal. The intestinal hormone *secretin*, which is released in response to acid in the duodenum, enhances aqueous alkaline secretion by the liver. Secretin has no effect on the secretion of bile salts. During the cephalic phase of digestion, before food even reaches the stomach or intestine, *parasympathetic stimulation*, by way of the vagus nerve, promotes bile secretion from the liver.

18.9 Gallbladder

During a meal, bile enters the duodenum from the common bile duct through the *Sphincter of Oddi*. Between meals, this sphincter is closed to prevent bile from entering the small intestine. As a result, much of the bile secreted from the liver is backed up the common bile duct into the *cystic duct* and the *gallbladder*. The gallbladder is located on the inferior surface of the liver. Within the gallbladder, sodium is actively removed from the bile. Chloride follows the sodium down its electrical gradient and water follows osmotically. As a result, the organic constituents of bile are concentrated 5- to 10-fold. During a meal, when bile is needed for digestion, the gallbladder contracts and the bile is squeezed out and into the duodenum. Contraction is elicited by *cholecystokinin*, an intestinal hormone released in response to the presence of chyme, especially lipids, in the duodenum.

18.10 Pancreas

Exocrine glands within the pancreas secrete an aqueous fluid referred to as pancreatic juice. This fluid is alkaline and contains a high concentration of bicarbonate ion; it is transported to the duodenum by the pancreatic duct.

Pancreatic juice neutralizes the acidic chyme entering the duodenum from the stomach. Neutralization not only prevents damage to the duodenal mucosa, but also creates a neutral or slightly alkaline environment optimal for the function of pancreatic enzymes. The pancreas also secretes several enzymes involved in the digestion of carbohydrates, proteins, and lipids.

The three major phases of pancreatic secretion are:

- Cephalic phase: approximately 20% of pancreatic secretory response to a meal
- Gastric phase: 5 to 10% of pancreatic secretory response to a meal
- Intestinal phase: approximately 80% of pancreatic secretory response to a meal

As with gastric secretion, nervous stimulation and hormones regulate secretion from the pancreas. During the *cephalic phase* and *gastric phase*, the pancreas secretes a low-volume, enzyme-rich fluid mediated by the vagus nerve.

Most pancreatic secretion takes place during the *intestinal phase*. The intestinal hormone *secretin* stimulates release of a large volume of pancreatic juice with a high concentration of bicarbonate ion. Secretin is released in response to acidic chyme in the duodenum (maximal release at pH ≤ 3.0). The intestinal hormone *cholecystokinin* is released in response to the presence of the products of protein and lipid digestion. Cholecystokinin then stimulates the release of digestive enzymes from the pancreas.

18.11 Transport of bile and pancreatic juice to small intestine

Bile is secreted by the liver, stored in the gallbladder, and used in the small intestine. It is transported toward the small intestine by the *hepatic duct* (from the liver) and the *cystic duct* (from the gallbladder), which join to form the *common bile duct*. Pancreatic juice is transported toward the small intestine by the *pancreatic duct*. The common bile duct and the pancreatic duct join to form the *hepatopancreatic ampulla*, which empties into the duodenum. The entrance to the duodenum is surrounded by the *Sphincter of Oddi*. This sphincter is closed between meals in order to prevent bile and pancreatic juice from entering the small intestine; it relaxes in response to the intestinal hormone cholecystokinin, thus allowing biliary and pancreatic secretions to flow into the duodenum.

18.12 Small intestine

The small intestine is the longest (>6 m) and most convoluted organ in the digestive system. It is divided into three segments:

- Duodenum: first 20 cm
- Jejunum: next 2.5 m

- Ileum: remaining 3.5 m

Most digestion and absorption take place in the small intestine, the mucosa of which is well adapted for these functions with certain anatomical modifications:

- Plicae circulares
- Villi
- Microvilli

The *plicae circulares*, or circular folds, form internal rings around the circumference of the small intestine that are found along the length of the small intestine. They are formed from inward foldings of the mucosal and submucosal layers of the intestinal wall. The plicae circulares are particularly well developed in the duodenum and jejunum and increase the absorptive surface area of the mucosa about threefold. Each plica is covered with millions of smaller projections of mucosa referred to as *villi*. Two types of epithelial cells cover the villi:

- Goblet cells
- Absorptive cells

The *goblet cells* produce mucus. The *absorptive cells*, found in a single layer covering the villi, are far more abundant. Taken together, the villi increase the absorptive surface area another 10-fold.

Microvilli are microscopic projections found on the luminal surface of the absorptive cells. Each absorptive cell may have literally thousands of microvilli forming the *brush border*. These structures increase the surface area for absorption another 20-fold. Together, these three anatomical adaptations of the intestinal mucosa — plicae circulares, villi, and microvilli — increase the surface area as much as 600-fold, which has a profound positive effect on the absorptive process.

Motility of the small intestine. Segmentation and peristalsis take place in the small intestine. *Segmentation* mixes chyme with digestive juices and exposes it to the intestinal mucosa for absorption. This form of motility causes only a small degree of forward movement of the chyme along the small intestine. *Peristalsis*, the wave-like form of muscle contraction, primarily moves chyme along the intestine and causes only a small amount of mixing. These contractions are weak and slow in the small intestine so that time is sufficient for complete digestion and absorption of the chyme as it moves forward. Intestinal peristaltic contractions are normally limited to short distances.

Segmentation contractions occur as a result of the *basic electrical rhythm* (*BER*) of pacemaker cells in the small intestine. This form of muscular activity is slight or absent between meals. The motility of the small intestine may be enhanced during a meal by:

- Distension of the small intestine
- Gastrin
- Extrinsic nerve stimulation

During a meal, segmentation occurs initially in the duodenum and the ileum. The movement of chyme into the intestine and the *distension of the duodenum* elicit segmentation contractions in this segment of the small intestine. Segmentation of the empty ileum is caused by *gastrin* released in response to distension of the stomach. This mechanism is referred to as the *gastroileal reflex. Parasympathetic stimulation*, by way of the vagus nerve, further enhances segmentation. *Sympathetic stimulation* inhibits this activity.

Digestion and absorption in the small intestine. Most digestion and absorption of carbohydrates, proteins, and lipids occurs in the small intestine. A summary of the digestive enzymes involved in these processes is found in Table 18.3.

Carbohydrates. Approximately 50% of the human diet is composed of starch. Other major dietary carbohydrates include the disaccharides, sucrose (table sugar, composed of glucose and fructose) and lactose (milk sugar, composed of glucose and galactose). Starch is initially acted upon by amylase. *Salivary amylase* breaks down starch molecules in the mouth and stomach. *Pancreatic amylase* carries on this activity in the small intestine. Amylase fragments polysaccharides into disaccharides (maltose, composed of two glucose molecules). The disaccharide molecules, primarily maltose, are presented to the brush border of the absorptive cells. As the disaccharides are absorbed, *disaccharidases* (maltase, sucrase, and lactase) split these nutrient molecules into monosaccharides (glucose, fructose, and galactose).

Glucose and galactose enter the absorptive cells by way of *secondary active transport*. Cotransport carrier molecules associated with the disaccharidases in the brush border transport the monosaccharide and a Na+ ion from the lumen of the small intestine into the absorptive cell. This process is referred to as "secondary" because the cotransport carriers operate passively and do not require energy. However, they do require a concentration gradient for the transport of Na+ ions into the cell. This gradient is established by the active transport of Na+ ions out of the absorptive cell at the basolateral surface. Fructose enters the absorptive cells by way of facilitated diffusion. All monosaccharide molecules exit the absorptive cells by way of facilitated diffusion and enter the blood capillaries.

Proteins. Protein digestion begins in the stomach by the action of the gastric enzyme *pepsin*. This enzyme fragments large protein molecules into smaller peptide chains. Digestion is continued in the small intestine by the pancreatic enzymes *trypsin, chymotrypsin,* and *carboxypeptidase,* which hydrolyze the peptide chains into amino acids, dipeptides, and tripeptides. Similar to glucose and galactose, amino acids enter the absorptive cells by way of secondary active transport. Once again, energy is expended to pump Na+ ions out of the absorptive cells, creating a concentration gradient for the cotransport of amino acids and Na+ ions into the cell.

Table 18.3 Digestive Enzymes

Nutrient molecule	Enzyme	Enzyme action	Enzyme source	Action site
Carbohydrate				
Polysaccharide (starch)	Amylase	Fragment polysaccharides into disaccharides (maltose)	Salivary glands; pancreas	Mouth; stomach; small intestine
Disaccharides	Disaccharidases (maltase, lactase, sucrase)	Hydrolyze disaccharides into monosaccharides (glucose, galactose, fructose)	Absorptive cells of small intestine	Brush border of absorptive cells
Protein				
Protein (long peptide chain)	Pepsin	Fragment proteins into smaller peptides	Stomach chief cells	Stomach
Peptides	Trypsin; chymotrypsin carboxypeptidase	Hydrolyze peptides into di- and tripeptides	Pancreas	Small intestine
Di- and tripeptides	Aminopeptidases	Hydrolyze di- and tripeptides into amino acids	Absorptive cells of small intestine	Brush border of absorptive cells
Lipid				
Triglyceride	Lingual lipase	Hydrolyze triglycerides into monoglycerides and free fatty acids	Salivary glands	Mouth; stomach
	Pancreatic lipase	Hydrolyze triglycerides into monoglycerides and free fatty acids	Pancreas	Small intestine

Note: The role of lingual lipase in the digestion of dietary lipids is minor because it accounts for less than 10% of the enzymatic breakdown of triglycerides.

Dipeptides and tripeptides are also presented to the brush border of the absorptive cells. As the nutrient molecules are absorbed, aminopeptidases split them into their constituent amino acids. The activity of *aminopeptidases* accounts for approximately 60% of protein digestion. The amino acid molecules then exit the absorptive cells by way of facilitated diffusion and enter the blood capillaries.

Lipids. Dietary fat consists primarily of triglycerides. Fat digestion begins in the mouth and stomach by the action of the salivary enzyme *lingual lipase*. However, the role of this enzyme is minor because it accounts for less than 10% of enzymatic breakdown of triglycerides. Lipids are digested primarily in the small intestine. The first step in this process involves the action of *bile salts* contained in the bile. Bile salts cause *emulsification*, which is the dispersal of large fat droplets into a suspension of smaller droplets (<1 mm). This process creates a significantly increased surface area upon which fat-digesting enzymes can act.

Because intact triglycerides are too large to be absorbed, *pancreatic lipase* acts on the lipid droplets to hydrolyze the triglyceride molecules into *monoglycerides* and *free fatty acids*. These water-insoluble constituent molecules would tend to float on the surface of the aqueous chyme; therefore, they need to be transported to the absorptive surface — a process carried out by *micelles* formed by the amphipathic bile salts. The bile salts associate with each other such that the polar region of the molecule is oriented outward, making them water soluble. The nonpolar region faces inward away from the surrounding water; the monoglycerides and free fatty acids are carried in this interior region of the micelle. Upon reaching the brush border of the absorptive cells, they leave the micelles and enter the cells by simple diffusion. Because they are nonpolar, these molecules move passively through the lipid bilayer of the cell membrane. This process takes place primarily in the jejunum and proximal ileum. The bile salts are absorbed in the distal ileum by way of passive diffusion or secondary active transport.

Within the absorptive cells, the monoglycerides and free fatty acids are transported to the endoplasmic reticulum, which contains the necessary enzymes to resynthesize these substances into triglycerides. The newly synthesized triglycerides then move to the Golgi apparatus. Within this organelle, they are packaged in a lipoprotein coat consisting of phospholipids, cholesterol, and apoproteins. These protein-coated lipid globules, referred to as *chylomicrons*, are now water soluble. Approximately 90% of the chylomicron consists of triglycerides.

Chylomicrons leave the absorptive cell by way of exocytosis. Because they are unable to cross the basement membrane of the blood capillaries, the chylomicrons enter the *lacteals*, which are part of the lymphatic system. The vessels of the lymphatic system converge to form the thoracic duct that drains into the venous system near the heart. Therefore, unlike products of carbohydrate and protein digestion that are transported directly to the liver by way of the hepatic portal vein, absorbed lipids are diluted in the blood of the circulatory system before they reach the liver. This dilution of the lipids prevents the liver from being overwhelmed with more fat than it can process at one time.

Water and electrolytes. Each day in an average adult, about 5.5 l of food and fluids move from the stomach to the small intestine as chyme. An additional 3.5 l of pancreatic and intestinal secretions produce a total of 9 l of material in the lumen. Most of this (≥7.5 l) is absorbed from the small intestine. The absorption of nutrient molecules, which takes place primarily in the duodenum and jejunum, creates an osmotic gradient for the passive absorption of water. Sodium may be absorbed passively or actively. Passive absorption occurs when the electrochemical gradient favors the movement of Na^+ between the absorptive cells through "leaky" tight junctions. Sodium is actively absorbed by way of transporters in the absorptive cell membrane. One type of transporter carries a Na^+ ion and a Cl^- ion into the cell. Another carries a Na^+ ion, a K^+ ion, and two Cl^- ions into the cell.

18.13 Large intestine

The *large intestine* is the region of the digestive tract from the ileocecal valve to the anus. Approximately 1.5 m in length, this organ has a larger diameter than the small intestine. The mucosa of the large intestine is composed of absorptive cells and mucus-secreting goblet cells. However, in contrast to the small intestine, the mucosa in this organ does not form villi. The large intestine consists of the following structures:

- Cecum
- Appendix
- Colon
- Rectum

The *cecum*, which is the most proximal portion of the large intestine, receives chyme from the ileum of the small intestine through the *ileocecal valve*. The *appendix*, a small projection at the bottom of the cecum, is a lymphoid tissue. This tissue contains lymphocytes and assists in defense against bacteria that enter the body through the digestive system. The largest portion of the large intestine is the *colon*. It consists of four regions: ascending colon (travels upward toward the diaphragm on the right side of the abdomen), transverse colon (crosses the abdomen under the diaphragm), descending colon (travels downward through the abdomen on the left side), and sigmoid colon (S-shaped region found in the lower abdomen). The sigmoid colon is continuous with the *rectum*, which leads to the external surface of the body through the *anus*.

The large intestine typically receives 500 to 1500 ml of chyme per day from the small intestine. As discussed, most digestion and absorption have already taken place in the small intestine. In fact, the large intestine produces no digestive enzymes. At this point in the human digestive tract, chyme consists of indigestible food residues (e.g., cellulose), unabsorbed biliary components, and any remaining fluid. Therefore, the two major functions of the large intestine are:

- Drying
- Storage

The colon's absorption of most of the water and salt from the chyme results in this *"drying"* or concentrating process. As a result, only about 100 ml of water is lost through this route daily. The remaining contents, now referred to as *feces*, are *"stored"* in the large intestine until it can be eliminated by way of defecation.

The longitudinal layer of smooth muscle in the small intestine is continuous. In the large intestine, this layer of muscle is concentrated into three flat bands referred to as *taniae coli*. Furthermore, the large intestine appears to be subdivided into a chain of pouches or sacs referred to as *haustra*. The haustra are formed because the bands of taniae coli are shorter than the underlying circular layer of smooth muscle and cause the colon to bunch up, forming the haustra.

Motility of the large intestine. Movements through the large intestine are typically quite sluggish. It will often take 18 to 24 h for materials to pass through its entire length. The primary form of motility in the large intestine is *haustral contractions*, or *haustrations*. These contractions are produced by the inherent rhythmicity of smooth muscle cells in the colon. Haustrations, which result in the pronounced appearance of the haustra, are similar to segmentation contractions in the small intestine. *Nonpropulsive*, haustrations serve primarily to move the contents slowly back and forth, exposing them to the absorptive surface.

In contrast to segmentation contractions in the small intestine (9 to 12 per minute), haustral contractions occur much less frequently (up to 30 min between contractions). These very slow movements allow for the growth of *bacteria* in the large intestine. Normally, the bacterial flora in this region is harmless. In fact, some of the bacteria produce absorbable vitamins, especially vitamin K.

A second form of motility in the large intestine is *mass movement*. Three or four times per day, typically after a meal, a strong propulsive contraction occurs that moves a substantial bolus of chyme forward toward the distal portion of the colon. Mass movements may result in the sudden distension of the rectum that elicits the defecation reflex.

Secretion of the large intestine. The large intestine produces an *alkaline mucus secretion*, the function of which is to protect the mucosa from mechanical or chemical injury. *Mucus* provides lubrication to facilitate the movement of the contents of the lumen. *Bicarbonate ion* neutralizes the irritating acids produced by local bacterial fermentation; colonic secretion increases in response to mechanical or chemical stimuli. The mechanism of the enhanced secretion involves intrinsic and vagal nerve reflexes.

Bibliography

1. Brown, J.H. and Taylor, P., Muscarinic receptor agonists and antagonists, in *Goodman and Gilman's: The Pharmacological Basis of Therapeutics*, 9th ed., Hardman, J.G. and Limbird, L.E., Eds., McGraw–Hill, New York, 1996, chap. 7.

2. Brunton, L., Agents for control of gastric acidity and treatment of peptic ulcers, in *Goodman and Gilman's: The Pharmacological Basis of Therapeutics*, 9th ed., Hardman, J.G. and Limbird, L.E., Eds., McGraw–Hill, New York, 1996, chap. 37.

3. Brunton, L., Agents affecting gastrointestinal water flux and motility; emesis and antiemetics; bile acids and pancreatic enzymes, in *Goodman and Gilman's: The Pharmacological Basis of Therapeutics*, 9th ed., Hardman, J.G. and Limbird, L.E., Eds., McGraw–Hill, New York, 1996, chap. 38.

4. Ganong, W.F., *Review of Medical Physiology*, 19th ed., Appleton & Lange, Stamford, CT, 1999.

5. Guyton, A.C. and Hall, J.E., *Textbook of Medical Physiology*, 10th ed., W.B. Saunders, Philadelphia, 2000.

6. Johnson, L.R., Salivary secretion, in *Gastrointestinal Physiology*, 6th ed., Johnson, L.R., Ed., C.V. Mosby, St. Louis, 2001, chap. 7.

7. Johnson, L.R., Gastric secretion, in *Gastrointestinal Physiology*, 6th ed., Johnson, L.R., Ed., C.V. Mosby, St. Louis, 2001, chap. 8.

8. Lichtenberger, L.M., Gastrointestinal physiology, in *Physiology Secrets*, Raff, H., Ed., Hanley and Belfus, Inc., Philadelphia, 1999, chap. 5.

9. Pappano, A.J. and Katzung, B.G., Cholinergic-blocking drugs, in *Basic and Clinical Pharmacology*, 8th ed., Katzung, B.G., Ed., Lange Medical Books/McGraw–Hill, New York, 2001, chap. 8.

10. Sherwood, L., *Human Physiology from Cells to Systems*, 4th ed., Brooks/Cole, Pacific Grove, CA, 2001.

11. Silverthorn, D.U., *Human Physiology: An Integrated Approach*, 2nd ed., Prentice- Hall, Upper Saddle River, NJ, 2001.

12. Weisbrodt, N.W., Swallowing, in *Gastrointestinal Physiology*, 6th ed., Johnson, L.R., Ed., C.V. Mosby, St. Louis, 2001, chap. 3.

13. Weisbrodt, N.W., Gastric emptying, in *Gastrointestinal Physiology*, 6th ed., Johnson, L.R., Ed., C.V. Mosby, St. Louis, 2001, chap. 4.

14. Weisbrodt, N.W., Bile production, secretion, and storage, in *Gastrointestinal Physiology*, 6th ed., Johnson, L.R., Ed., C.V. Mosby, St. Louis, 2001, chap. 10.

chapter nineteen

The renal system

Study objectives

- List vascular components of the nephron and describe their function
- List tubular components of the nephron and describe their function
- Distinguish between a cortical nephron and a juxtamedullary nephron
- Define the three basic renal processes
- Describe the components of the filtration barrier
- Explain how the filtration coefficient and net filtration pressure determine glomerular filtration
- Describe the mechanisms by which sodium, chloride, and water are reabsorbed
- Describe how each segment of the tubule handles sodium, chloride, and water
- Distinguish between the vertical osmotic gradient and the horizontal osmotic gradient
- Describe the functions of the vasa recta
- Describe the process by which potassium ions are secreted and the mechanism that regulates this process
- Define plasma clearance
- Explain how plasma clearance of inulin is used to determine glomerular filtration rate
- Explain how plasma clearance of para-aminohippuric acid is used to determine the effective renal plasma flow
- Explain how the myogenic mechanism and tubuloglomerular feedback are responsible for autoregulation of renal blood flow
- Explain how sympathetic nerves, angiotensin II, and prostaglandins affect the resistance of the afferent arteriole
- Describe factors that regulate the release of renin
- Explain how the control of sodium excretion regulates plasma volume
- Describe the mechanisms by which sodium excretion is controlled

- Explain how the control of water excretion regulates plasma osmolarity
- Describe the mechanisms by which water balance is maintained

19.1 Introduction

The kidneys are organs specialized to filter the blood. As such, they make an important contribution to the removal of metabolic waste products as well as to maintenance of fluid and electrolyte balance. Specific functions of the kidneys include:

- Regulation of extracellular fluid volume
- Regulation of inorganic electrolyte concentration in extracellular fluid
- Regulation of the osmolarity of extracellular fluid
- Removal of metabolic waste products
- Excretion of foreign compounds
- Maintenance of acid-base balance
- Hormone and enzyme production

The *regulation of extracellular fluid volume,* in particular, plasma volume, is important in the long-term regulation of blood pressure. An increase in plasma volume leads to an increase in blood pressure and a decrease in plasma volume leads to a decrease in blood pressure. Plasma volume is regulated primarily by altering the excretion of sodium in the urine. Other *inorganic electrolytes* regulated by the kidneys include chloride, potassium, calcium, magnesium, sulfate, and phosphate.

The kidneys also *regulate the osmolarity of extracellular fluid,* in particular plasma osmolarity. The maintenance of plasma osmolarity close to 290 mOsm prevents any unwanted movement of fluid into or out of the body's cells. An increase in plasma osmolarity causes water to leave the cells, leading to cellular dehydration; a decrease in plasma osmolarity causes water to enter the cells, leading to cellular swelling and possibly lysis. Plasma osmolarity is regulated primarily by altering the excretion of water in the urine.

As the major excretory organs in the body, the kidneys are responsible for the *removal of many metabolic waste products.* These include urea and uric acid, which are nitrogenous waste products of amino acid and nucleic acid metabolism, respectively; creatinine, a breakdown product of muscle metabolism; and urobilinogen, a metabolite of hemoglobin that gives urine its yellow color. *Foreign compounds* excreted by the kidneys include drugs (e.g., penicillin, nonsteroidal anti-inflammatory drugs); food additives (e.g., saccharin, benzoate); pesticides; and other exogenous nonnutritive materials that have entered the body. If allowed to accumulate, these substances become quite toxic.

Along with the respiratory system, the renal system *maintains acid-base balance* by altering the excretion of hydrogen and bicarbonate ions in the urine. When the extracellular fluid becomes acidic and pH decreases, the kidneys excrete H^+ ions and conserve HCO_3^- ions. Conversely, when the extracellular fluid becomes alkaline and pH increases, the kidneys conserve H^+ ions and excrete HCO_3^- ions. Normally, the pH of arterial blood is 7.4.

Although the kidneys are not considered endocrine glands per se, they are involved in *hormone production*. Erythropoietin is a peptide hormone that stimulates red blood cell production in bone marrow. Its primary source is the kidneys. Erythropoietin is secreted in response to renal hypoxia. Chronic renal disease may impair the secretion of erythropoietin, leading to development of anemia. The kidneys also *produce enzymes*. The enzyme renin is part of the renin–angiotensin–aldosterone system. As will be discussed, these substances play an important role in the regulation of plasma volume and therefore blood pressure. Other renal enzymes are needed for the conversion of vitamin D into its active form, 1,25-dihydroxyvitamin D_3, which is involved with calcium balance.

19.2 Functional anatomy of kidneys

The kidneys lie outside the peritoneal cavity in the posterior abdominal wall, one on each side of the vertebral column, slightly above the waistline. In the adult human, each kidney is approximately 11 cm long, 6 cm wide, and 3 cm thick. These organs are divided into two regions: the inner *renal medulla* and the outer *renal cortex*. The functional unit of the kidney is the *nephron* (see Figure 19.1 and Figure 19.2). Approximately 1 million nephrons are in each kidney. The nephron has two components:

- Vascular
- Tubular

Vascular component. Filtration of the plasma takes place at the *glomerulus* (i.e., *glomerular capillaries*) located in the cortical region of the kidney. Water and solutes exit the vascular compartment through these capillaries to be processed by the tubular component of the nephron. Blood is delivered to the glomerulus by *afferent arterioles*. The glomerular capillaries then join together to form a second group of arterioles referred to as *efferent arterioles*. All cellular elements of the blood (red blood cells, white blood cells, and platelets) as well as the unfiltered plasma continue through these vessels. The efferent arterioles then lead to a second set of capillaries, the *peritubular capillaries*. These capillaries provide nourishment to the renal tissue and return the substances reabsorbed from the tubule to the vascular compartment. Peritubular capillaries are closely associated with all portions of the renal tubules and wrap around them. These capillaries then join together to form venules and progressively larger veins that remove blood from the kidneys.

Tubular component. Approximately 180 l of filtrate is processed by the kidneys each day. Depending upon the volume of fluid intake, about 99% of this filtrate must be reabsorbed from the renal tubule back into the vascular

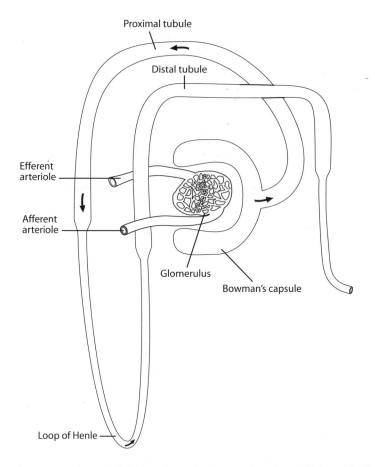

Figure 19.1 The nephron. The functional unit of the kidney is the nephron, which has two components. The vascular component includes the afferent arteriole, which carries blood toward the glomerulus where filtration of the plasma takes place. The efferent arteriole carries the unfiltered blood away from the glomerulus. The tubular component of the nephron includes Bowman's capsule, which receives the filtrate; the proximal tubule; the Loop of Henle; and the distal tubule. The tubule processes the filtrate, excreting waste products and reabsorbing nutrient molecules, electrolytes, and water.

compartment. The movement of substances out of the tubule is facilitated by its structure, which consists of *a single layer of epithelial cells*. As will be discussed, each region of the tubule plays a different role in the reabsorption process.

Upon leaving the glomerular capillaries, the filtrate enters the first portion of the tubule, *Bowman's capsule*. The glomerulus is pushed into Bowman's capsule, much like a fist pushed into a balloon or a catcher's mitt. From Bowman's capsule, the filtrate passes through the *proximal tubule*,

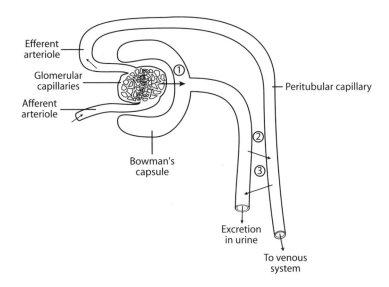

Figure 19.2 Basic renal processes. These processes include filtration, reabsorption, and secretion. (1) Filtration is the movement of fluid and solutes from the glomerular capillaries into Bowman's capsule. (2) Reabsorption, which takes place throughout the nephron, is the movement of filtered substances out of the tubule and into the surrounding peritubular capillaries. (3) Secretion is the movement of selected unfiltered substances from the peritubular capillaries into the renal tubule for excretion. Any substance that is filtered or secreted, but not reabsorbed, is excreted in the urine.

which is also located in the cortex of the kidney. The next segment of the tubule is the *Loop of Henle* found in the medulla of the kidney. The descending limb penetrates into the medulla and the ascending limb returns toward the cortex. From the Loop of Henle, the filtrate passes through the *distal tubule* in the cortex of the kidney. Finally, up to eight distal tubules empty into a *collecting duct* that runs downward through the medulla. Any filtrate remaining within the tubule at the end of the collecting duct drains through the renal pelvis to the ureters and is excreted as urine.

Two types of nephrons are distinguished by their anatomical characteristics:

- Cortical nephron
- Juxtamedullary nephron

The glomerulus of each *cortical nephron* is located in the outer region of the cortex. Furthermore, the Loop of Henle in these nephrons is short and does not penetrate deeply into the medulla. In humans, 70 to 80% of the nephrons are cortical.

In contrast, the glomerulus of each *juxtamedullary nephron* is located in the inner region of the cortex, close to the medulla. The Loop of Henle in these nephrons is significantly longer, penetrating to the innermost region of the medulla. Within the medulla, the peritubular capillaries of the nephrons are modified to form the *vasa recta*, or straight vessels. Similar to the Loop of Henle, the vasa recta descend deep into the medulla, form a hairpin loop, and then ascend back toward the cortex. In fact, these vessels run parallel and in close association with the Loop of Henle and the collecting ducts. The remaining 20 to 30% of nephrons in the human kidney are juxtamedullary.

19.3 Basic renal processes

The nephron performs three basic renal processes (see Figure 19.2):

- Filtration
- Reabsorption
- Secretion

Filtration is the movement of fluid and solutes from the glomerular capillaries into Bowman's capsule. Filtration is a *nonselective* process, so everything in the plasma except for the plasma proteins is filtered. Approximately 20% of the plasma is filtered as it passes through the glomerulus. On average, this results in a *glomerular filtration rate (GFR)* of 125 ml/min or 180 l of filtrate per day. *Reabsorption* is the movement of filtered substances from the renal tubule into the peritubular capillaries for return to the vascular compartment. This process takes place throughout the tubule. Approximately 178.5 l of filtrate are reabsorbed, resulting in an average urine output of 1.5 l per day. *Secretion* is the movement of selected unfiltered substances from the peritubular capillaries into the renal tubule for excretion. Any substance that is filtered or secreted, but not reabsorbed, is excreted in the urine.

The maintenance of plasma volume and plasma osmolarity occurs through regulation of the *renal excretion* of sodium, chloride, and water. Each of these substances is freely filtered from the glomerulus and reabsorbed from the tubule; none is secreted. Because salt and water intake in the diet may vary widely, the renal excretion of these substances is also highly variable. In other words, the kidneys must be able to produce a wide range of urine concentrations and urine volumes. The most dilute urine produced by humans is 65 to 70 mOsm/l and the most concentrated the urine can be is 1200 mOsm/l (recall that the plasma osmolarity is 290 mOsm/l). The volume of urine produced per day depends largely upon fluid intake. As fluid intake increases, urine output increases to excrete the excess water. Conversely, as fluid intake decreases or as an individual becomes dehydrated, urine output decreases in order to conserve water.

On average, 500 mOsm of waste products must be excreted in the urine per day. The minimum volume of water in which these solutes can be dissolved is determined by the ability of the kidney to produce a maximally concentrated urine of 1200 mOsm/l:

$$\frac{500 \ \text{mOsm} / \text{day}}{1200 \ \text{mOsm} / \text{L}} = 420 \ \text{ml} \ \text{water} / \text{day}$$

This volume, referred to as *obligatory water loss,* is 420 ml water/day. In other words, 420 ml of water will be lost in the urine each day in order to excrete metabolic waste products regardless of water intake.

19.4 Glomerular filtration

The first step in the formation of urine is glomerular filtration. The barrier to filtration is designed to facilitate the movement of fluid from the glomerular capillaries into Bowman's capsule without any loss of cellular elements or plasma proteins. Maximizing GFR has two advantages:

* Waste products are rapidly removed from the body.
* All body fluids are filtered and processed by the kidneys several times per day, resulting in precise regulation of volume and composition of these fluids.

Filtration barrier. The *filtration barrier* is composed of three structures:

* Glomerular capillary wall
* Basement membrane
* Inner wall of Bowman's capsule

Like the walls of other capillaries, the *glomerular capillary wall* consists of a single layer of endothelial cells. However, these cells are specialized in that they are *fenestrated.* The presence of large pores in these capillaries makes them 100 times more permeable than the typical capillary. These pores are too small, however, to permit the passage of blood cells through them.

The *basement membrane* is an acellular meshwork consisting of collagen and glycoproteins. The *collagen* provides structural support and the negatively charged *glycoproteins* prevent the filtration of plasma proteins into Bowman's capsule.

The *inner wall of Bowman's capsule* consists of specialized epithelial cells referred to as *podocytes.* This layer of epithelial cells is not continuous; instead, the podocytes have foot-like processes that project outward. The processes of one podocyte interdigitate with the processes of an adjacent podocyte, forming narrow *filtration slits.* These slits provide an ample route for the filtration of fluid.

In summary, the filtrate moves through the pores of the capillary endothelium, the basement membrane, and, finally, the filtration slits between the podocytes. This route of filtration is completely acellular.

Determinants of filtration. The glomerular filtration rate is influenced by two factors:

- Filtration coefficient
- Net filtration pressure

The *filtration coefficient* is determined by the *surface area* and *permeability* of the filtration barrier. An increase in the filtration coefficient leads to an increase in GFR; if the filtration coefficient decreases, then GFR decreases. However, this factor does not play a role in the daily regulation of GFR because its value is relatively constant under normal physiological conditions. On the other hand, chronic, uncontrolled hypertension and diabetes mellitus lead to gradual thickening of the basement membrane and therefore to a decrease in the filtration coefficient and GFR, and impaired renal function.

The *net filtration pressure* is determined by the following forces (see Figure 19.3):

- Glomerular capillary blood pressure
- Plasma colloid osmotic pressure
- Bowman's capsule pressure

Glomerular capillary pressure (P_{GC}) is a hydrostatic pressure that pushes blood out of the capillary. The blood pressure in these capillaries is markedly different from that of typical capillaries. In capillaries elsewhere in the body, blood pressure at the arteriolar end is about 30 mmHg and at the venular end is about 10 mmHg (see Chapter 15). These pressures lead to the net filtration of fluid at the inflow end of the capillary and net reabsorption of fluid at the outflow end.

In contrast, blood pressure in the glomerular capillaries is significantly higher and essentially nondecremental. At the inflow end of the capillary near the afferent arteriole, P_{GC} is about 60 mmHg and at the outflow end near the efferent arteriole, it is about 58 mmHg. Interestingly, the diameter of the afferent arteriole is larger than that of the efferent arteriole; therefore, the vascular resistance in the afferent arteriole is comparatively low and blood flows readily into the glomerular capillaries resulting in higher pressure. Furthermore, the smaller diameter of the efferent arteriole results in an increase in vascular resistance, which limits the flow of blood through this vessel. Consequently, the blood dams up in the glomerular capillaries, resulting in a sustained, elevated hydrostatic pressure that promotes the net filtration of fluid along the entire length of the glomerular capillaries.

Plasma colloid osmotic pressure (π_{GC}) is generated by the plasma proteins. These proteins exert an osmotic force on the fluid, which opposes filtration

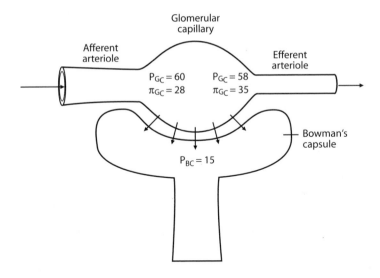

Figure 19.3 Forces determining net filtration pressure. Three forces contribute to net filtration pressure in the glomerulus. Glomerular capillary blood pressure (P_{GC}) is higher than that of a typical capillary (60 vs. 30 mmHg). Furthermore, P_{GC} remains high throughout the length of the capillary because of the comparatively small diameter of the efferent arteriole, which causes the blood to dam up within the glomerular capillaries. Glomerular capillary pressure promotes filtration along the entire length of the glomerular capillaries. Plasma colloid osmotic pressure (π_{GC}) generated by the plasma proteins opposes filtration. This force increases from 28 mmHg at the inflow end of the glomerular capillary to 35 mmHg at the outflow end, due to the concentration of plasma proteins as filtration of plasma fluid progresses. Bowman's capsule pressure (P_{BC}) is generated by the presence of filtered fluid within Bowman's capsule. This pressure opposes filtration with a force of 15 mmHg.

and draws the fluid into the capillary. The π_{GC} is approximately 28 mmHg at the inflow end of the glomerular capillaries. Because 20% of the fluid within the capillaries is filtered into Bowman's capsule, the plasma proteins become increasingly concentrated. Therefore, at the outflow end of the glomerular capillaries, π_{GC} is approximately 35 mmHg.

Bowman's capsule pressure (P_{BC}) is a hydrostatic pressure generated by the presence of filtered fluid within Bowman's capsule. This pressure pushes the fluid out of the capsule and forward toward the remainder of the renal tubule for processing. Bowman's capsule pressure also tends to oppose filtration. On average, P_{BC} is approximately 15 mmHg.

The net filtration pressure may be summarized as follows:

$$\text{Net filtration pressure} = P_{GC} - \pi_{GC} - P_{BC}$$

Therefore, at the inflow end of the glomerular capillaries:

$$\text{Net filtration pressure} = 60 \text{ mmHg} - 28 \text{ mmHg} - 15 \text{ mmHg}$$

$$= 17 \text{ mmHg}$$

At the outflow end of the glomerular capillaries:

$$\text{Net filtration pressure} = 58 \text{ mmHg} - 35 \text{ mmHg} - 15 \text{ mmHg}$$

$$= 8 \text{ mmHg}$$

Under physiological conditions, values for π_{GC} and P_{BC} vary little. In other words, when plasma protein synthesis is normal and in the absence of any urinary obstruction that would cause urine to back up and increase P_{BC}, the primary factor that affects glomerular filtration is P_{GC}. An increase in P_{GC} leads to an increase in GFR and a decrease in P_{GC} leads to a decrease in GFR.

Glomerular capillary pressure is determined primarily by *renal blood flow (RBF)*. As RBF increases, P_{GC} and therefore GFR increase. On the other hand, as RBF decreases, P_{GC} and GFR decrease. Renal blood flow is determined by mean arterial pressure (MAP) and the resistance of the afferent arteriole (aff art):

$$RBF = \frac{MAP}{R_{aff\ art}}$$

19.5 Tubular reabsorption

The process of *tubular reabsorption* is essential for the conservation of plasma constituents important to the body, in particular electrolytes and nutrient molecules. This process is highly selective in that waste products and substances with no physiological value are not reabsorbed, but instead excreted in the urine. Furthermore, reabsorption of many substances, such as Na^+, H^+, and Ca^{++} ions, and water is physiologically controlled. Consequently, volume, osmolarity, composition, and pH of the extracellular fluid are precisely regulated.

Throughout its length, the tubule of the nephron is composed of a single layer of epithelial cells. Furthermore, the tubule is close to the peritubular capillaries, so reabsorption involves movement of a substance along the following pathway:

Filtrate within tubular lumen
↓
Across the luminal membrane of the epithelial cell
↓
Through the cytoplasm of the epithelial cell
↓
Across the basolateral membrane of the epithelial cell

↓

Through the interstitial fluid

↓

Across the capillary endothelium

↓

Peritubular capillary blood

This pathway is referred to as *transepithelial transport.*
There are two types of tubular reabsorption:

- Passive
- Active

Tubular reabsorption is considered *passive* when each of the steps in transepithelial transport takes place without the expenditure of energy. In other words, the movement of a given substance is from an area of high concentration to an area of low concentration by way of passive diffusion. Water is passively reabsorbed from the tubules back into the peritubular capillaries.

Active reabsorption occurs when the movement of a given substance across the luminal surface or the basolateral surface of the tubular epithelial cell requires energy. Substances that are actively reabsorbed from the tubule include glucose; amino acids; and Na^+, PO_4^{-3}, and Ca^{++} ions. Three generalizations can be made regarding the tubular reabsorption of sodium, chloride, and water:

- Reabsorption of *Na^+ ions* is an *active* process; 80% of the total energy expended by the kidneys is used for sodium transport out of the tubular epithelial cell.
- Reabsorption of *Cl^- ions* is a *passive* process; Cl^- ions are reabsorbed according to the electrical gradient created by the reabsorption of Na^+ ions.
- Reabsorption of *water* is a *passive* process; water is reabsorbed according to the osmotic gradient created by reabsorption of Na^+ ions.

In other words, when sodium is reabsorbed, chloride and water follow it.

Sodium reabsorption. Sodium is reabsorbed by different mechanisms as the filtrate progresses through the tubule. Sodium ions leave the filtrate and enter the tubular epithelial cell by way of the following processes (see Figure 19.4):

- Na^+–glucose, Na^+–amino acid, Na^+–phosphate, and Na^+–lactate symporter mechanisms; Na^+–H^+ antiporter mechanism: first half of the proximal tubule
- Coupled with Cl^- reabsorption by way of transcellular (through the epithelial cell) and paracellular (in between the epithelial cells) pathways: second half of the proximal tubule

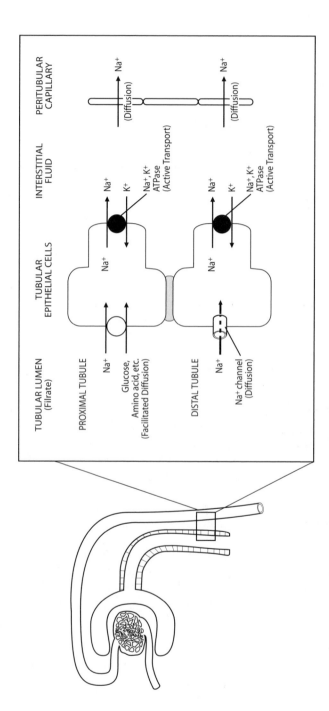

Figure 19.4 Tubular reabsorption of sodium. Sodium ions are actively transported out of the tubular epithelial cell through the basolateral membrane by the Na⁺, K⁺–ATPase pump. These ions then passively diffuse from interstitial fluid into blood of the peritubular capillaries. The active removal of Na⁺ ions from the tubular epithelial cells establishes a concentration gradient for passive diffusion of Na⁺ ions into cells from the tubular lumen. Potassium ions actively transported into epithelial cells of the proximal tubule as a result of this process simply diffuse back into interstitial fluid through channels located in the basolateral membrane. In the distal tubule and collecting duct, the K⁺ ions diffuse through channels in the luminal membrane into the tubular fluid and are excreted in the lumen. The diffusion of sodium may be coupled to reabsorption of organic molecules such as glucose or amino acids in the proximal tubule and the Loop of Henle. It may also occur through Na⁺ channels in the distal tubule and collecting duct.

- Na^+, K^+, $2Cl^-$ symporter mechanism: ascending limb of the Loop of Henle
- Na^+, Cl^- symporter mechanism: distal tubule
- Na^+ channels: distal tubule, collecting duct

More simply, in the early regions of the tubule (proximal tubule and Loop of Henle), Na^+ ions leave the lumen and enter the tubular epithelial cells by way of passive *facilitated transport mechanisms*. The diffusion of Na^+ ions is coupled with organic molecules or with other ions that electrically balance the flux of these positively charged ions. In the latter regions of the tubule (distal tubule and collecting duct), Na^+ ions diffuse into the epithelial cells through Na^+ channels.

An essential requirement for diffusion of Na^+ ions is the creation of a concentration gradient for sodium between the filtrate and intracellular fluid of the epithelial cells. This is accomplished by the *active transport of Na^+ ions* through the basolateral membrane of the epithelial cells (see Figure 19.4). Sodium is moved across this basolateral membrane and into the interstitial fluid surrounding the tubule by the *Na^+, K^+–ATPase pump*. As a result, the concentration of Na^+ ions within the epithelial cells is reduced, facilitating the diffusion of Na^+ ions into the cells across the luminal membrane. Potassium ions transported into the epithelial cells as a result of this pump diffuse back into the interstitial fluid (proximal tubule and Loop of Henle) or into the tubular lumen for excretion in the urine (distal tubule and collecting duct).

The amount of sodium reabsorbed from the proximal tubule and the Loop of Henle is held constant:

- Proximal tubule: 65% of the filtered sodium is reabsorbed
- Ascending limb of the Loop of Henle: 25% of the filtered sodium is reabsorbed

This reabsorption occurs regardless of the sodium content of the body. In order to make adjustments in the *sodium load*, the reabsorption of the remaining 10% of filtered Na^+ ions from the distal tubule and collecting duct is physiologically controlled by two hormones:

- Aldosterone
- Atrial natriuretic peptide

Aldosterone released from the adrenal cortex *promotes the reabsorption of sodium* from the distal tubule and collecting duct. The mechanisms of action of aldosterone include:

- Formation of Na⁺ channels in the luminal membrane of the tubular epithelial cells (facilitates passive diffusion of Na⁺ ions into the cell)
- Formation of Na⁺, K⁺–ATPase carrier molecules in the basolateral membrane of the tubular epithelial cells (promotes extrusion of Na⁺ ions from the cells and their movement into plasma by way of peritubular capillaries; enhances the concentration gradient for passive diffusion through Na⁺ channels in the luminal membrane)

Atrial natriuretic peptide (*ANP*) released from myocardial cells in the atria of the heart *inhibits the reabsorption of sodium* from the collecting duct. The mechanisms of action of ANP include:

- Inhibition of aldosterone secretion
- Inhibition of Na⁺ channels in the luminal membrane of the tubular epithelial cells

Recall that the reabsorption of Na⁺ ions is accompanied by reabsorption of Cl⁻ ions, which diffuse down their electrical gradient, and by reabsorption of water, which diffuses down its osmotic gradient. The net result is an expansion of plasma volume and consequently an increase in blood pressure. Therefore, the regulation of sodium reabsorption is important in the long-term regulation of blood pressure. As such, aldosterone and ANP, as well as the factors involved in their release, are discussed further in subsequent sections.

Chloride reabsorption. Chloride ions are reabsorbed passively according to the electrical gradient established by the active reabsorption of sodium. Chloride ions move from the tubular lumen back into the plasma by two pathways:

- Transcellular; through the tubular epithelial cells
- Paracellular; in-between the tubular epithelial cells

Most of the Cl⁻ ions diffuse between the tubular epithelial cells.

Water reabsorption. Water is reabsorbed passively by way of osmosis from many regions of the tubule. As with sodium and chloride, 65% of the filtered water is reabsorbed from the proximal tubule. An additional 15% of the filtered water is reabsorbed from the descending limb of the Loop of Henle. This reabsorption occurs regardless of the water content of the body. The water enters the tubular epithelial cells through *water channels*, also referred to as *aquaporins*. These channels are always open in the early regions of the tubule.

In order to make adjustments in the water load, the reabsorption of the remaining 20% of the filtered water from the distal tubule and the collecting duct is physiologically controlled by *antidiuretic hormone* (*ADH*), also referred to as *vasopressin*. Antidiuretic hormone, synthesized in the hypothalamus and released from the neurohypophysis of the pituitary gland, *promotes the reabsorption of water* from the distal tubule and collecting duct. The mechanism of action of ADH involves an increase in permeability of the water channels in the luminal membrane of tubular epithelial cells. Water diffuses into these cells and is ultimately reabsorbed into the plasma by way of the peritubular capillaries.

Recall that reabsorption of water is important in the regulation of plasma osmolarity. As the levels of ADH increase and more water is reabsorbed from the kidneys, the plasma is diluted and plasma osmolarity decreases. Conversely, as the levels of ADH decrease and more water is lost in the urine, plasma becomes more concentrated and plasma osmolarity increases. Factors involved in the release of ADH are discussed further in subsequent sections.

Production of urine of varying concentrations. In order to regulate plasma volume and osmolarity effectively, the kidneys must be able to alter the volume and concentration of the urine that is eliminated. Accordingly, the concentration of urine may be varied over a very wide range depending upon the body's level of hydration. The most dilute urine produced by the kidneys is 65 to 70 mOsm/l (when the body is overhydrated) and the most concentrated urine is 1200 mOsm/l (when the body is dehydrated). (Recall that plasma osmolarity is 290 to 300 mOsm/l.)

An essential factor in the ability to excrete urine of varying concentrations is the presence of a *vertical osmotic gradient* in the medullary region of the kidney (see Figure 19.5). The osmolarity of the interstitial fluid in the cortical region of the kidney is about 300 mOsm/l; however, the osmolarity of interstitial fluid in the medulla increases progressively, from 300 mOsm/l in the outer region near the cortex to 1200 mOsm/l in the innermost region of the medulla. The increase in osmolarity is due to the accumulation of Na^+ and Cl^- ions in the interstitial fluid. This vertical osmotic gradient is created by the Loops of Henle of the juxtamedullary nephrons. Recall that the Loop of Henle in these nephrons penetrates deeply into the medulla. The gradient is then utilized by the collecting ducts, along with ADH, to alter the concentration of urine. The following is a summary of the reabsorption of sodium, chloride, and water by each region of the nephron.

Plasma is freely filtered from the *glomerulus* so that everything in the plasma, except for the plasma proteins, is filtered. Therefore, the initial osmolarity of the filtrate is no different from that of the plasma and is about 300 mOsm/l (see Figure 19.5). Approximately 125 ml/min of the plasma is filtered. As the filtrate flows through the *proximal tubule*, 65% of the filtered Na^+ ions are actively reabsorbed, and 65% of the filtered Cl^- ions and water are passively reabsorbed. Because the water follows the sodium by way of osmosis, no change takes place in the osmolarity of the filtrate — only a change in volume. At the end of the proximal tubule, approximately 44 ml of filtrate with an osmolarity of 300 mOsm/l remain in the tubule.

The *descending limb of the Loop of Henle* is permeable to water only. As this region of the tubule passes deeper into the medulla, water leaves the filtrate down its osmotic gradient until it equilibrates with the increasingly concentrated interstitial fluid (see Figure 19.5). As a result, the filtrate also

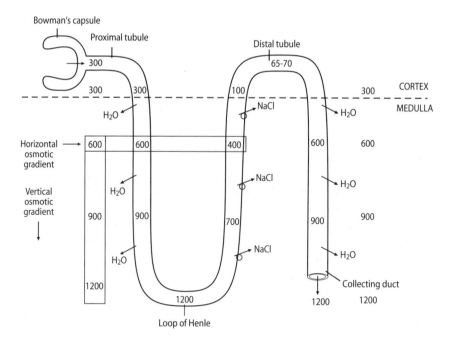

Figure 19.5 Production of varying concentrations of urine. The kidneys are capable of producing urine as diluted as 65 to 70 mOsm/l and as concentrated as 1200 mOsm/l. The concentration of urine is determined by the body's level of hydration. Sodium ions are actively transported from the ascending limb of the Loop of Henle into interstitial fluid —an active process used to accumulate Na $^+$ and Cl$^-$ ions in the medulla. As a result, a vertical osmotic gradient is established in which interstitial fluid becomes increasingly concentrated. This gradient is necessary for reabsorption of water from the collecting duct. Furthermore, a horizontal osmotic gradient of 200 mOsm/l is developed between filtrate of the ascending limb of the Loop of Henle and interstitial fluid. Consequently, osmolarity of the filtrate at the end of the Loop of Henle is 100 mOsm/l and the kidney may now excrete a urine significantly more diluted than plasma. In this way, when the body is overhydrated, excess water is eliminated. The presence of aldosterone promotes additional reabsorption of Na $^+$ ions from the distal tubule and collecting duct, further diluting the filtrate to 65 to 70 mOsm/l. The presence of ADH promotes reabsorption of water from the distal tubule and collecting duct. Water diffuses out of the collecting duct down its concentration gradient into interstitial fluid. High levels of ADH may concentrate the filtrate to 1200 mOsm/l so that, when the body is dehydrated, water is conserved.

becomes increasingly concentrated. At the tip of the Loop of Henle, the filtrate has an osmolarity of 1200 mOsm/l.

The *ascending limb of the Loop of Henle* is permeable to NaCl only. As the filtrate flows upward through this region of the tubule back toward the cortex, Na$^+$ ions are continuously and actively pumped out of the filtrate and into the interstitial fluid; chloride ions passively follow the sodium. As a result, the filtrate becomes increasingly dilute. At the end of the ascending limb of the Loop of Henle, approximately 25 ml of filtrate with an osmolarity of 100 mOsm/l remain in the tubule.

Because the transport of sodium is an active process, it is used to accumulate NaCl in the interstitial fluid of the medulla. In fact, this activity is involved in the initial establishment of the vertical osmotic gradient. Furthermore, sodium is actively transported out of the tubular epithelial cells up its concentration gradient until the filtrate is 200 mOsm/l less concentrated than the surrounding interstitial fluid. This difference between the filtrate and the interstitial fluid is referred to as the *horizontal osmotic gradient*. Because the filtrate at the end of the Loop of Henle has an osmolarity of 100 mOsm/l, the kidneys have the ability to produce urine that is significantly more dilute than the plasma.

As the filtrate progresses through the *distal tubule* and the *collecting duct*, the remaining NaCl (10% of that which was filtered) and water (20% of that filtered) are handled. As discussed, the presence of aldosterone enhances the reabsorption of sodium from these regions. Consequently, the filtrate becomes as dilute as 65 to 70 mOsm/l. The presence of ADH enhances the reabsorption of water from these regions; in particular, as the filtrate flows through the collecting duct, it enters a region of increasing osmolarity. The increased permeability of water due to ADH allows it to diffuse out of the collecting duct and into the interstitial fluid down its concentration gradient. When the levels of ADH are high, the water may continue to leave the tubule until the filtrate equilibrates with the surrounding interstitial fluid. In this case, the filtrate becomes as concentrated as 1200 mOsm/l and a small volume of urine is produced. When the levels of ADH are low, water remains in the collecting duct and a large volume of urine is produced.

Pharmacy application: physiological action of diuretics

Diuretics are drugs that cause an increase in urine output. It is important to note that, except for the osmotic diuretics, these drugs typically enhance the excretion of solute and water. Therefore, the net effect of most diuretics is to decrease plasma volume, but cause little change in plasma osmolarity. Five classes of diuretics and their major sites of action are:

- Osmotic diuretics: proximal tubule and descending limb of the Loop of Henle
- Loop diuretics: ascending limb of the Loop of Henle
- Thiazide diuretics: distal tubule
- Potassium-sparing diuretics: cortical collecting duct
- Carbonic anhydrase inhibitors: proximal tubule

Osmotic diuretics such as mannitol act on the proximal tubule and, in particular, the descending limb of the Loop of Henle — portions of the tubule permeable to water. These drugs are freely filtered at the glomerulus, but not reabsorbed; therefore, the drug remains in the tubular filtrate, increasing the osmolarity of this fluid. This increase in osmolarity keeps the water within the tubule, causing water diuresis. Because they primarily affect water and not sodium, the net effect is a reduction in total body water content more than cation content. Osmotic diuretics are poorly absorbed and must be administered intravenously. These drugs may be used to treat patients in acute renal failure and with dialysis disequilibrium syndrome. The latter disorder is caused by the excessively rapid removal of solutes from the extracellular fluid by hemodialysis.

Loop diuretics such as furosemide act on the ascending limb of the Loop of Henle, a portion of the tubule permeable to sodium and chloride. The mechanism of action of these diuretics involves inhibition of the Na^+, K^+, $2Cl^-$ symporter in the luminal membrane. By inhibiting this transport mechanism, loop diuretics reduce the reabsorption of NaCl and K^+ ions. Recall that reabsorption of NaCl from the ascending limb of the Loop of Henle generates and maintains the vertical osmotic gradient in the medulla. Without the reabsorption of NaCl, this gradient is lost and the osmolarity of the interstitial fluid in the medulla is decreased. When the osmolarity of the medulla is decreased, the reabsorption of water from the descending limb of the Loop of Henle and the collecting duct is significantly reduced. The net result of the loop diuretics includes reduced NaCl and water reabsorption and, therefore, enhanced NaCl and water loss in the urine. The most potent diuretics available (up to 25% of the filtered Na^+ ions may be excreted) — the loop diuretics — may cause hypovolemia. These drugs are often used to treat acute pulmonary edema, chronic congestive heart failure, and the edema and ascites of liver cirrhosis.

Thiazide diuretics such as chlorothiazide act on the distal tubule, a portion of the tubule that is permeable to sodium. The mechanism of action of these diuretics involves inhibition of NaCl reabsorption by blocking the Na^+, Cl^- symporter in the luminal membrane. The thiazide diuretics are only moderately effective due to the location of their site of action. Approximately 90% of the filtered Na^+ ions have already been reabsorbed when the filtrate reaches the distal tubule. These drugs may be used for treatment of edema associated with heart, liver, and renal disease. Thiazide diuretics are also widely used for the treatment of hypertension.

Potassium-sparing diuretics act on the late portion of the distal tubule and on the cortical collecting duct. As a result of their site of action, these diuretics also have a limited effect on diuresis compared to the loop diuretics (3% of the filtered Na^+ ions may be excreted). However, the clinical advantage of these drugs is that the reabsorption of K^+ ions is enhanced, reducing the risk of hypokalemia.

Two types of potassium-sparing diuretics have different mechanisms of action. Agents of the first type, which include spironolactone, are also known as aldosterone antagonists. These drugs bind directly to the aldosterone receptor and prevent this hormone from exerting its effects. Agents of the second type, which include amiloride, are inhibitors of the tubular epithelial Na^+ channels. Acting on the Na^+ channels in the luminal membrane, these drugs prevent movement of Na^+ ions from the filtrate into the epithelial cell. Because this transport of Na^+ ions into the cell is coupled to the transport of K^+ ions out of the cell, less potassium is lost to the filtrate and therefore the urine.

Potassium-sparing diuretics are often coadministered with thiazide or loop diuretics in the treatment of edema and hypertension. In this way, edema fluid is lost to the urine while K^+ ion balance is better maintained. The aldosterone antagonists are particularly useful in the treatment of primary hyperaldosteronism.

Carbonic anhydrase inhibitors such as acetazolamide act in the proximal tubule. These drugs prevent the formation of H^+ ions, which are transported out of the tubular epithelial cell in exchange for Na^+ ions. These agents have limited clinical usefulness because they result in development of metabolic acidosis.

19.6 Vasa recta

The *vasa recta* are modified peritubular capillaries. As with the peritubular capillaries, the vasa recta arise from efferent arterioles. However, these vessels are associated only with the juxtamedullary nephrons and are found only in the medullary region of the kidney. The vasa recta pass straight through to the inner region of the medulla, form a hairpin loop, and return straight toward the cortex. This structure allows these vessels to lie parallel to the Loop of Henle and collecting ducts.

The vasa recta perform several important functions, including:

- Providing nourishment to tubules of the medullary region of the kidneys
- Returning NaCl and water reabsorbed from the Loop of Henle and collecting ducts back to the general circulation

- Maintaining the vertical osmotic gradient within the interstitial fluid of the medulla

Blood entering the vasa recta has an osmolarity of about 300 mOsm/l. As the vessels travel through the increasingly concentrated medulla, the osmolarity of the blood within them equilibrates with that of the surrounding interstitial fluid. In other words, the blood also becomes increasingly concentrated. Water leaves the vasa recta down its concentration gradient and NaCl enters the vasa recta down its concentration gradient. Therefore, at the innermost region of the medulla, the osmolarity of the blood is 1200 mOsm/l. If the process were to be interrupted at this point, all the NaCl that had initially created the vertical gradient would eventually be washed away, or removed from the medulla, by the blood flowing through it. However, like the Loop of Henle, the vasa recta form a hairpin loop and travel back toward the cortex through an increasingly dilute interstitial fluid. Once again, the osmolarity of the blood within them equilibrates with that of the surrounding interstitial fluid. In other words, the blood now becomes increasingly dilute. Water enters the vasa recta down its concentration gradient and NaCl leaves the vasa recta down its concentration gradient. Consequently, when this blood has reached the cortex, its osmolarity has returned to 300 mOsm/l. Therefore, the blood leaving the vasa recta has an osmolarity similar to that of the blood that entered it. What does change is the volume of blood that leaves the vasa recta. Once again, the excess NaCl and water reabsorbed from the tubules within the medulla have been picked up by these vessels and returned to general circulation. It is important to note that this process has been performed without disrupting the vertical medullary gradient.

19.7 Tubular secretion

Tubular secretion is the transfer of substances from the peritubular capillaries into the renal tubule for excretion in urine. This process is particularly important for the regulation of potassium and hydrogen ions in the body; it is also responsible for removal of many organic compounds from the body. These may include metabolic wastes as well as foreign compounds, including drugs such as penicillin. Most substances are secreted by secondary active transport.

Potassium ion secretion. *Potassium ions* are secreted in the distal tubule and the collecting duct. These ions diffuse down their concentration gradient from the peritubular capillaries into the interstitial fluid. They are then actively transported up their concentration gradient into the tubular epithelial cells by way of the Na^+, K^+ pump in the basolateral membrane. Finally, potassium ions exit the epithelial cells by passive diffusion through K^+ channels in the luminal membrane and enter tubular fluid to be excreted in the urine.

Potassium secretion is enhanced by aldosterone. As the concentration of K^+ ions in the extracellular fluid increases, the secretion of aldosterone from the adrenal cortex also increases. The mechanism of action of aldosterone involves an increase in the activity of the Na^+, K^+ pump in the basolateral membrane. Furthermore, aldosterone enhances formation of K^+ channels in the luminal membrane.

Hydrogen ion secretion. Hydrogen ions are secreted in the proximal tubule, distal tubule, and collecting duct. The secretion of hydrogen ions is an important mechanism in acid-base balance. The normal pH of the arterial blood is 7.4. When the plasma becomes acidic, H^+ ion secretion increases and when it becomes alkalotic, H^+-ion secretion is reduced.

19.8 Plasma clearance

Plasma clearance is defined as the volume of plasma from which a substance is completely cleared by the kidneys per unit time (ml/min). Calculation of the plasma clearance of certain substances can be used to determine:

- GFR: volume of plasma filtered per minute
- ERPF: effective renal plasma flow

In order to measure plasma clearance of a substance, the following variables must be determined:

- Rate of urine formation (V; ml/min)
- Concentration of the substance in the urine (U; mg/ml)
- Concentration of the substance in the arterial plasma (P; mg/ml)

The plasma clearance of a substance is calculated as follows:

$$\text{Plasma clearance} = \frac{V \ (ml/min) \times U \ (mg/ml)}{P \ (mg/ml)}$$

In order to use the *plasma clearance of a substance to determine GFR*, the following criteria regarding the substance must be met:

- Freely filtered at the glomerulus
- Not reabsorbed
- Not secreted
- Not synthesized or broken down by the tubules

A substance that fulfills these criteria is *inulin*, a polysaccharide found in plants. Inulin is administered intravenously to a patient at a rate that results in a constant plasma concentration over the course of at least 1 h. The urine is collected and its volume and concentration of inulin are measured.

Consider the following example in which, at the end of 1 h, 60 ml of urine are produced; the concentration of inulin in the urine is 20 mg/ml; and the concentration of inulin in the plasma is 0.16 mg/ml:

$$\text{Plasma clearance of inulin} = \frac{1 \text{ ml/min} \times 20 \text{ mg/ml}}{0.16 \text{ mg/ml}}$$

$$= 125 \text{ ml/min}$$

Because inulin is neither reabsorbed nor secreted, all of the inulin in the urine was filtered at the glomerulus. Therefore, the plasma clearance of inulin is equal to the GFR.

Although the measurement of GFR with inulin is quite accurate, it is inconvenient because it requires the continuous infusion of this exogenous substance for several hours. More often, in clinical situations, the plasma clearance of *creatinine* is used to estimate GFR. Creatinine, an end-product of muscle metabolism, is released into the blood at a fairly constant rate. Consequently, only a single blood sample and a 24-h urine collection are needed. Measurement of the plasma clearance of creatinine provides only an *estimate* of GFR; in fact, this measurement slightly overestimates it. A small amount of creatinine is secreted into the urine (about 10% on average). In other words, the concentration of creatinine in the urine is the result of the amount filtered (as determined by GFR) *plus* the amount secreted.

In order to use the *plasma clearance of a substance to determine the effective rate of plasma flow (ERPF)* through the kidneys, the following criteria regarding the substance must be met:

- Freely filtered at the glomerulus
- Not reabsorbed
- Secreted into the tubules

A substance that fulfills these criteria is *para-aminohippuric acid (PAH)*. All of the PAH not filtered at the glomerulus is secreted by the proximal tubule. The net effect is that all of the plasma flowing through the nephrons is completely cleared of PAH. It is important to note that about 10 to 15% of the total renal plasma flow supplies regions of the kidneys that are not involved with filtration or secretion. Consequently, this plasma cannot be cleared of PAH. Therefore, the plasma clearance of PAH provides a measurement of the *effective* renal plasma flow, that is, the volume of plasma that actually flows through the nephrons. The ERPF is normally about 625 ml/min. (This value is based on a renal blood flow of about 1.1 l/min and a hematocrit of about 42.)

The *filtration fraction* is the percent of the plasma flowing through the nephrons that is filtered into the tubules. It is calculated using the plasma clearance of inulin (GFR) and the plasma clearance of PAH (ERPF):

$$\text{Filtration fraction} = \frac{\text{GFR}}{\text{ERPF}}$$

$$= \frac{125 \ \text{ml/min}}{625 \ \text{ml/min}}$$

$$= 20\%$$

On average, 20% of the plasma that flows through the glomerulus is filtered into the tubules.

19.9 Renal blood flow

The kidneys receive a disproportionate fraction of cardiac output. Although the combined weight of the kidneys accounts for less than 1% of total body weight, these organs receive 20 to 25% of the cardiac output. This magnitude of blood flow, which is in profound excess to their metabolic needs, enables them to carry out their multiple homeostatic functions more efficiently. Assuming a resting cardiac output of 5 l/min, the renal blood flow (RBF) is approximately 1.1 l/min.

Renal blood flow has a direct effect on GFR, which in turn has a direct effect on urine output. As RBF increases, GFR and urine output increase. Conversely, as RBF decreases, GFR and urine output decrease. Furthermore, any change in urine output affects plasma volume and blood pressure. Therefore, the regulation of RBF and GFR are important considerations. According to Ohm's law ($Q = \Delta P/R$), RBF is determined by mean arterial pressure (MAP) and the resistance of the afferent arteriole ($R_{aff \ art}$):

$$\text{RBF} = \frac{\text{Mean Arterial Pressure}}{R_{aff \ art}}$$

Autoregulation. The equation for RBF predicts that an increase in MAP will increase blood flow through the kidneys and a decrease will decrease blood flow through them. Physiologically, this response is not always desired. For example, during exercise, MAP increases in order to increase blood flow to the working skeletal muscles. A corresponding increase in RBF would lead to an increase in GFR and an undesired loss of water and solutes in the urine. On the other hand, a profound decrease in MAP could decrease RBF and GFR. In this case, elimination of wastes would be impaired. Maintaining a constant RBF and GFR, even when MAP changes, is advantageous in some physiological conditions.

Interestingly, RBF remains relatively constant when MAP changes in the range of 85 to 180 mmHg. This ability to maintain a constant blood flow in spite of changes in MAP is referred to as *autoregulation*. The mechanism of autoregulation involves corresponding changes in the resistance of the afferent arteriole. For example, when MAP increases, the resistance of the afferent arteriole increases proportionately so that RBF remains unchanged. It is important to note that the major site of autoregulatory changes is the *afferent arteriole*. As this arteriole constricts, glomerular capillary pressure and therefore the GFR are reduced toward their normal values.

Autoregulation of RBF is an *intrarenal response*. In other words, the mechanisms responsible for autoregulation function entirely within the kidney and rely on no external inputs. Two mechanisms elicit this response:

- Myogenic mechanism
- Tubuloglomerular feedback

Myogenic mechanism. As discussed in Chapter 16 on the circulatory system, the *myogenic mechanism* involves contraction of vascular smooth muscle in response to stretch. For example, an increase in MAP would tend to increase RBF, leading to an increase in pressure within the afferent arteriole and distension, or stretch, of the vessel wall. Consequently, the vascular smooth muscle of the afferent arteriole contracts, increases the resistance of the vessel, and decreases RBF toward normal.

Tubuloglomerular feedback. *Tubuloglomerular feedback* involves the activity of the *juxtaglomerular apparatus* (see Figure 19.1). This structure is located where the distal tubule comes into contact with the afferent and efferent arterioles adjacent to the glomerulus. The juxtaglomerular apparatus is composed of the following:

- Macula densa
- Granular cells

The *macula densa* consists of specialized cells of the distal tubule adapted to monitor GFR. In other words, they are sensitive to changes in the rate of filtrate flow through the distal tubule. *Granular cells* are specialized smooth muscle cells of the arterioles, in particular the afferent arteriole. These cells are adapted to monitor RBF — they are sensitive to changes in blood flow and blood pressure in the afferent arteriole. As such, they are also referred to as *intrarenal baroreceptors*. It is the granular cells of the juxtaglomerular apparatus that secrete renin. Further discussion of granular cell function is found in a subsequent section. Tubuloglomerular feedback involves the function of the macula densa. This mechanism may be summarized with the following example in which MAP increases:

↑ Mean arterial pressure
↓
↑ Renal blood flow
↓
↑ Glomerular capillary pressure

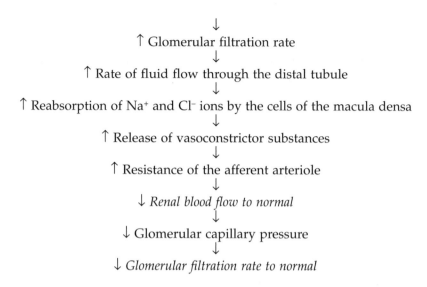

$\downarrow$

$\uparrow$ Glomerular filtration rate

$\downarrow$

$\uparrow$ Rate of fluid flow through the distal tubule

$\downarrow$

$\uparrow$ Reabsorption of Na^+ and Cl^- ions by the cells of the macula densa

$\downarrow$

$\uparrow$ Release of vasoconstrictor substances

$\downarrow$

$\uparrow$ Resistance of the afferent arteriole

$\downarrow$

$\downarrow$ *Renal blood flow to normal*

$\downarrow$

$\downarrow$ Glomerular capillary pressure

$\downarrow$

$\downarrow$ *Glomerular filtration rate to normal*

An increase in MAP leads to an increase in RBF, P_{GC}, and GFR. As a result, the rate of fluid flow through the distal tubule increases, leading to an increase in reabsorption of Na^+ and Cl^- ions by the cells of the macula densa in the distal tubule. Consequently, these cells release vasoconstrictor substances, primarily adenosine. The subsequent increase in the resistance of the nearby afferent arteriole decreases RBF to normal and, as a result, P_{GC} and therefore GFR decrease to normal. In this way, the distal tubule regulates its own filtrate flow.

Resistance of the afferent arteriole. Many physiological conditions warrant a change in RBF and GFR, even when MAP is within the autoregulatory range. For example, volume overload is resolved with an increase in RBF, GFR, and urine output so that excess water and solutes are eliminated. Conversely, volume depletion, such as that which occurs with hemorrhage or dehydration, is resolved with decreased RBF, GFR, and urine output; in this way, water and solutes are conserved.

The resistance of the afferent arteriole is influenced by several factors, including (see Table 19.1):

- Sympathetic nerves
- Angiotensin II
- Prostaglandins

Sympathetic nerves. The afferent and efferent arterioles are densely innervated with sympathetic nerves. Norepinephrine released directly from the nerves or circulating epinephrine released from the adrenal medulla stimulates α_1 adrenergic receptors to cause vasoconstriction. The predominant site of regulation is the afferent arteriole. Under normal resting conditions, there is little sympathetic tone to these vessels so that RBF is comparatively high. As discussed previously, this facilitates glomerular filtration.

However, the degree of sympathetic stimulation to the kidneys is altered under various physiological and pathophysiological conditions. For example, consider a case in which an individual is volume depleted due to hemorrhage or dehydration:

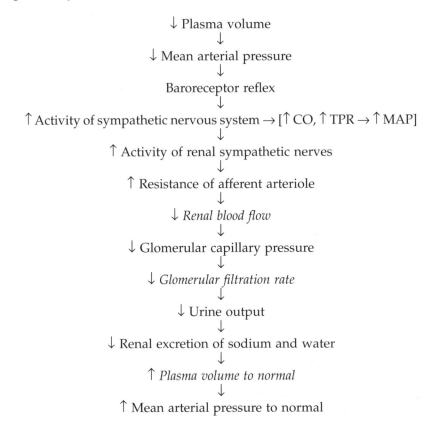

↓ Plasma volume
↓
↓ Mean arterial pressure
↓
Baroreceptor reflex
↓
↑ Activity of sympathetic nervous system → [↑ CO, ↑ TPR → ↑ MAP]
↓
↑ Activity of renal sympathetic nerves
↓
↑ Resistance of afferent arteriole
↓
↓ *Renal blood flow*
↓
↓ Glomerular capillary pressure
↓
↓ *Glomerular filtration rate*
↓
↓ Urine output
↓
↓ Renal excretion of sodium and water
↓
↑ *Plasma volume to normal*
↓
↑ Mean arterial pressure to normal

Loss of plasma volume leads to a decrease in MAP. Baroreceptors located in the aortic and carotid sinuses detect this fall in MAP and elicit reflex responses that include an increase in the overall activity of the sympathetic nervous system. Sympathetic stimulation of the heart and blood vessels leads to an increase in cardiac output (CO) and increased total peripheral resistance (TPR). These adjustments, which increase MAP, are responsible for the *short-term regulation of blood pressure*. Although increases in CO and TPR are effective in temporary maintenance of MAP and blood flow to the vital organs, these activities cannot persist indefinitely. Ultimately, plasma volume must be returned to normal (see Table 19.1).

An overall increase in sympathetic nerve activity includes an increase in sympathetic input to the kidneys. Consequently, resistance of the afferent arteriole increases, leading to a decrease in RBF. As discussed, this results in a decrease in P_{GC}, GFR, and urine output. As such, the renal excretion of sodium and water is decreased. In other words, sodium and water are conserved by the body, which increases plasma volume and MAP toward normal. These changes are responsible for the *long-term regulation of blood pressure* (see Table 19.1).

Sympathetic stimulation also increases the resistance of the efferent arteriole, leading to a decrease in blood pressure in the peritubular capillaries. This fall in pressure facilitates movement of sodium and water from the tubules into these capillaries.

Angiotensin II. Angiotensin II also increases the resistance of the renal arterioles and consequently decreases RBF and GFR. Angiotensin II is synthesized by the following pathway:

$$Angiotensinogen$$
$$\downarrow$$
$$Angiotensin\ I$$
$$\downarrow$$
$$Angiotensin\ II$$

Angiotensinogen, which is synthesized by the liver, is an inactive plasma protein. *Renin*, a hormone secreted by the granular cells of the juxtaglomerular apparatus, promotes the conversion of circulating angiotensinogen into *angiotensin I*. As angiotensin I travels in the blood through the lungs, it is exposed to the *angiotensin-converting enzyme* (*ACE*) located in the endothelial cells lining the blood vessels of the pulmonary circulation. This enzyme converts angiotensin I into *angiotensin II*.

Angiotensin II has multiple effects throughout the body, all of which directly or indirectly increase MAP. For example, angiotensin II causes the secretion of aldosterone, which enhances sodium reabsorption; expands plasma volume; and increases MAP. Angiotensin II is also a potent vasoactive substance that causes widespread vasoconstriction and therefore an increase in TPR, which increases MAP. Furthermore, angiotensin II causes powerful vasoconstriction in the renal arterioles in particular, which leads to decreased RBF and GFR. Consequently, urine output is reduced and water and solutes are conserved by the body, leading to an increase in plasma volume and therefore MAP. Taken together, these effects demonstrate that the production of angiotensin II is beneficial when blood pressure or blood volume has fallen.

Formation of angiotensin II requires the release of renin from the granular cells. Therefore, the factors affecting renin release must be considered:

- Renal sympathetic nerves
- Intrarenal baroreceptors
- Macula densa
- Atrial natriuretic peptide
- Angiotensin II

The sympathetic nervous system increases blood pressure through multiple mechanisms including an increase in cardiac activity and vasoconstriction. Furthermore, stimulation of *β₁ adrenergic receptors* on the granular cells through the activity of *renal sympathetic nerves* or by circulating epinephrine has a *direct stimulatory effect on renin secretion*. The enhanced formation of angiotensin II also increases blood pressure through the mechanisms outlined previously. Specifically, angiotensin II constricts the afferent arteriole, decreases RBF, decreases GFR, decreases urine output, and increases plasma volume and blood pressure. Conversely, a decrease in sympathetic activity results in decreased secretion of renin.

The granular cells that secrete renin also serve as *intrarenal baroreceptors*, monitoring blood volume and blood pressure in the afferent arterioles. Arteriolar pressure and renin secretion have an inverse relationship; in other words, an increase in blood volume causes an increase in arteriolar blood pressure; increased stimulation of the intrarenal baroreceptors; and *decreased secretion of renin*. With less angiotensin II-induced vasoconstriction of the afferent arteriole, RBF, GFR, and urine output will increase so that blood volume returns to normal.

The *macula densa*, which is involved in tubuloglomerular feedback, is also a factor in the regulation of renin secretion. In fact, this mechanism involving the macula densa is thought to be important in the maintenance of arterial blood pressure under conditions of decreased blood volume. For example, a decrease in blood volume leads to a decrease in RBF, GFR, and filtrate flow through the distal tubule. The resulting decrease in the delivery of NaCl to the macula densa *stimulates the secretion of renin*. Increased formation of angiotensin II serves to increase MAP and maintain blood flow to the tissues.

Atrial natriuretic peptide is released from myocardial cells in the atria of the heart in response to an increase in atrial filling, or an increase in plasma volume. This hormone *inhibits the release of renin*. With less angiotensin II-induced vasoconstriction of the afferent arteriole, RBF, GFR, and urine output increase. The increased loss of water and solutes decreases blood volume toward normal.

Angiotensin II directly *inhibits the secretion of renin* from the granular cells. This negative feedback mechanism enables angiotensin II to limit its own formation.

Prostaglandins. The third important factor influencing the resistance of afferent arterioles is the *prostaglandins*, specifically, *PGE_2* and *PGI_2*. Produced by the kidney, these prostaglandins function as local *vasodilators* that decrease arteriole resistance and increase RBF and GFR. Interestingly, the synthesis of PGE_2 and PGI_2 is stimulated by increased activity of the renal sympathetic nerves and by angiotensin II. The vasodilator prostaglandins then oppose the vasoconstrictor effects of norepinephrine and angiotensin II, resulting in a smaller increase in the resistance of the afferent arterioles. This "dampening" effect is important in that it prevents an excessive reduction in RBF that could lead to renal tissue damage.

Table 19.1 Summary of Factors Affecting Cardiovascular and Renal Systems

Sympathetic nervous activity

↑ Cardiac output

↑ Total peripheral resistance

↑ Resistance of afferent arteriole → ↓ renal blood flow → ↓ glomerular filtration rate → ↓ Na^+ filtration
↓ H_2O filtration

↑ Renin → ↑ angiotensin II → ↑ aldosterone → ↑ Na^+ reabsorption
Net effects: ↓ urine output; ↑ blood volume; ↑ mean arterial pressure

Angiotensin II

↑ Total peripheral resistance

↑ Resistance of afferent arteriole → ↓ renal blood flow → ↓ glomerular filtration rate → ↓ Na^+ filtration
↓ H_2O filtration

↑ Aldosterone → ↑ Na^+ reabsorption

↑ Antidiuretic hormone → ↑ H_2O reabsorption

↑ Thirst → ↑ H_2O intake
Net effects: ↓ urine output; ↑ blood volume; ↑ mean arterial pressure

Atrial natriuretic peptide

↓ Renin

↓ Aldosterone

↓ Total peripheral resistance
Net effects: ↑ urine output; ↓ blood volume; ↓ mean arterial pressure

19.10 Control of sodium excretion: regulation of plasma volume

Sodium is the major extracellular cation. Because of its osmotic effects, changes in sodium content in the body have an important influence on extracellular fluid volume, including plasma volume. For example, excess sodium leads to the retention of water and an increase in plasma volume. Increased plasma volume then causes an increase in blood pressure. Conversely, sodium deficit leads to water loss and decreased plasma volume. A decrease in plasma volume then causes a decrease in blood pressure. Therefore, homeostatic mechanisms involved in the regulation of plasma volume and blood pressure involve regulation of sodium content, or *sodium balance*, in the body.

Sodium balance is achieved when salt intake is equal to salt output. The intake of salt in the average American diet (10 to 15 g/day) far exceeds what is required physiologically. Only about 0.5 g/day of salt is lost in sweat and feces. The remaining ingested salt must be excreted in the urine. The *amount of sodium excreted* by the renal system is determined by:

- Amount of sodium filtered at the glomerulus
- Amount of sodium reabsorbed from the tubules

Sodium is freely filtered at the glomerulus. Therefore, any factor that affects GFR will also affect sodium filtration. As discussed previously, GFR is directly related to RBF. In turn, RBF is determined by blood pressure and the resistance of the afferent arteriole (RBF = $\Delta P/R$). For example, an increase in blood pressure or a decrease in resistance of the afferent arteriole will increase RBF, GFR, and, consequently, filtration of sodium. The *amount of sodium reabsorbed* from the tubules is physiologically regulated, primarily by aldosterone and, to a lesser extent, by ANP. Aldosterone promotes reabsorption and ANP inhibits it. The alterations in sodium filtration and sodium reabsorption in response to decreased plasma volume are illustrated in Figure 19.6.

A decrease in plasma volume leads to decreased MAP, which is detected by baroreceptors in the carotid sinuses and the arch of the aorta. By way of the vasomotor center, the baroreceptor reflex results in an overall increase in sympathetic nervous activity. This includes stimulation of the heart and vascular smooth muscle, which causes an increase in cardiac output and total peripheral resistance. These changes are responsible for the short-term regulation of blood pressure, which temporarily increases MAP toward normal.

Changes in sodium filtration and sodium reabsorption, which lead to a change in sodium excretion, are responsible for the long-term regulation of blood pressure. These changes are brought about by increased activity of the renal sympathetic nerves. Sympathetic stimulation of α_1 adrenergic receptors on renal vascular smooth muscle leads to an increase in the resistance of the afferent arteriole. This causes a decrease in RBF, in glomerular filtration

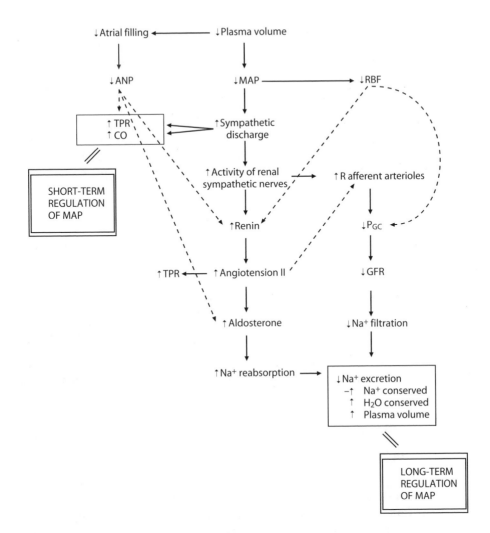

Figure 19.6 Renal handling of sodium.

pressure, in GFR, and a *decrease in sodium filtration*. If less sodium is filtered, then less sodium is lost in the urine.

Sympathetic stimulation of β_1 adrenergic receptors on the granular cells of the juxtaglomerular apparatus promotes secretion of renin and, consequently, formation of angiotensin II. Angiotensin II then causes:

- Widespread vasoconstriction
- Increased resistance of the afferent arteriole
- Increased secretion of aldosterone

Widespread vasoconstriction supplements the increase in TPR induced by the sympathetic nervous system. Angiotensin II also causes vasoconstriction of the afferent arteriole in particular, which enhances the decrease in RBF and sodium filtration. Finally, angiotensin II promotes secretion of aldosterone from the adrenal cortex. Aldosterone then acts on the distal tubule and collecting duct to increase *sodium reabsorption*.

Sodium reabsorption is also influenced by ANP. The original decrease in plasma volume leads to a decrease in atrial filling and a decrease in the release of ANP from the myocardium. Atrial natriuretic peptide, which acts on vascular smooth muscle, granular cells of the kidney, and the adrenal cortex, normally causes the following:

- Vasodilation
- Decreased renin release
- Decreased aldosterone secretion

Therefore, inhibition of ANP release leads to vasoconstriction and increased MAP. Furthermore, less ANP promotes the release of renin and secretion of aldosterone, which further enhance sodium reabsorption.

Taken together, the homeostatic responses elicited by the initial decrease in plasma volume serve to decrease sodium filtration, increase sodium reabsorption, and, consequently, decrease sodium excretion in the urine. This conservation of sodium leads to conservation of water and an expansion of plasma volume toward normal.

19.11 Control of water excretion: regulation of plasma osmolarity

Regulation of the osmolarity of extracellular fluid, including that of the plasma, is necessary in order to avoid osmotically induced changes in intracellular fluid volume. If the extracellular fluid were to become hypertonic (too concentrated), water would be pulled out of the cells; if it were to become hypotonic (too dilute), water would enter the cells. The osmolarity of extracellular fluid is maintained at 290 mOsm/l by way of the physiological regulation of water excretion. As with sodium, *water balance* in the body is achieved when water intake is equal to water output. Sources of water input include:

- Fluid intake
- Water in food
- Metabolically produced water

Sources of water output include:

- Loss from the lungs and nonsweating skin
- Sweating
- Feces
- Urine

The two factors controlled physiologically in order to maintain water balance include fluid intake and urine output. *Fluid intake* is largely influenced by the subjective feeling of *thirst*, which compels an individual to ingest water or other fluids. Urine output is largely influenced by the action of ADH, which promotes the reabsorption of water from the distal tubule and the collecting duct. Thirst and ADH secretion are regulated by the hypothalamus, of which three functional regions are involved:

- Osmoreceptors
- Thirst center
- ADH-secreting cells

The *osmoreceptors* of the hypothalamus monitor the osmolarity of extracellular fluid. These receptors are stimulated primarily by an increase in *plasma osmolarity*; they then provide excitatory inputs to the *thirst center* and the *ADH-secreting cells* in the hypothalamus. The stimulation of the thirst center leads to increased fluid intake. The stimulation of the ADH-secreting cells leads to release of ADH from the neurohypophysis and, ultimately, an increase in reabsorption of water from the kidneys and a decrease in urine output. These effects increase the water content of the body and dilute the plasma back toward normal. Plasma osmolarity is the major stimulus for thirst and ADH secretion; two additional stimuli include:

- Decreased extracellular volume
- Angiotensin II

A more moderate stimulus for thirst and ADH secretion is a *decrease in extracellular fluid, or plasma volume*. This stimulus involves low-pressure receptors in the atria of the heart as well as baroreceptors in the large arteries. A decrease in plasma volume leads to a decrease in atrial filling, which is detected by low-pressure receptors, and a decrease in MAP, which the baroreceptors detect. Each of these receptors then provides excitatory inputs to the thirst center and to the ADH-secreting cells.

Angiotensin II also stimulates the thirst center to increase the urge to ingest fluids, and ADH secretion to promote reabsorption of water from the kidneys. Other factors influencing ADH-secreting cells (but not the thirst center) include pain, fear, and trauma, which increase ADH secretion, and alcohol, which decreases it.

Pharmacy application: drug-related nephropathies

Drug-related nephropathies involve functional or structural changes in the kidneys following the administration of certain drugs. The nephrons are subject to a high rate of exposure to substances in the blood due to the high rate of renal blood flow and the substantial glomerular filtration rate. Furthermore, the kidneys may be involved in the metabolic transformation of some drugs and therefore exposed to their potentially toxic end-products.

Elderly patients are particularly susceptible to kidney damage due to their age-related decrease in renal function. Also, the potential for nephrotoxicity is increased when two or more drugs capable of causing renal damage are administered at the same time. Drugs and toxic end-products of drug metabolism may damage the kidneys by way of the following mechanisms:

- Decrease in renal blood flow
- Direct damage to the tubulointerstitial structures
- Hypersensitivity reactions

Nonsteroidal anti-inflammatory drugs (NSAIDs) may damage renal structures, in particular, the interstitial cells of the medulla. Prostaglandins E_2 and I_2 are vasodilators that help to regulate renal blood flow under normal physiological conditions. Because NSAIDs inhibit the synthesis of prostaglandins, renal damage likely results from an inappropriate decrease in renal blood flow. Chronic analgesic nephritis (inflammation of the nephrons) is associated with analgesic abuse; ingredients such as aspirin and acetaminophen have been implicated in this disorder.

Acute drug-related hypersensitivity reactions (allergic responses) may cause tubulointerstitial nephritis, which will damage the tubules and interstitium. These reactions are most commonly observed with administration of methicillin and other synthetic antibiotics as well as furosemide and the thiazide diuretics. The onset of symptoms occurs in about 15 days. Symptoms include fever, eosinophilia, hematuria (blood in the urine), and proteinuria (proteins in the urine). Signs and symptoms of acute renal failure develop in about 50% of the cases. Discontinued use of the drug usually results in complete recovery; however, some patients, especially the elderly, may experience permanent renal damage.

Bibliography

Costanzo, L., *Physiology*, W.B. Saunders, Philadelphia, 1998.

Guyton, A.C. and Hall, J.E., *Textbook of Medical Physiology*, 10th ed., W.B. Saunders, Philadelphia, 2000.

Jackson, E.K., Diuretics, in *Goodman and Gilman's: The Pharmacological Basis of Therapeutics*, 9th ed., Hardman, J.G. and Limbird, L.E., Eds., McGraw–Hill, New York, 1996, chap. 29.

Koeppen, B.M. and Stanton, B.A., *Renal Physiology*, 3rd ed., C.V. Mosby, St. Louis, 2001.

Porth, C.M., *Pathophysiology: Concepts of Altered Health States*, 5th ed., Lippincott, Philadelphia, 1998.

Sherwood, L., *Human Physiology from Cells to Systems*, 4th ed., Brooks/Cole, Pacific Grove, CA, 2001.

Silverthorn, D.U., *Human Physiology: An Integrated Approach*, 2nd ed., Prentice-Hall, Upper Saddle River, NJ, 2001.

Vander, A.J., *Renal Physiology*, 5th ed., McGraw–Hill, New York, 1995.

Index

A

Absolute refractory period, 26, 28, 173
Absorptive cells, 299
Acetaminophen, 88
Acetazolamide, 325
Acetylcholine, 98, 101, 143, 253
Acetylcholinesterase, 99
Acidosis, 41
Actin, 143, 153
Action potentials
  absolute refractory period of, 28
  after-hyperpolarization of, 28
  cardiac, 170, 173
  conduction of, 28–32
  definition of, 25
  features of, 24
  initiation of, 29
  propagated, 143
  relative refractory period of, 28
  unidirectional conduction of, 32
  voltage-gated ion channels, 25, 27
Activated factor XII, 236
Activation gate, 27
Active hyperemia, 217–218
Active transport, 14
A-delta fibers, 78, 80
Adenohypophysis
  description of, 120, 122
  hormones of, 126–129
Adenosine diphosphate, 145
Adenosine triphosphate
  muscle contraction and, 145–146
  sources of, 146–147
Adjuvant analgesics, 88
Adrenal cortex
  anatomy of, 132
  androgens of, 136
  glucocorticoids, 134–135

hormones produced by, 123, 132–135
  mineralocorticoids, 123, 133–134
Adrenal medulla
  description of, 99, 107–109, 132
  hormones produced by, 123, 132
Adrenalin, 99
Adrenergic fibers, 99
β_2-Adrenergic receptor agonists, 253–254
Adrenergic receptors, 101–102
Adrenocorticotropic hormone, 115, 122, 127
Afferent arterioles
  angiotensin II effects on, 333–334
  description of, 330–331
  prostaglandins effect on, 334
  sympathetic nerves effect on, 331–333
Afferent division, of peripheral nervous system, 46
Afferent neurons, 46, 67, 73
After-hyperpolarization, 28
Afterload, 189
Agglutination, 230, 234
Agonist, 11, 42
Agranulocytes, 232
Airway(s)
  collapse of, 252
  description of, 241–242
  obstruction of, 251–252, 262
  radius of, 251–252
Airway resistance, 251–253
Albumin, 129, 228
Aldosterone
  description of, 123, 133
  sodium reabsorption and, 319–320
Alkalosis, 41
Alpha motor neurons, 67

343